575/-

GE[illegible]OMY

3 VOLUME SERIES

Vishram Singh

TEXTBOOK OF ANATOMY UPPER LIMB AND THORAX

Volume I

1. Introduction to the Upper Limb
2. Bones of the Upper Limb
3. Pectoral region
4. Axilla (Armpit)
5. Back of the Body and Scapular Region
6. Shoulder Joint Complex (Joints of Shoulder Girdle)
7. Cutaneous Innervation, Venous Drainage and Lymphatic Drainage of the Upper Limb
8. Arm
9. Forearm
10. Elbow and Radio-ulnar Joints
11. Hand
12. Joints and Movements of the Hand
13. Major Nerves of the Upper Limb
14. Introduction to Thorax and Thoracic Cage
15. Bones and Joints of the Thorax
16. Thoracic Wall and Mechanism of Respiration
17. Pleural Cavities
18. Lungs (Pulmones)
19. Mediastinum
20. Pericardium and Heart
21. Superior Vena Cava, Aorta, Pulmonary Trunk, and Thymus
22. Trachea and Esophagus
23. Thoracic Duct, Azygos and Hemiazygos Veins, and Thoracic Sympathetic Trunks

Multiple Choice Questions

TEXTBOOK OF ANATOMY ABDOMEN AND LOWER LIMB

Volume II

1. Introduction and Overview of the Abdomen
2. Osteology of the Abdomen
3. Anterior Abdominal Wall
4. Inguinal Region/Groin
5. Male External Genital Organs
6. Abdominal Cavity and Peritoneum
7. Abdominal Part of Esophagus, Stomach, and Spleen
8. Liver and Extrahepatic Biliary Apparatus
9. Duodenum, Pancreas, and Portal Vein
10. Small and Large Intestines
11. Kidneys, Ureters, and Suprarenal Glands
12. Posterior Abdominal Wall and Associated Structures
13. Pelvis
14. Pelvic Walls and Associated Soft Tissue Structures
15. Perineum
16. Urinary Bladder and Urethra
17. Male Genital Organs
18. Female Genital Organs
19. Rectum and Anal Canal
20. Introduction to the Lower Limb
21. Bones of the Lower Limb
22. Front of the Thigh
23. Medial Side of the Thigh
24. Gluteal Region
25. Back of the Thigh and Popliteal Fossa
26. Hip Joint
27. Front of the Leg and Dorsum of the Foot
28. Lateral and Medial Sides of the Leg
29. Back of the Leg
30. Sole of the Foot
31. Arches of the Foot
32. Joints of the Lower Limb
33. Venous and Lymphatic Drainage of the Lower Limb
34. Innervation of the Lower Limb

Multiple Choice Questions

TEXTBOOK OF ANATOMY HEAD, NECK AND BRAIN

Volume III

1. Living Anatomy of the Head and Neck
2. Osteology of the Head and Neck
3. Scalp, Temple, and Face
4. Skin, Superficial Fascia, and Deep Fascia of the Neck
5. Side of the Neck
6. Anterior Region of the Neck
7. Back of the Neck and Cervical Spinal Column
8. Parotid Region
9. Submandibular Region
10. Infratemporal Fossa, Temporomandibular Joint, and Pterygopalatine Fossa
11. Thyroid and Parathyroid Glands, Trachea, and Esophagus
12. Pre- and Paravertebral Regions and Root of the Neck
13. Oral Cavity
14. Pharynx and Palate
15. Larynx
16. Blood Supply and Lymphatic Drainage of the Head and Neck
17. Nose and Paranasal Air Sinuses
18. Ear
19. Orbit and Eyeball
20. Vertebral Canal and Its Contents
21. Cranial Cavity
22. Cranial Nerves
23. General Plan and Membranes of the Brain
24. Brainstem
25. Cerebellum and Fourth Ventricle
26. Diencephalon and Third Ventricle
27. Cerebrum
28. Basal Nuclei and Limbic System
29. Blood Supply of the Brain

Multiple Choice Questions

GENERAL ANATOMY

WITH

SYSTEMIC ANATOMY
RADIOLOGICAL ANATOMY
MEDICAL GENETICS

Second Edition

Vishram Singh, MS, PhD, FASI
Professor and Head, Department of Anatomy, Santosh Medical College
Member, Academic Council and Core Committee PhD Course, Santosh University, Ghaziabad
Editor-in-Chief, Journal of the Anatomical Society of India
Member, Editorial Board, Indian Journal of Otology
Medicolegal Advisor, ICPS, India
Consulting Editor, ABI, North Carolina, USA

Formerly at: GSVM Medical College, Kanpur
King George's Medical College, Lucknow
Al-Arab Medical University, Benghazi (Libya)
All India Institute of Medical Sciences, New Delhi

ELSEVIER

ELSEVIER

RELX India Private Limited (Formerly Reed Elsevier India Private Limited)
Registered Office: 818, 8th Floor, Indraprakash Building, 21, Barakhamba Road, New Delhi 110001
Corporate Office: 14th Floor, Building No. 10B, DLF Cyber City, Phase II, Gurgaon-122 002, Haryana, India

General Anatomy with Systemic Anatomy, Radiological Anatomy, Medical Genetics, Vishram Singh

Previous edition 2008, Reprinted 2011, 2012, 2014

ISBN: 978-81-312-3463-1
e-book ISBN: 978-81-312-4255-1

First Printed in India 2015, Reprinted 2015, 2016, 2017

Content Strategist: Renu Rawat
Senior Project Manager-Education Solutions: Shabina Nasim
Project Manager: Prasad Subramanian
Content Development Specialist: Goldy Bhatnagar
Senior Operations Manager: Sunil Kumar
Sr Production Executive: Ravinder Sharma
Sr Graphic Designer: Milind Majgaonkar

Laser typeset by GW India

Printed in India by Repro India Ltd., Navi Mumbai

Dedicated to

My Mother

Late Smt Ganga Devi Singh Rajput

an ever guiding force in my life for achieving knowledge through education

My Wife

Mrs Manorama Rani Singh

for tolerating my preoccupation happily during the preparation of this book

My Children

Dr Rashi Singh and **Dr Gaurav Singh**

for helping me in preparing the manuscript

My Teachers

Late Professor (Dr) AC Das

for inspiring me to be multifaceted and innovative in life

Professor (Dr) A Halim

for imparting to me the art of good teaching

My Students, Past and Present

for appreciating my approach to teaching anatomy and
transmitting the knowledge through this book

Preface to the Second Edition

It is with great pleasure that I express my gratitude to all students and teachers who appreciated, used, and recommended the first edition of this book. It is because of their support that the book was reprinted three times since its first publication in 2008.

The huge success of this book reflects appeal of its clear, uncluttered presentation of the anatomical text supplemented by perfect simple line diagrams, which could be easily reproduced by students in the exam and clinical correlations providing the anatomical, embryological, and genetic basis of medical problems seen in day-to-day life in clinical practice.

Based on a large number of suggestions from students and fellow academicians, the text has been extensively revised. Many new line diagrams and halftone images have been added and earlier diagrams have been updated.

I greatly appreciate the constructive suggestions that I received from past and present students and colleagues for improvement of the content of this book. I do not claim to absolute originality of the text and figures other than the new mode of presentation and expression.

Once again, I whole heartedly thank students, teachers, and fellow anatomists for inspiring me to carry out the revision. I sincerely hope that readers will find this edition more interesting and useful than the previous one. I would highly appreciate comments and suggestions from students and teachers for further improvement of this book.

"To learn from previous experience and improve accordingly, makes you a successful man."

Vishram Singh

Preface to the Second Edition

Preface to the First Edition

There has been a long felt need of a comprehensive book on general anatomy which would systematically explain not only the basic principles of anatomical structures, but also the relationships and functions of these structures within the human body in both healthy and diseased states.

The explosion in knowledge of diseases and the technological advances associated with diagnosis and treatment in the past decade or so has necessitated a radical restructuring of the anatomy curriculum for medical, dental, nursing and paramedical students. As a result, the present-day curriculum of anatomy is more integrated, clinically oriented and system based. This has also created the need for a new textbook reflecting these changes.

This book is prepared in the light of the recent curriculum changes keeping in view the time allotted for anatomy teaching. Throughout the preparation of this book, the basic theme kept in mind is that anatomical knowledge is required for performing physical examination and diagnostic procedures. Thus, while anatomical details of little clinical relevance have been omitted, clinically oriented topographic anatomy relating to diagnostic and surgical procedures is included. The histological features and developmental aspects have been mentioned wherever they facilitate an appreciation of gross structure/functions of organs and occurrence of congenital anomalies.

In the present-day scenario, there is an alarming increase in problems associated with the spine (vertebral column). Unfortunately, most books do not deal with it as an independent entity. In this book, therefore, a separate chapter has been provided on the vertebral column. Further, important advances have taken place in genetics and radiodiagnosis and it has become imperative for medical students to have an overview of medical genetics and imaging anatomy before going through their clinical courses. For this reason, fundamentals of medical genetics and imaging anatomy are included in this volume.

Most medical colleges and centers follow the regional approach to teach gross anatomy in order to make it surgically relevant. As a result, students often fail to develop the systemic concept to understand medical problems. This volume, therefore, provides an overview of systemic anatomy and lays the foundation for the study of gross anatomy through the regional approach in the subsequent volumes.

The chapters of this volume have been so structured to make the text user friendly, facilitating ready access to the required material and smooth flow of knowledge. The chapters are organized in terms of the following components:

- *Chapter Outline:* broadly provides the contents of each chapter.
- *Learning Objectives:* indicate the level of competency a student is supposed to attain.
- *Text:* provides accurate and up-to-date information on the subject, in a visually appealing, interesting and simple manner.
- *Clinical Correlations:* offer clinical facts of practical value and reinforce the importance of theoretical learning in day-to-day clinical situations.
- *N.B.:* presents concepts of high academic value in a simple way.
- *Golden Facts to Remember:* lists important facts needed for appearing in PG entrance examinations, PLAB, USMLE, etc.
- *Multiple Choice Questions:* at the end of each chapter would help the reader assess his understanding and learning.
- *Tables and Flowcharts:* summarize the information and present complex data in a simpler manner.
- *Illustrations:* form the backbone of the book, anatomy being a descriptive science. All illustrations have been carefully drawn–for conceptual clarity and accuracy. They have been designed to integrate well with the text to maximize learning.

The standard color scheme, applicable to anatomical drawings is used throughout the book. Broadly, the color scheme followed is:

Structures	Color
Arteries	Red
Veins	Blue
Nerves	Yellow
Lymph vessels/Lymph nodes	Violet
Muscles	Pinkish brown
Bone	Creamy yellow
Cartilage	Sky blue

In addition, real life three dimensional radiographs and images are provided to enhance understanding of currently used diagnostic imaging techniques.

General Anatomy is intended to serve as an introduction to human anatomy for students pursuing the first course in anatomy in medical, dental, nursing and allied health institutes.

I hope both teachers and students find this book interesting and useful. I would greatly welcome comments and suggestions from readers for the further improvement of the book.

Vishram Singh

Acknowledgments

At the outset, I express my gratitude to Dr P Mahalingam, CMD; Dr Sharmila Anand, MD; Dr Ashwyn Anand, CEO; Dr Yogesh Tripathi, Hon Chancellor; Dr VK Arora, Hon Vice Chanceller, Santosh University, Ghaziabad, UP, for providing an appropriate academic atmosphere and encouragement, which helped me in preparing this book. I am also grateful to Dr Usha Dhar, Dean and Dr VK Sharma, Dean Research, Santosh Medical College for their cooperation.

- I highly appreciate the good gesture shown by Dr Preeti Srivastava, Dr Rohini Rahate, Dr Deepa Singh and Mr Krishna Chaitanya for going through the proofs sincerely and suggesting corrections wherever necessary.
- I sincerely thank the colleagues of my Department, Dr Nisha Kaul, Dr Latika Arora, Dr Ruchira Sethi, Dr Rohini Rahate, and Dr LK Pathy for their cooperation and help.
- I am highly thankful to Mr Krishna Chaitanya, PhD Scholar in the Department for providing most of the histology illustrations. I gratefully acknowledge the feedback and support of fellow colleagues in Anatomy, particularly,
- Professors AK Srivastava (Head of the Department), PK Sharma, and Punita Manik, King George's Medical College, Lucknow, UP.
- Professor NC Goel (Head of the Department), Hind Institute of Medical Sciences, Barabanki, Lucknow, UP.
- Professor Kuldeep Singh Sood (Head of the Department), SGT Medical College, Budhera, Gurgaon, Haryana.
- Professor Poonam Kharb, Sharda Medical College, Greater Noida, UP.
- Professor Ramesh Babu, Muzaffarnagar Medical College, Muzaffarnagar, UP.
- Professors RK Suri (Head of the Department), Gayatri Rath, and Dr Hitendra Lohiya, Vardhman Mahavir Medical College and Safdarjang Hospital, New Delhi.
- Professor Veena Bharihoke (Head of the Department), Rama Medical College, Hapur, Ghaziabad.
- Professors SL Jethani (Dean and Head of the Department) and RK Rohtagi, Himalayan Institute of Medical Sciences, Jolly Grant, Dehradun, Uttarakhand.
- Professors Anita Tuli (Head of the Department), Shipra Paul, and Shashi Raheja, Lady Harding Medical College, New Delhi.
- Professor SD Joshi (Dean and Head of the Department), Sri Aurobindo Institute of Medical Sciences, Indore, MP.
- Professor TC Singel, Government Medical College, Ahmedabad, Gujarat.
- Professors Pritha, S Bhuiyan (Head of the Department), M Natarajan, Anjali Dhamangaonkar, Lakshmi Rajgopal, K Shyam Kishore and Yuvraj Bhosale, Seth GS Medical College, Parel, Mumbai, Maharashtra.
- Professors N Imphal Damayanti Devi (Head of the Department) and Narainbabu Singh, RIMS, Imphal, Manipur.
- Professors AK Asthana (Dean) and Satyam Khare, Subharti Medical College, Meerut, UP.
- Professor SK Jain (Head of the Department), Teerthankar Mahaveer Medical College, Moradabad, UP.

Lastly, I eulogize the patience of my wife Mrs Manorama Rani Singh, daughter Dr Rashi Singh, and son Dr Gaurav Singh for helping me in the preparation of this manuscript.

I would also like to acknowledge with gratitude and pay my regards to my teachers Prof AC Das and Prof A Halim and other renowned anatomists of India, viz. Prof Shamer Singh, Prof Inderbir Singh, Prof Mahdi Hasan, Prof AK Dutta, Prof Inder Bhargava, etc. who inspired me during my student life.

I gratefully acknowledge the help and cooperation received from the staff of Elsevier, a division of Reed Elsevier India Pvt. Ltd., especially Ganesh Venkatesan (Director Editorial and Publishing Operations), Shabina Nasim (Senior Project Manager-Education Solutions), Renu Rawat (Content Strategist), and Goldy Bhatnagar (Project Coordinator).

Vishram Singh

Contents

CHAPTER 1

Introduction and History of Anatomy

Learning Objectives

After studying this chapter, the student should be able to:

- define anatomy and learn its subdivisions
- discuss why understanding human anatomy is essential to the science of medicine
- presents historical perspective of main contributors to the science of human anatomy through life and achievements of Hippocrates, Herophilus, Aristotle, Galen, Leonardo da Vinci and Vesalius
- correctly solve the review questions given at the end of the chapter

INTRODUCTION

Anatomy is the science which deals with the structure of the body from macroscopic to the microscopic level. Human anatomy has for long been studied through dissection of cadavers (preserved dead bodies), which served as the basis for understanding the structure and functions of the human body. The understanding of structural organization of the human body is essential so that the doctor knows which structure is affected in disease, which structure is being examined by him and which structure is being cut by him during operation.

The term anatomy is derived from the Greek word *anatome* meaning *to cut up*. The term dissection is the Latin equivalent of the Greek term *anatome* and in the past the word *anatomize* was more commonly used than the word *dissect*.

Earlier, the human anatomy was a descriptive science primarily concerned with identifying and naming the body structures, but today the importance of anatomy lies in its functional approach and clinical applications. Therefore, presently, human anatomy is a practical applied science that forms the firm foundation of the practice of medicine (i.e. art of healing).

SUBDIVISIONS OF ANATOMY

In the past, anatomy was studied mainly by dissection, but nowadays, it is studied by all possible ways and techniques like imaging, microscopy, etc. Different approaches have been adopted to study anatomy. Based on this, anatomy is divided into following types:

1. Gross anatomy/topographical anatomy
2. Microscopic anatomy (histology)
3. Surface anatomy
4. Comparative anatomy
5. Physical anthropology
6. Living anatomy
7. Clinical anatomy
8. Radiological anatomy
9. Developmental anatomy/embryology
10. Genetics
11. Experimental anatomy

1. **Gross (topographical) anatomy:** study on cadavers by dissection and observation of structures by naked eye. In gross anatomy the structures are either studied region-wise (**regional anatomy**) or system-wise (**systemic anatomy**).
   (a) ***Regional anatomy:*** approach in which all the structures in a particular region of the body are studied at the same time. The body is dissected region-wise. Since the regional anatomy deals with several systems located in a particular region of the body, this approach of studying anatomy is most useful to the clinicians, particularly the surgeons who need to concentrate mostly on a limited region during surgery. Therefore, regional approach is the most preferred method of anatomy all over the world.

Conventionally, the body is divided into the following six regions (Fig. 1.1):

1. Head and neck
2. Brain
3. Thorax
4. Abdomen
5. Upper limb
6. Lower limb

(b) ***Systemic anatomy:*** approach in which all the structures forming a particular system are studied together at the same time. A system consists of related organs which have a common function. The systemic anatomy provides comprehensive knowledge of a particular system throughout the body; hence, it is most useful for the physicians. In Indian subcontinent the gross anatomy is generally taught by regional approach. Therefore, a brief overview of all the systems is dealt in the book.

The various systems of the body (Fig. 1.2) are as follows:

(a) Integumentary system (study of skin and its appendages)
(b) Skeletal system (study of bones)
(c) Articular system/arthrology/syndesmology (study of joints)

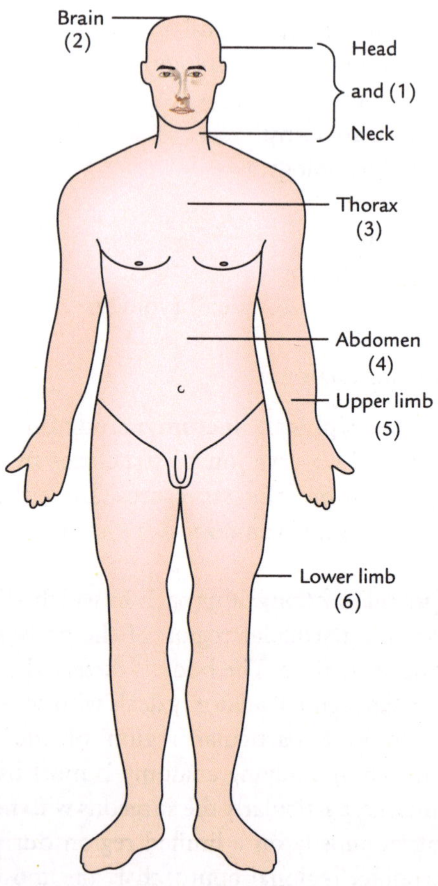

Fig. 1.1 Various regions of the body.

(d) Muscular system (study of muscles)
(e) Nervous system (study of neural tissue)
(f) Cardiovascular system (deals with heart and associated blood vessels)
(g) Lymphatic system (study of lymphoid tissue and lymph vessels)
(h) Endocrine system (study of ductless glands)
(i) Digestive system (study of structures concerned with digestion)
(j) Respiratory system (study of structures concerned with respiration)
(k) Reproductive system (study of structures concerned with reproduction)
(l) Urinary system (study of structures concerned with the formation and disposal of urine)

N.B.

- The term ***locomotor system*** includes osteology, arthrology and myology.
- The term ***splanchnology*** deals with the study of the visceral organs of respiratory, digestive, urinary, reproductive and endocrine systems.

2. **Microscopic anatomy (histology):** study of body structures with the help of microscope (light/electron microscope). Microscopic anatomy provides structural details of tissues and cells, which otherwise are not visible to the naked eye.
3. **Surface anatomy:** study of the relationship of deeper structures with skin surface; some of these structures can be seen, whereas others can be palpated on the body surface. These structures are sometimes used as surface (anatomical) landmarks for surface-marking of the much deeper structures with the help of 'skin-pencil'.

   The main aim of surface anatomy is visualization in the *mind's eye* of structures that lie beneath the skin. It can be learned on cadavers as well as on living subjects. Surface anatomy provides the basis for physical examination and the knowledge is of paramount importance for surgical operations.
4. **Comparative anatomy:** study of changes in the form, structure and function of the different parts of the body that have taken place in the Animal Kingdom during the course of evolution (phylogeny).
5. **Physical anthropology:** study of physical characteristics of the human beings and their ancestors, and of variability of these characteristics among and within different racial groups. The knowledge of physical anthropology helps to solve medicolegal problems of identification of individuals.
6. **Living anatomy:** study of the structures of the body of the living human beings by inspection, palpation, percussion, auscultation and with the help of various medical procedures like bronchoscopy, gastroscopy, cystoscopy and imaging techniques.

7. **Clinical anatomy:** use of anatomical knowledge for diagnosis and treatment of various diseases. It also provides the anatomical basis of various diseases.
8. **Radiological anatomy:** visualization of the structures and their relations with the neighboring structures inside the body by taking radiographs using x-rays. Recently, new imaging techniques like computerized axial tomography (CAT scan), magnetic resonance imaging (MRI) and ultrasound are frequently being used to study the deeper structures with greater accuracy and with little or no harmful effects.
9. **Developmental anatomy/embryology:** study of intrauterine development of an individual, which begins with fertilization and ends with birth. Much can be learned about the structure and function of adults by studying changes that occur during development.
10. **Genetics:** study of the principles of heredity and variation.
    (a) Heredity is the study of similar traits passed from the parents to their offspring, hence resemblance of family members.
    (b) Variation is the study of traits influenced by internal and external forces so that no individual is exact replica of the other.

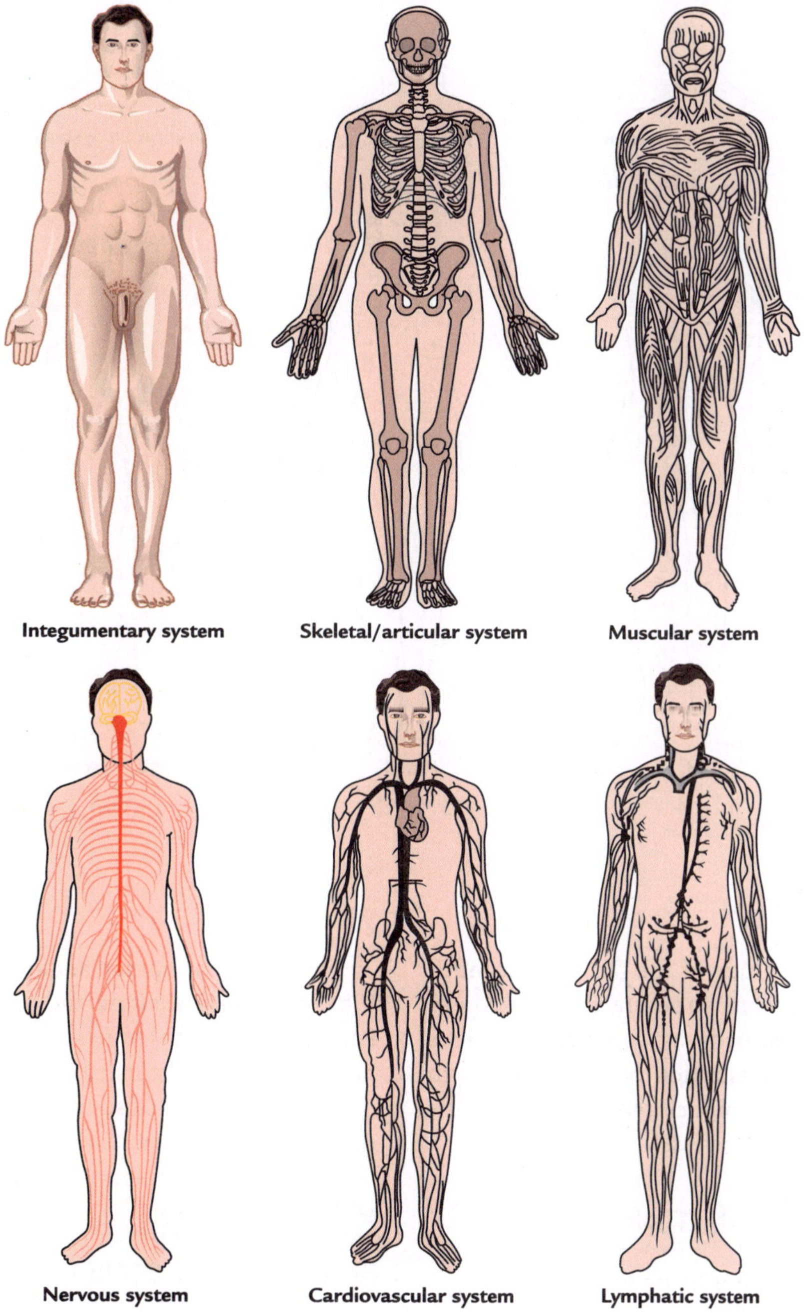

Fig. 1.2 Various systems of the body.

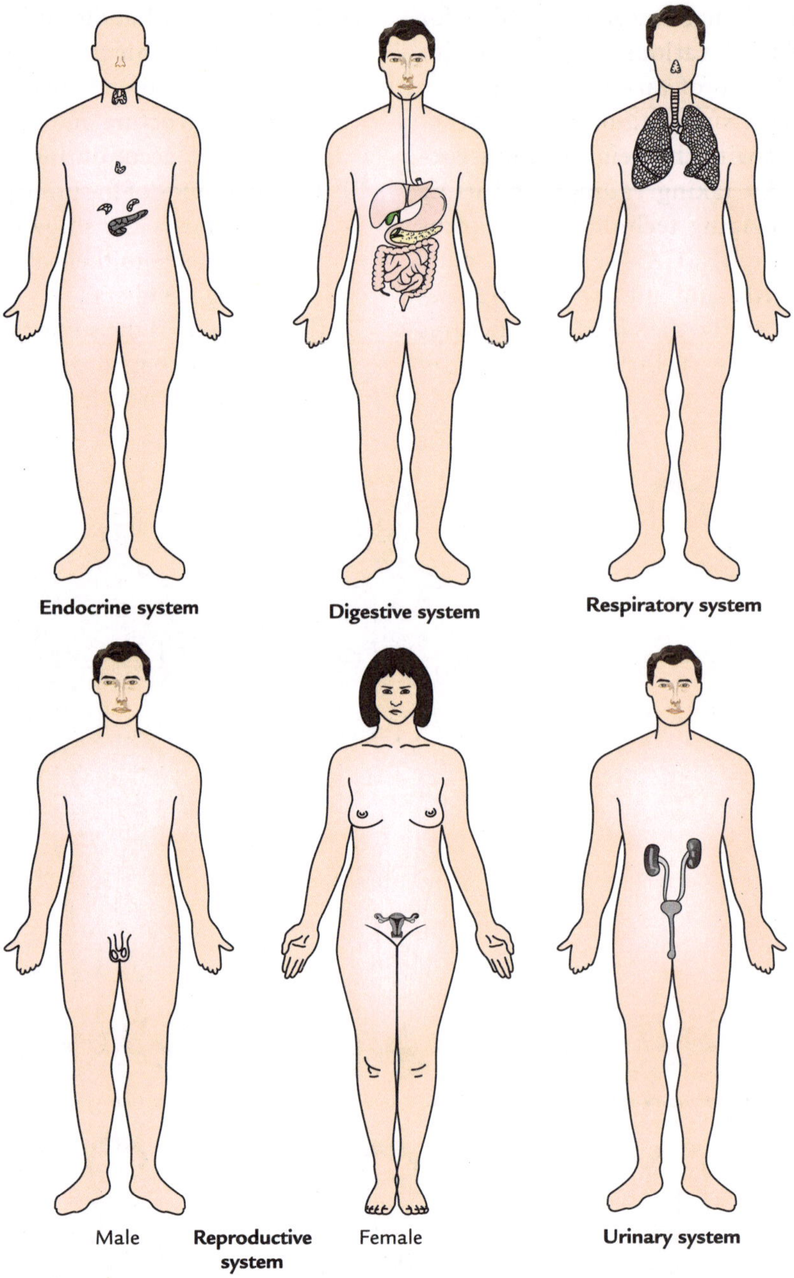

Fig. 1.2, cont'd

11. **Experimental anatomy:** study of the factors that influence and determine the form, structure and function of the different parts of the body by conducting various experiments such as demonstration of sites of valves in the veins by applying a tourniquet and determining the direction of blood flow in the vessel.

HISTORY OF ANATOMY

'The past is not dead history, it is living material out of which man builds for the future'.

Rene Dubos (1901–1982)

The history of human anatomy parallels that of medicine. It has rich, long, exciting and a frequently troubled heritage. People who made significant contributions to the science of human anatomy are listed in Table 1.1.

A brief account of some of the main contributors corresponding to different historical times is as follows:

GRECIAN PERIOD

Hippocrates (460–377 BC), Fig. 1.3

He was a famous Greek physician who is regarded as the **Father of Medicine** because of the sound principles of

Table 1.1 Contributors to the science of anatomy: historical perspective

Contributor	Period	Contribution
Menes	About 3400 BC	Wrote the first anatomy manual
Sushruta	About 1000 BC	Recorded weight of tongue and length of the intestine
Hippocrates	About 460–377 BC	Hippocratic oath. Called the Father of Medicine
Aristotle	384–322 BC	Comparative anatomist, first recorded illustration of anatomy, wrote first ever account of embryology
Herophilus	About 325 BC	Remarkable work on nervous system. Recognized brain as the center of nervous system and the site of intelligence
Galen	AD 130–201	Most influential writer of all time on medical subjects including anatomy
Leonardo da Vinci	1452–1519	Drew outstanding anatomical sketches Made wax cast of ventricles of the brain
Vesalius	1514–1564	Refuted misconceptions of Galen. Authored *De humani corporis fabrica.* Called the Father of Anatomy
Harvey	1578–1657	Demonstrated motion of blood in heart and vessels
Leeuwenhoek	1632–1723	Refined microscope. Described cells and tissues
Malpighi	1628–1694	Regarded as the Father of Histology
Robert Hooke	1665	Coined the term 'cell'
Schleiden and Schwann	1838–1839	Formulated Cell Theory
John Hunter	1728–1793	Established Hunterian museums in London. Discovered Hunter's canal
Mendel	1822–1884	Regarded as the Father of Genetics
Röentgen	1895	Discovered x-rays
Henry Gray	1827–1861	Authored the most accepted book on anatomy titled *Gray's Anatomy*
Watson and Crick	1953	Discovered the structure of DNA

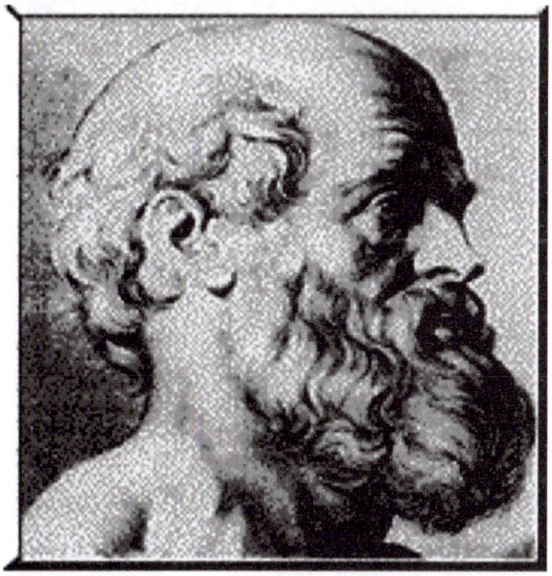

Fig. 1.3 Hippocrates.

medical practice that he had established. His name is memorialized in the *Hippocratic oath*, which the graduating students take before entering into medical practice.

Hippocrates had a limited exposure to human dissection, but he was well disciplined in proclaiming his popular theory of body organization called the *humoral theory*. According to this theory four body humors (i.e. four elements of body fluids) form the physiologic and pathologic basis of health and disease. These humors are blood, phlegm, yellow bile and black bile. He associated these humors with a particular body organ, *viz.* blood with the liver, yellow bile with the gallbladder, phlegm with the lungs and black bile with the spleen. A healthy person was thought to have balance of these four humors. The concept of humors has long since been discarded, but it had dominated medical thought for over 2000 years. Perhaps the greatest contribution of Hippocrates was that he attributed diseases to natural causes than to the displeasure of Gods. His application of logic and reason to the disease was the beginning of the present day scientific medicine.

Aristotle (384–322 BC), Fig. 1.4

A great Greek philosopher, Aristotle, was a zoologist, a renowned teacher and an accomplished writer. He made careful examinations on all kinds of animals, including references to humans. He wrote the first ever account of embryology, in which he described the development of the heart in an embryo. He named the aorta and differentiated the arteries and the veins.

In spite of his tremendous achievements, Aristotle perpetuated some erroneous views of anatomy. For example, according to him heart and not brain was the seat of intelligence and that function of brain, which is bathed in fluid, was to cool the blood that was pumped from the heart.

Herophilus (About 325 BC), Fig. 1.5

He was a great teacher of anatomy in the school of medicine at Alexandria, then the capital of Egypt. Through vivisections* (dissections of living humans) and dissections of human cadavers, Herophilus provided great descriptions of the skull, eye, various visceral organs and their relationships. He also described functional relationship of the spinal cord to the brain. Herophilus regarded the brain as the seat of intelligence and described many of its structures such as cerebrum, cerebellum and the fourth ventricle. He was the first to identify that nerves are either sensory or motor. Two monumental works of Herophilus were titled *On anatomy* and *On the eyes*.

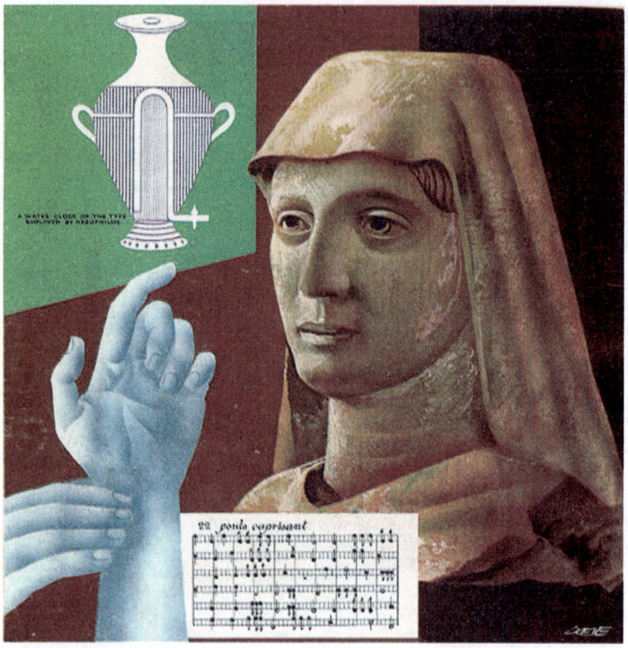

Fig. 1.5 Herophilus.

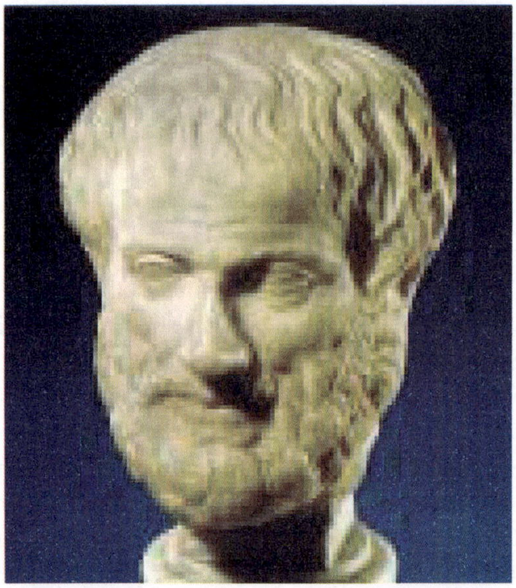

Fig. 1.4 Aristotle.

*The study of anatomy flourished in the school of medicine at Alexandria because of acceptance of dissections of human cadavers and of living human beings (vivi-sections). The vivi-sections were performed on condemned criminals by the permission of King 'Ptolemy Soter'. The people reasoned that the functions of the human body can be best understood if they were studied while the person was alive and a condemned man could repay society through the use of his body for vivi-section.

ROMAN PERIOD

Claudius Galen (AD 130–201), Fig. 1.6

Galen was perhaps the best physician since Hippocrates. He was the foremost practitioner of his days in Rome and was called the *Prince of Physicians*. He was certainly the most

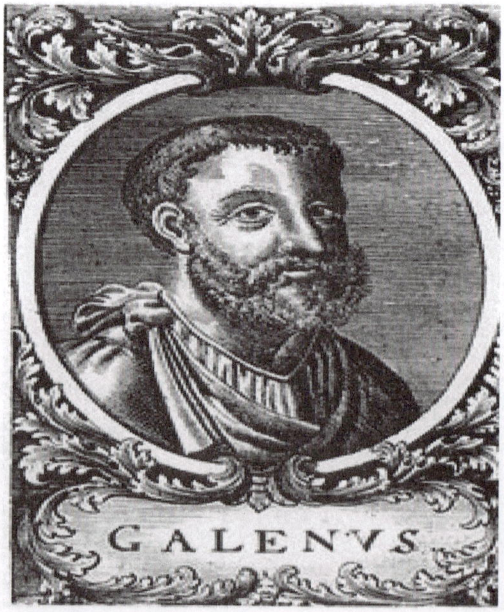

Fig. 1.6 Claudius Galen.

influential writer of all time on medical subjects. He wrote voluminously and theorized on many medical subjects like, anatomy, physiology, pathology, symptomatology and treatment. Galen's work was mainly based on the data on nonhuman animals and, therefore, contained many errors. He did, however, provide some accurate anatomical details that are still regarded as classics. For 1500 years (known as Galenic age) his writings were taken as unquestionable authority on anatomy and medical treatment.

RENAISSANCE PERIOD

It is the period when both arts and science were revived. It lasted from 14th century to the 16th century and was a transitional period from the middle ages to the modern age of science. The middle ages were frequently referred to as **dark ages** because there was no progress in arts and science during this period in Europe. It began with the fall of Rome in AD 476 and lasted for nearly 1000 years.

Leonardo da Vinci (1452–1519), Fig. 1.7

He was a great Italian genius who displayed his abilities as a painter, sculptor, architect, musician and anatomist. He is best known for his artistic works, such as *Mona Lisa*.

As an anatomist he observed dissections on cadavers very carefully and intended to publish a textbook on anatomy with the Pavian Professor, Marcantonio della Torre. His plan failed due to the untimely death of della Torre at the age of 31. When Leonardo died, his anatomical sketches were lost and remained undiscovered for over four centuries. His 60 notebooks containing nearly 500 diagrams were later published—in the year 1898. He was intent on accuracy and his illustrations showed the structural relationships of many organs. The advancement of anatomy would have accelerated by many years if Leonardo's notebooks had been available to the world at the time of his death.

He is considered as an originator of cross-sectional anatomy and was the first to describe the moderator band of the right ventricles. He constructed the models of the heart valves to demonstrate their actions.

SIXTEENTH CENTURY

Vesalius (1514–1654), Fig. 1.8

The contribution of Andreas Vesalius to the science of human anatomy is immeasurable. Vesalius was born in Brussels to a family of physicians. He was Professor of anatomy at the University of Padua in Italy. He performed human dissections and initiated the use of live models to determine the surface landmarks for internal structures. His masterpiece anatomical treatise, *De humani corporis fabrica* (*On the Workings of the Human Body*), written in seven volumes at the age of 28 years revolutionized the teaching of anatomy and remained an authoritative text for two centuries. The various body systems and individual organs were beautifully illustrated and described in the fabrica. In his book he boldly challenged hundreds of Galen's erroneous concepts that were taught as facts. Bitter controversies ensued between Vesalius and Galenic anatomists. Vesalius became so incensed by the relentless attacks that he destroyed much of his unpublished work and stopped doing dissections. However, by freeing anatomy from many of the Galen's errors, Vesalius laid the foundation on which many subsequent advances in medicine and surgery could take place.

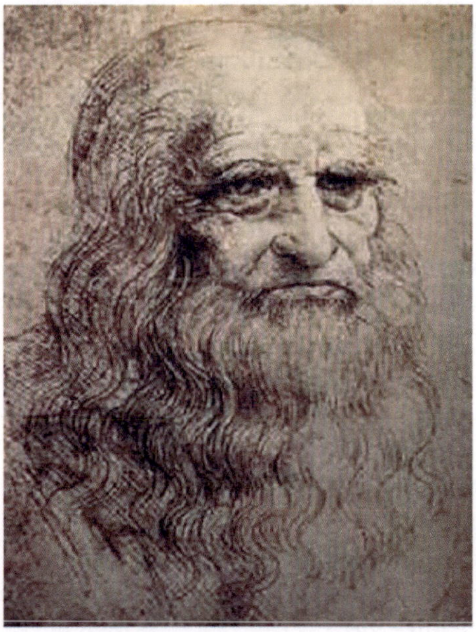

Fig. 1.7 Leonardo da Vinci.

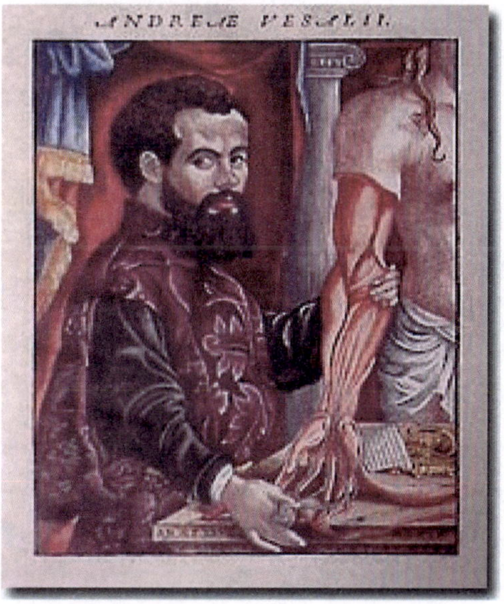

Fig. 1.8 Andreas Vesalius.

Another credit of Vesalius is that unlike other anatomists of his time (*viz.* Sylvius, Fallopius, Eustachius, etc.), Vesalius chose not to have his name attached to the parts of the body that he described. He remained a teacher of anatomy and bachelor throughout his life.

Vesalius was the greatest anatomist of his time and is now regarded as the **Father of Modern Anatomy**. He is also called the '**reformer of anatomy**'.

SEVENTEENTH AND EIGHTEENTH CENTURY

During the seventeenth and eighteenth centuries, the science of anatomy attained unparalleled acceptance and theatrical status. The human dissections were demonstrated to public. Two of the most important contributions during this period were:

(a) Explanation of blood flow
(b) Development of microscope

William Harvey (1578–1657)

In 1628, William Harvey, an English anatomist, conducted experiments *on the motion of the heart and blood in animals* and published the data. His technique of investigation is still regarded as a classic example of the scientific method of conducting research. He established a brilliant proof of the continuous circulation of blood within the vessels. He demonstrated that blood circulates and does not flow back and forth through the same vessels. Like Vesalius, he was also severely criticized for his deviation from Galenic philosophy.

William Harvey is credited for providing physiological (functional) orientation to anatomy.

Antonie van Leeuwenhoek (1632–1723), Fig. 1.9

He was a Dutch lens grinder, who improved the microscope tremendously and achieved a magnification of 270 times. The development of the microscope added an entire new dimension to the study of anatomy. His many contributions include:

(a) Development of techniques for examining tissues
(b) Description of blood cells, spermatozoa and skeletal muscle

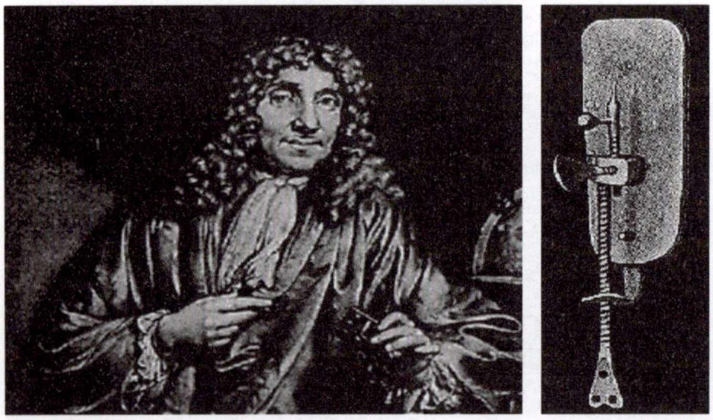

Fig. 1.9 Antonie van Leeuwenhoek.

Malpighi (1628–1634)

An Italian anatomist, Malpighi, has been referred to as the **Father of Histology** because he propounded microscopic anatomy and displayed fine details of the body tissues. His name is associated with malpighian corpuscles of the kidney and malpighian bodies of spleen.

John Hunter (1728–1793), Fig. 1.10

He was not only one of the foremost surgeons of all time, but the most versatile of scientists. He developed the Hunterian museums in London and Glasgow. He was the brother of William Hunter (1682–1771), who was the founder of anatomical theatre in London in the year 1768. The name of John Hunter is associated with Hunter's canal (adductor canal). It was John Hunter's study of the capillary system of deer which led to his treatment for aneurysm which is still in use today.

Wilhelm Konrad Von Röentgen (1845–1923), Fig. 1.11

He was a German physicist. He accidentally discovered x-rays in 1895 that opened new channels of observations in clinical anatomy that are used in medicine. The x-rays were first used by Röentgen to detect bone fractures and assess the extent of tuberculosis. He was awarded the first noble prize in physics in the year 1901.

N.B.

In 1750–1832, the selling of dead bodies flourished immensely in Great Britain and Ireland to interested parties, and people even went to the extent that they resorted to murder for obtaining dead bodies. In 1928 W Burke and W Hare were convicted for 16 murders. This led to the enactment of the *Anatomy Act* in London in 1832.

Gregor Johann Mendel (1822–1884)

Mendel performed experiments on plant's hybridization. He is known as the **Father of Genetics**.

The other anatomists who made contributions during this period were:

1. **De Graaf:** described ovaries.
2. **Spallanzani:** showed that both the sperm and ovum were necessary for conception.
3. **Francis Glisson:** described the liver, gallbladder, stomach and the intestine.
4. **Thomas Willis:** published summary of nervous system.

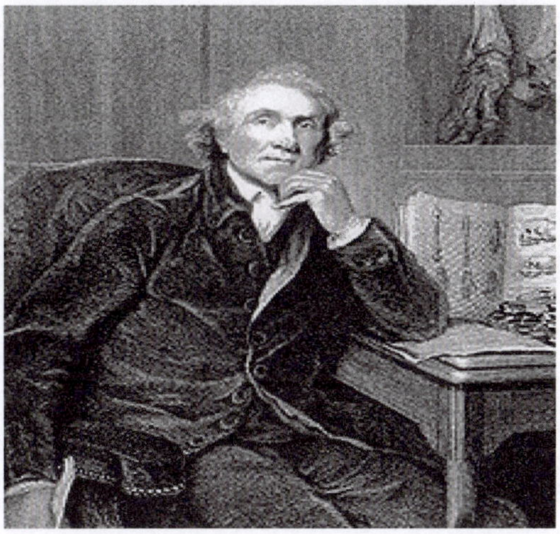

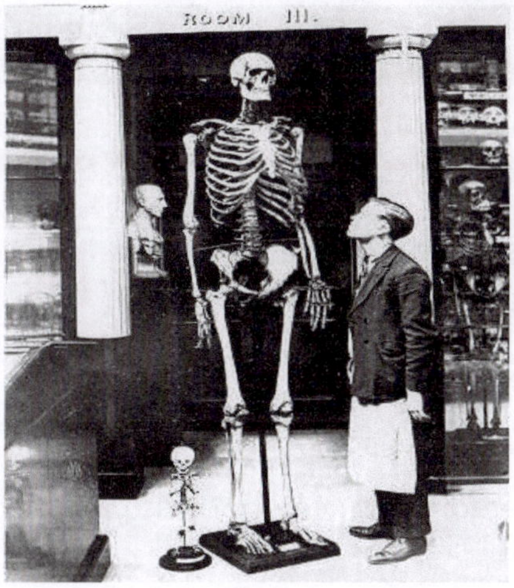

Fig. 1.10 John Hunter.

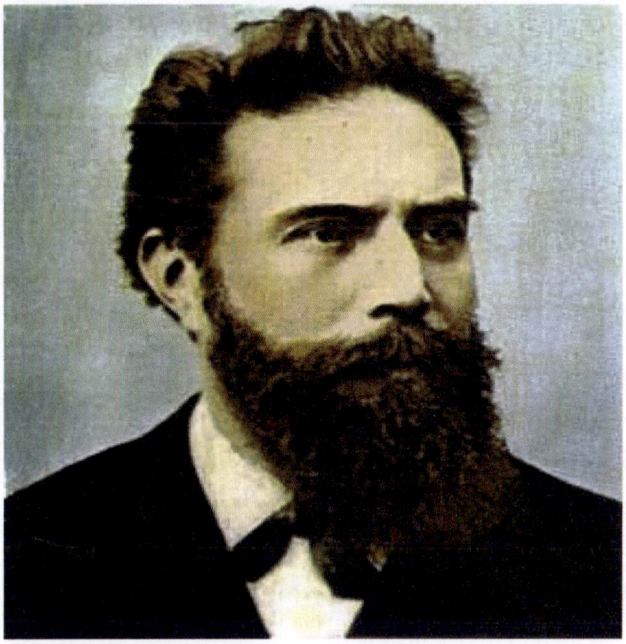

Fig. 1.11 Wilhelm Conrad Röentgen.

NINETEENTH CENTURY

The major contribution in the 19th century was the formulation of the cell theory and its implications in the understanding of the structure and functioning of the body.

Anatomy became a comparative science during this period. Dissection was made compulsory to medical students during this period in Edinburgh and Maryland.

The noted anatomists of this century include:

1. Astley Cooper
2. Georges Cuvier
3. Meckel
4. Henry Gray

TWENTIETH CENTURY

With the advent of electron microscope, the study of anatomy during this period became specialized and research became more detailed and complex.

The other innovation that gained momentum early in the 20th century was the **simplification and standardization of nomenclature.**

During this century, with the advent of newer imaging techniques like CT scan, ultrasound, MRI, PET, etc. more and more importance is being given to the radiological anatomy.

TWENTY-FIRST CENTURY

New virtual reality is being used to perform dissection on cyber cadavers. Currently, the visible human project created by National Health Institute (NIH), USA, is an extraordinary digital image library which is highly useful in orienting and associating structures seen in cadaver in exact location in cross section of the body.

N.B.

As seen in medical curricula, prescribed all over the world, it appears that the main objective of learning anatomy today is to use anatomical knowledge in understanding and solving clinical problems.

Golden Facts to Remember

➢ Father of Anatomy	Herophilus
➢ Father of Modern Anatomy	Vesalius
➢ Father of Medicine	Hippocrates
➢ Father of Histology	Marcello Malpighi
➢ Father of Genetics	Gregor Johann Mendel
➢ Term *'Anatomy'* was coined by	Aristotle (2300 years back)
➢ Who considered the human body as God's most beautiful creation	Andreas Vesalius
➢ First to dissect human body	Herophilus
➢ Human vivi-sections (dissections of living human body) were allowed in	School of medicine in Alexandria (Egypt)
➢ Two monumental works of Herophilus are entitled	*On Anatomy* and *Of the Eyes*
➢ Light microscope was first constructed by	Robert Hooke
➢ Modern light microscope was first designed by	Abbe
➢ Term 'cell' was first coined by	Robert Hooke in 1665
➢ First outstanding work on the motion of the heart and blood in animals was done by	William Harvey in 1628
➢ Leonardo da Vinci is best known for	His artistic work *Mona Lisa*
➢ Person who had dissected as many as 600 living human beings	Herophilus (about 325 BC)
➢ An embalming technique was first developed by	Egyptians (about 3400 BC)
➢ People who regarded the liver as the source of human emotions	People of ancient Mesopotamia*
➢ First recorded anatomical observations made in early Mesopotamia on	Early Mesopotamia on clay models of sheep's liver over 3000 years ago
➢ Best known but least understood contribution of *Chinese* to Anatomy is	Acupuncture**
➢ First manual on Anatomy was written	In Egypt about 3400 BC (i.e. even before the pyramids were built)

*Mesopotamia was the name given to a long narrow wedge of land between the Tigris and Euphrates rivers, which is now a large part of present-day Iraq. This area was settled 4000 BC. Because of the recorded information and culture of the people, Mesopotamia is frequently called the 'cradle of civilization'.

**The Chinese identified 365 precise meridian sites or vital points that correspond to the number of days in a year. The needles inserted at these sites cure body ailments. The effectiveness of acupuncture has been documented.

Acupuncture has gained acceptance with some medical specialists in the United States as a technique of anesthesia.

Multiple Choice Questions

1. **The term anatomy is derived from the Greek word *anatome* meaning:**
   (a) To analyze
   (b) To cut up
   (c) To observe death
   (d) To cut anus

2. **What is not true about Hippocrates:**
   (a) He was a famous Greek physician
   (b) He had wide exposure to human dissections
   (c) He had attributed diseases to natural causes
   (d) He is regarded as the Father of Medicine

3. **The anatomical masterpiece *De Humani Corporis Fabrica* was written by:**
   (a) Galen
   (b) Herophilus
   (c) Leonardo da Vinci
   (d) Vesalius

4. **Who is regarded as the Father of Modern Anatomy:**
   (a) Aristotle
   (b) Herophilus
   (c) Galen
   (d) Vesalius

5. **Who is regarded as the Father of Histology:**
   (a) Leeuwenhoek
   (b) Malpighi
   (c) Schleiden and Schwann
   (d) Watson and Crick

6. **The x-rays were discovered by:**
   (a) Röentgen
   (b) Madam Curie
   (c) Hooke
   (d) Muller

7. **What is not true about Aristotle:**
   (a) He was a pupil of Plato
   (b) He wrote the first known account of embryology
   (c) He thought heart to be the seat of intelligence
   (d) He had written eight volumes of *De re medicina*

8. **A trend towards simplification of anatomical nomenclature began:**
   (a) In 17th century
   (b) In 18th century
   (c) In 19th century
   (d) In 20th century

Answers

1. *b*, **2.** *b*, **3.** *d*, **4.** *d*, **5.** *b*, **6.** *a*, **7.** *d*, **8.** *d*

CHAPTER

2 Anatomical Terminology

Learning Objectives

After studying this chapter, the student should be able to:
- explain why anatomy is a very precise science
- describe the anatomical position of the body and discuss its significance in the science of medicine
- describe the anatomical planes of the body
- recall the terms used to describe joint movements, bony features, muscles, blood vessels and lymph vessels
- explain why directional terms are relative and must be used in reference to body structure or a body in anatomical position
- outline the terms used in clinical anatomy
- present a brief account of anatomical nomenclature
- explain how anatomical terms are derived
- correctly solve the review questions provided at the end of the chapter

INTRODUCTION

Anatomy is a very precise science because of its universally accepted terminology for describing the body parts and their locations.

In order to understand this science, students must master the terms used to describe anatomical structures and features. A little analysis of these terms would not only be an exciting experience but would also provide a glimpse into our medical heritage.

The majority of anatomical terms are derived from Greek or Latin, but some of the more recent ones are of German, French and British origin.

Many terms refer to common plants or animals, *viz.* the word *vermis* means worm, *cochlea* stands for shell of a snail, *cancer* refers to crab, *uvula* means little grape and even *muscle* is derived from the Latin word *musculus*, which means mouse.

The other terms are derived from materials and means used during wars, *viz. thyroid* means shield, *xiphos* means sword, *thorax* means breast plates, *sella* means saddle and *stapes* means the strirrups, *malleus* means anvil and *tympanum* refers to drum.

Further, the students can learn these terms more easily if they understand the meaning of their prefixes and suffixes.

Unfortunately, some of the anatomical terms have been coined in honor of various anatomists, surgeons and physicians. Such terms have no descriptive basis and cannot be associated with anything, and therefore, they must simply be memorized.

POSITIONS OF THE BODY

ANATOMICAL POSITION

In anatomical position the body is erect, the eyes are directed forward and look straight, the upper limbs hang by the side of the body with palms of the hand turned forward and the fingers are pointed straight down, the lower limbs, including the feet, are parallel to one another with feet flat on the floor and toes pointing forwards (Fig. 2.1).

In medical profession the body parts and their relationships are always described presuming that the body is in anatomical position, although it may lie or be placed in any position. Although in anatomical position the position of forearms and hands is not a natural one, it does allow for accurate description.

This is the position assumed in all anatomical descriptions to ensure accuracy and consistency.

In medicine, all descriptions of the human body are made in anatomical position.

FUNDAMENTAL POSITION

It is same as the anatomical position except that the palms of the hand face the sides of the body (Fig. 2.2). This position is

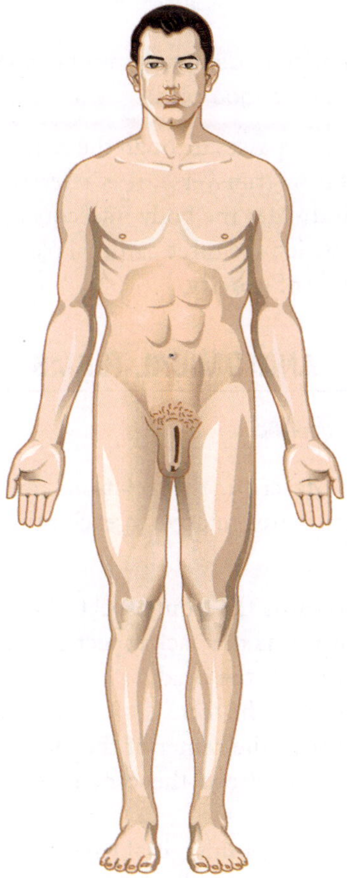

Fig. 2.1 Human body in anatomical position.

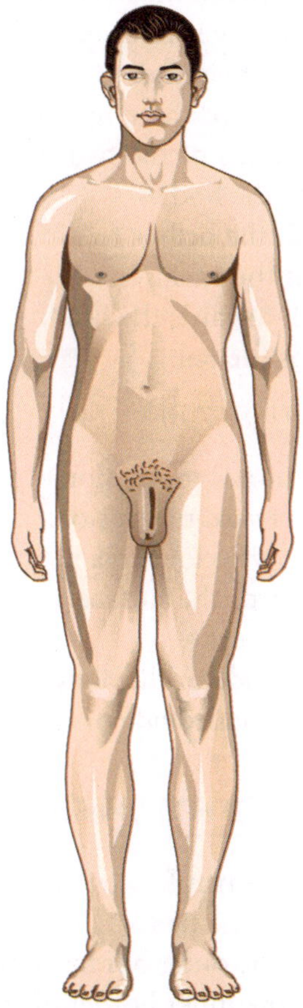

Fig. 2.2 Human body in fundamental position.

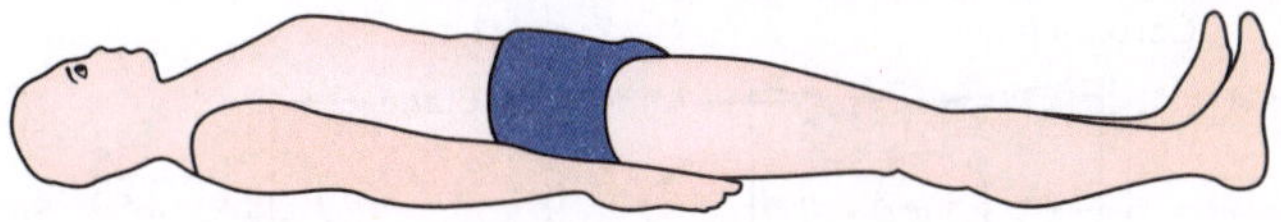

Fig. 2.3 Supine position.

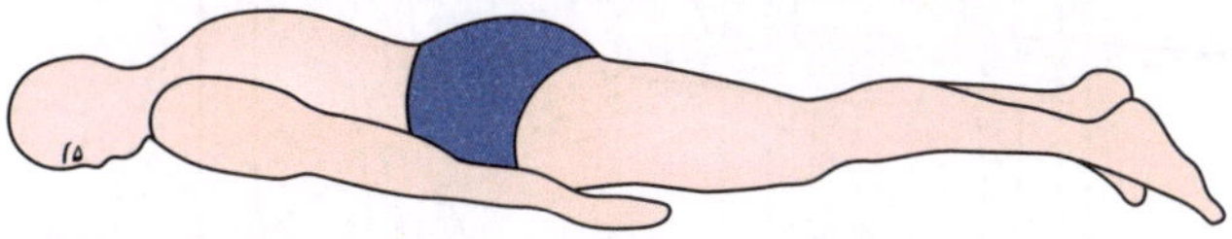

Fig. 2.4 Prone position.

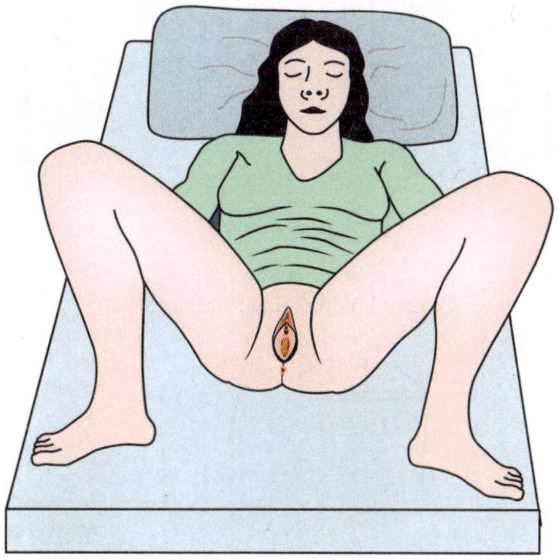

Fig. 2.5 Lithotomy position.

often used in discussing the rotation of the upper limbs, such as pronation and supination.

OTHER POSITIONS OF THE BODY

Some frequently used terms in clinical practice referring to body positions are as follows:

1. **Supine position:** the person lies on the back with face directed upwards (Fig. 2.3).
2. **Prone position**: the person lies on his belly (abdomen) with his face directed downwards (Fig. 2.4).
3. **Lithotomy position:** the person lies supine with buttocks at the edge of the table. The hips and knees are semiflexed and the thighs are abducted (Fig. 2.5). This position is used for adequate exposure for pelvis and vagina.

ANATOMICAL PLANES OF THE BODY

Four fundamental imaginary planes are frequently used to depict structural arrangement in the body (Fig. 2.6). These are:

1. **Midsagittal plane (or median plane):** It passes lengthwise, i.e. longitudinally through the sagittal suture (midline) and

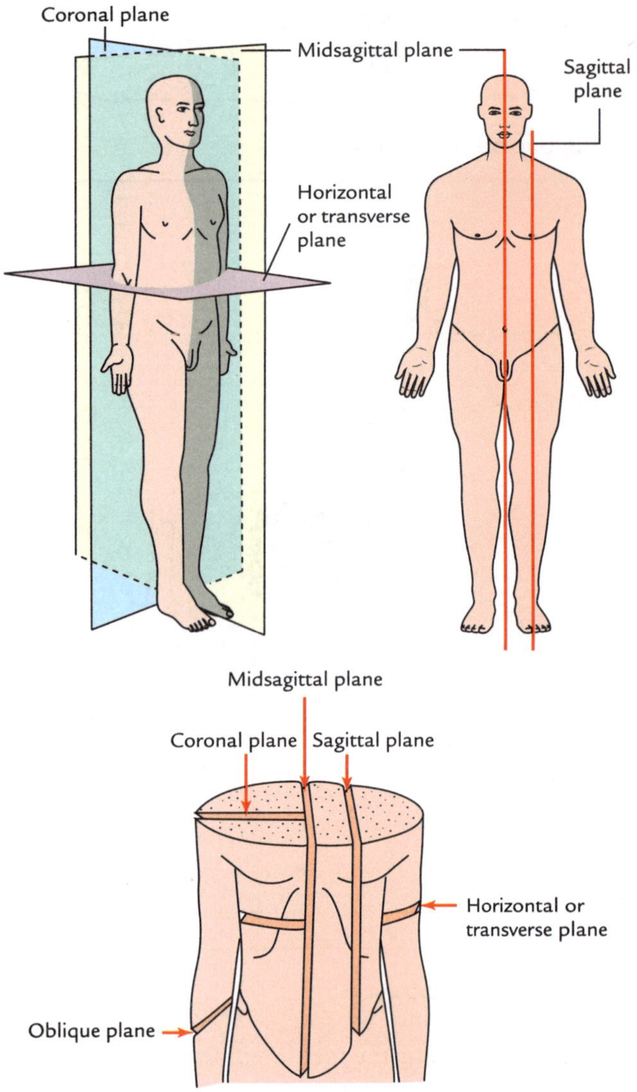

Fig. 2.6 Three fundamental planes of the human body in anatomical position.

divides the body into equal right and left halves. On the surface of the body, those halves are generally symmetrical in structure, yet the same symmetry does not apply to all internal structures.

2. **Sagittal plane:** Any plane parallel to midsagittal plane is termed sagittal plane. The sagittal plane also passes longitudinally but divides the body into unequal right and left halves.
3. **Coronal (or frontal) plane:** passes longitudinally at right angles to the median plane and divides the body into front and back portions. It corresponds to the coronal suture, hence the name coronal plane.
4. **Transverse plane (also called horizontal or cross-sectional plane):** passes parallel to the horizon (ground) and divides the body at any level into upper and lower portions. It is perpendicular to the median plane.

N.B.

Any plane other than midsagittal, sagittal, coronal and transverse is termed as *oblique plane*.

Whenever the plane passes through the center of the body, be it sagittal, frontal or transverse, it is referred to as **cardinal plane** because it divides the body into equal parts.

The point at which the three cardinal planes intersect each other is the **center of gravity**.

ANATOMICAL TERMS

DESCRIPTIVE TERMS

Terms used to describe the relationship between body parts and/or structures relative to each other are as follows (Fig. 2.7 A–D):

1. **Anterior:** towards the front aspect of the body.
2. **Posterior:** towards the back aspect of the body.
3. **Superior:** towards the head.
4. **Inferior:** towards the feet.
5. **Central:** towards the center of the mass of the body.
6. **Peripheral:** away from the center of the mass of the body.
7. **Median:** along the midsagittal (median) plane.
8. **Medial:** towards the median plane.
9. **Lateral:** away from the median plane.
10. **Intermediate:** between medial and lateral.
11. **External:** close to the surface of the body.
12. **Internal:** close to the center of the body.
13. **Superficial and deep:** these terms are used to describe the relative positions of the two structures with respect to the surface of the body.
14. **Ventral:** towards the belly.
15. **Dorsal:** towards the back.
16. **Cranial/rostral:** towards the head.
17. **Caudal:** towards the tail.

Some other terms (Fig. 2.7 E)

1. **Invagination:** inward protrusion.
2. **Evagination:** outward protrusion.
3. **Interior:** inside of hollow organ.
4. **Superficial:** towards the surface.
5. **Deep:** towards the center.
6. **Ipsilateral:** same side of the body.
7. **Contralateral:** opposite side of the body.

SPECIAL TERMS USED FOR LIMBS

1. **Proximal:** near the trunk.
2. **Distal:** away from the trunk.
3. **Radial:** towards the outer border of the upper limb.
4. **Ulnar:** towards the inner border of the upper limb.

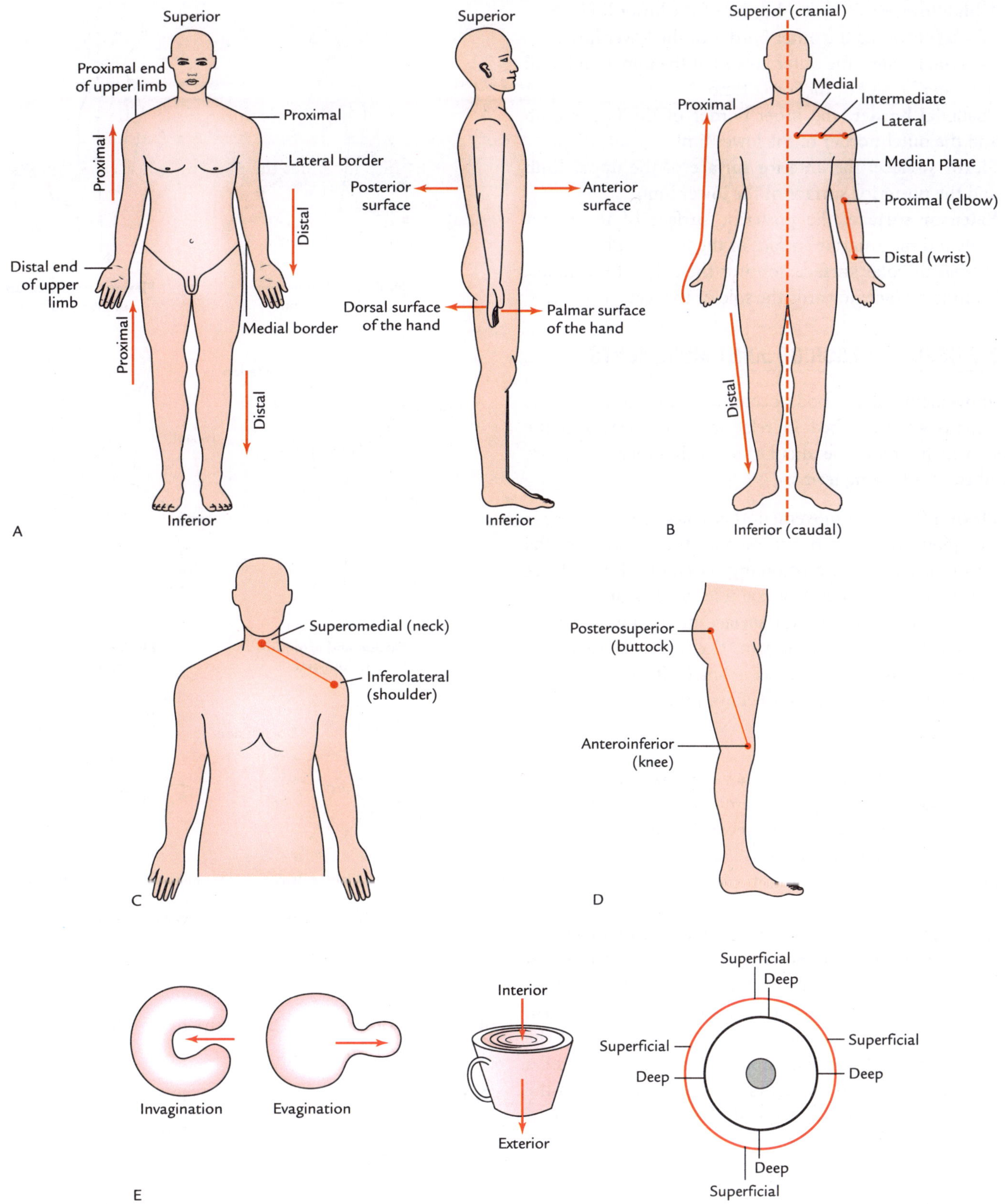

Fig. 2.7 A–E Relative relationship of body parts and/or structures with respect to each other: **A**, terms referring to direction of human body; **B**, relationship between location of three different points in thorax and median plane. It also shows relationship between elbow and wrist; **C**, relationship between neck and shoulder; **D**, relationship between buttock and knee; **E**, descriptions commonly used for referring to exterior/interior of body structures.

5. **Tibial:** towards the outer border of the lower limb.
6. **Fibular:** towards the outer border of the lower limb.
7. **Preaxial border:** the outer border of the upper limb and the inner border of the lower limb.
8. **Postaxial border:** the inner border of the upper limb and the outer border of the lower limb.
9. **Flexor surface:** the anterior surface of the upper limb and the posterior surface of the lower limb.
10. **Extensor surface:** the posterior surface of the upper limb and the anterior surface of the lower limb.
11. **Palmar or volar surface:** towards the palm of the hands.
12. **Plantar surface:** towards the sole of the feet.

TERMS USED TO DESCRIBE JOINT MOVEMENTS

The movements of the body occur at various joints. These movements are described in relation to the axis and the plane, which are perpendicular to each other. They are described in following terms:

1. **Flexion** (Fig. 2.5)**:** movement that takes place in the sagittal plane around a *transverse axis*. It approximates the flexor surfaces of the adjoining parts and thus reduces the angle of the joint. For example, the flexion of elbow approximates the anterior surface of the forearm with the anterior surface of the arm. The flexion is usually an anterior movement but occasionally it is a posterior movement, e.g. flexion of the knee joint.

N.B.

- In ankle joint, the flexion occurs when the dorsum of the foot is elevated and this movement is termed as *dorsiflexion*. Pressing the foot downward as in rising on the toes is called *plantar flexion*.
- *Lateral flexion* is movement of the trunk in coronal plane.

2. **Extension** (Fig. 2.8)**:** movement that approximates the extensor surfaces of the adjoining parts and thus increases the angle of the joint, e.g.: (a) extension of elbows approximate the extensor surface of the forearm with the extensor surface of the arm. Like flexion, the extension also takes place in the sagittal plane around a transverse axis, (b) extension of knee approximates the extensor surface of the leg with the extensor surface of the thigh.

N.B.

Hyperextension occurs when a part of body is extended beyond the anatomical position so that the angle of the joint is greater than 180°, e.g. when bending the head backward.

3. **Abduction** (Fig. 2.9)**:** movement of a limb away from the midline of the body in the coronal plane.

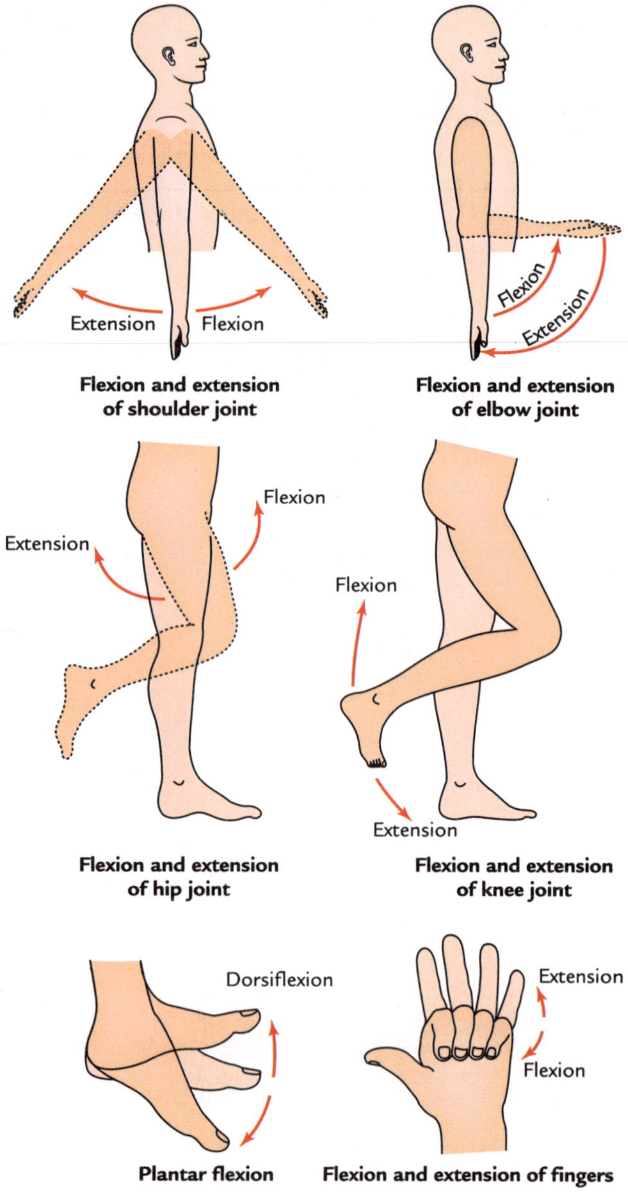

Fig. 2.8 Flexion and extension of joints and fingers.

4. **Adduction** (Fig. 2.9)**:** movement of a limb towards the midline of the body.

N.B.

- In case of fingers and toes, the term *abduction* is applied to spreading of these structures, whereas the term *adduction* for approximating these structures (Fig. 2.10).
- In case of thumb, the movements are little complicated (Fig. 2.10) and they are described in detail in *Textbook of Anatomy: Upper limb* (Volume 2).

5. **Rotation** (Fig. 2.11)**:** movements of a part of the body around its long/vertical axis:
   (a) *Medial rotation*: an inward rotation; results when anterior surface of the part faces medially.

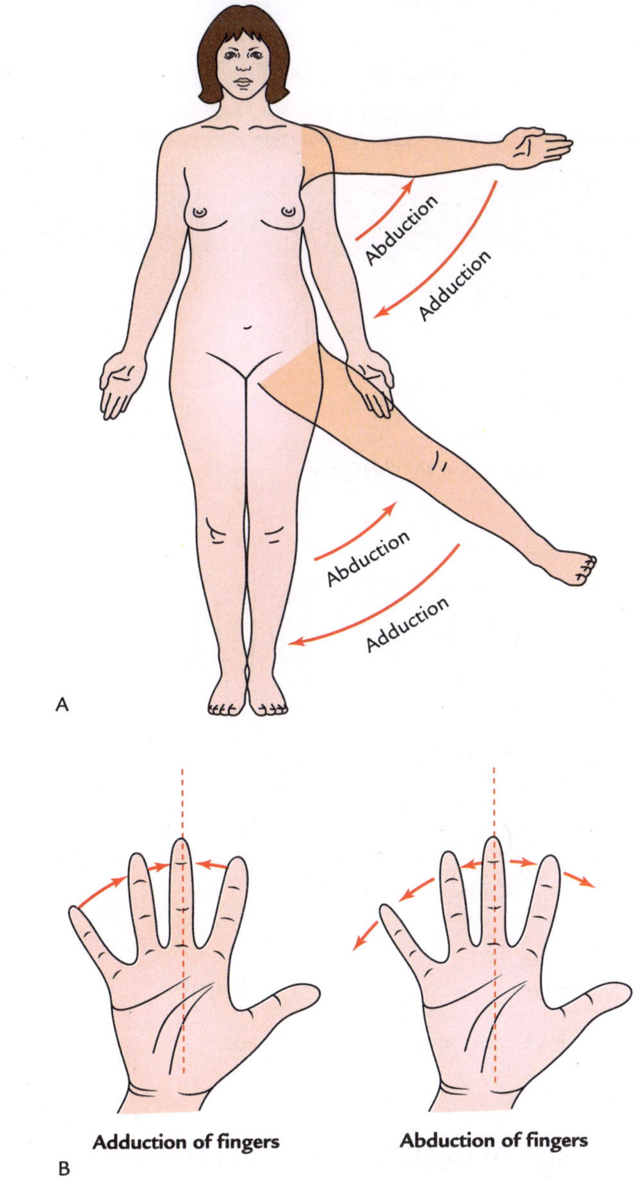

Fig. 2.9 Abduction and adduction of shoulder and hip joints **(A)** and fingers **(B)**.

(b) *Lateral rotation*: an outward rotation; results when the anterior surface of the part faces laterally.

6. **Circumduction** (Fig. 2.12)**:** circular cone-like movement of body segment which involves combination of angular movements in sequence, *viz.* flexion, extension, abduction and adduction. The base of the cone is formed by the distal end of the moving bone. Such type of movement is possible at the biaxial and polyaxial joints, *viz.* wrist, ankle, hip and shoulder joints. During bowling in cricket, there is a circumduction of upper limb at the shoulder joint where hand holding a cricket ball moves in a circle (Fig. 2.9).
7. **Supination** (Fig. 2.13)**:** rotation of the forearm and hand laterally from the midprone position around longitudinal axis so that the palm of the hand faces anteriorly.
8. **Pronation** (Fig. 2.13)**:** rotation of the forearm and hand medially from the midprone position around longitudinal axis so that the palm of the hand faces posteriorly.
9. **Inversion** (Fig. 2.14)**:** movement of the sole of the foot in which the sole faces inwards or medially.
10. **Eversion** (Fig. 2.14)**:** movement in which the sole of the foot faces outwards or laterally.
11. **Protraction:** movement in which a part of the body moves forward on a plane parallel to the ground, e.g. thrusting out the lower jaw or thrusting shoulder and arm forward.
12. **Retraction:** movement in which a part of the body moves backwards on a plane parallel to the ground, i.e. pulling back the protracted part.
13. **Elevation:** movement in which a part of the body is lifted upwards, e.g. elevation of the mandible to close the mouth or elevating the scapula to shrug the shoulder.
14. **Depression:** movement opposite to elevation.

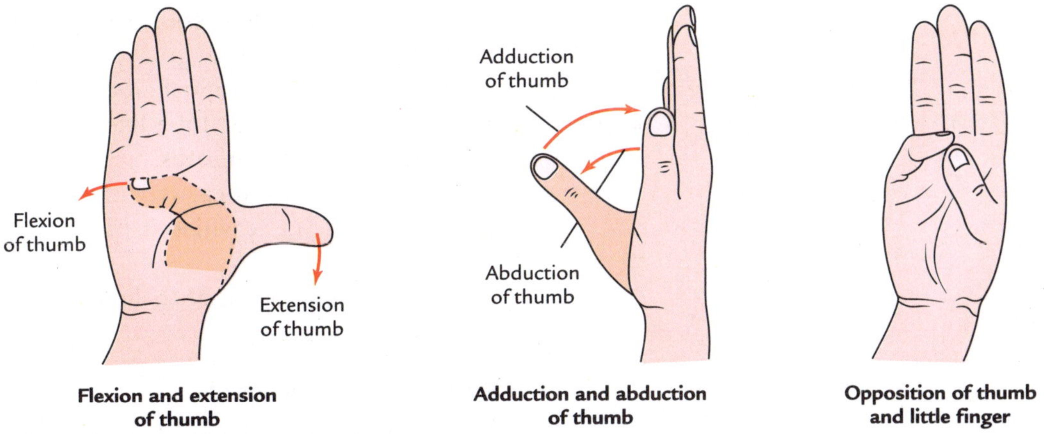

Fig. 2.10 Flexion–extension and abduction–adduction of thumb.

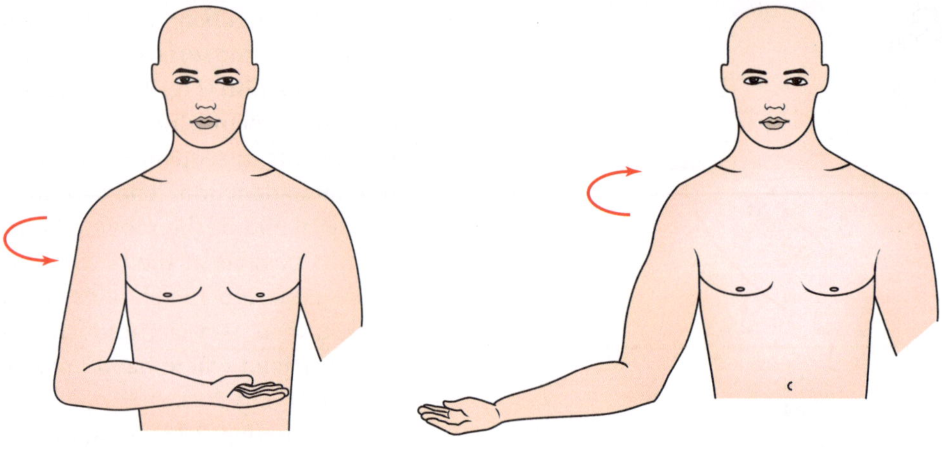

Fig. 2.11 Rotation movement of shoulder joint.

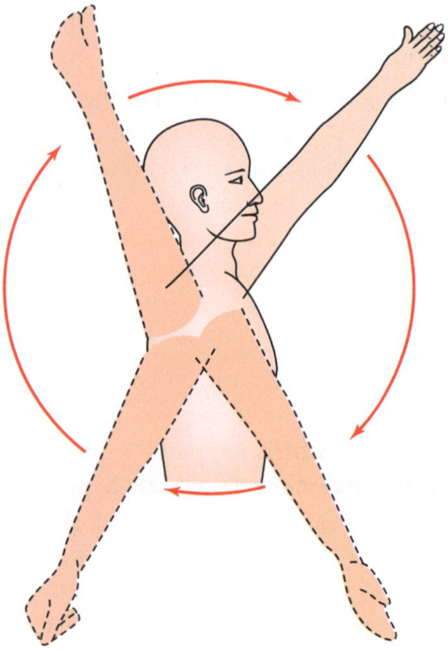

Fig. 2.12 Circumduction of shoulder joint.

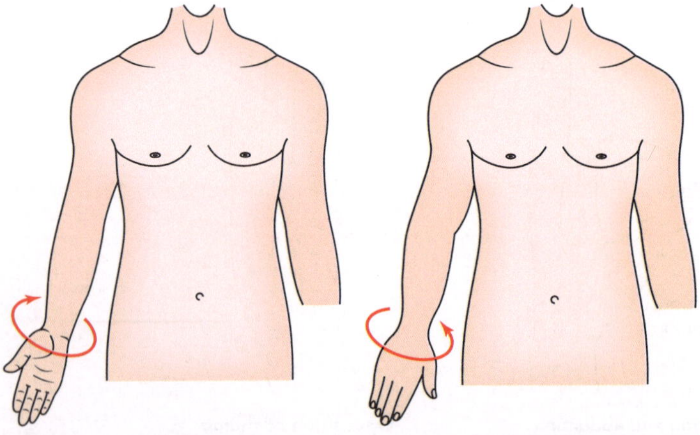

Fig. 2.13 Supination and pronation of forearm.

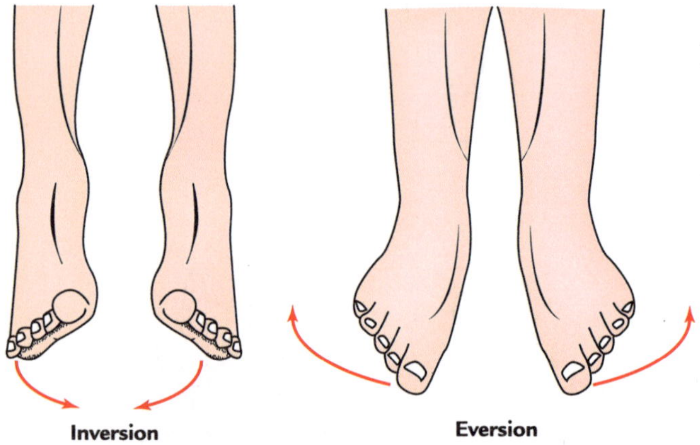

Fig. 2.14 Inversion and eversion of foot.

TERMS USED TO DESCRIBE BONY FEATURES

Depression and Openings

1. **Foramen:** a hole which provides passage to blood vessels and nerves, e.g. foramina in the transverse process of vertebra.
2. **Fossa:** a hollow depression, e.g. glenoid fossa of scapula.
3. **Groove:** a ditch-like groove containing a tendon or blood vessel, e.g. bicipital groove of humerus.
4. **Meatus:** a canal or tube-like opening in a bone, e.g. external auditory meatus.
5. **Sinus:** an air-filled cavity within a bone, e.g. paranasal air sinuses (i.e. cavities in the paranasal bones filled with air).
6. **Facet:** a smooth, flat or shallow area, e.g. articular facets of ribs.

Projections or Processes

1. **Condyle:** rounded knuckle-like projection, e.g. condyles of femur.

2. **Eminence:** projecting prominent part of bone, e.g. intercondylar eminence of tibia.
3. **Head:** rounded articular projection beyond a narrow neck-like portion of bone, e.g. head of femur, head of humerus.
4. **Crest:** sharp ridge or border.
5. **Epicondyle:** prominence above or on a condyle, e.g. medial and lateral epicondyles of humerus.
6. **Line:** less prominent ridge, e.g. linea aspera of femur.
7. **Spine:** long thin projection, e.g. spines of vertebrae.
8. **Trochanter:** very large prominence for muscle attachment, e.g. trochanters of femur.
9. **Tubercle:** small rounded projection, e.g. greater and lesser tubercles of humerus.
10. **Tuberosity:** large rounded projection, e.g. ischial tuberosity.

TERMS USED IN CLINICAL ANATOMY

1. **Analgesia:** loss of pain sensitivity.
2. **Analgesic:** an agent/drug causing loss of sensitivity to pain.
3. **Aplasia:** failure of development.
4. **Atrophy:** wasting or shrinking of a cell, tissue or organ.
5. **Anesthesia:** loss of sensation.
6. **Benign:** term used for illness or growth in which outcome is favorable (i.e. it does not endanger life).
7. **Coma:** loss of consciousness from which the patient cannot be roused (i.e. deep unconsciousness).
8. **Cancer:** in Latin, cancer = a crab. An uncontrollable proliferation of cells that usually destroys and invades adjacent tissues, metastasizes and usually follows a fatal course.
9. **Carcinoma:** cancerous growth arising from the epithelium (e.g. ectoderm or endoderm).
10. **Convalescence:** recovery period between the end of a disease and restoration of normal health.
11. **Diagnosis:** identification or determination of the nature of a disease.
12. **Degeneration:** physical alteration in a cell, tissue or organ consisting of a breaking down into a disorganized or less organized state. Degenerated structure may regenerate or end in necrosis.
13. **Dystrophy:** a degenerative disorder of the structure or organ due to improper nutrition resulting in diminution of size and function.
14. **Embolism:** occlusion of a vessel by a solid or gaseous matter which has been transported through the bloodstream, *viz.* detached thrombus (embolus).
15. **Gangrene:** necrosis (death) of a cell or tissue with liquefaction by bacteria and polymorphs (i.e. putrefaction).
16. **Hemiplegia:** paralysis of one-half of the body.
17. **Hypertrophy:** increase in size without any increase in the number of cells.
18. **Hematoma:** localized accumulation of blood in tissue or space. It is usually composed of clotted blood.
19. **Hyperplasia:** increase in size of tissue or organ due to increase in the number of cells.
20. **Hypoplasia:** underdevelopment of a tissue or organ. It implies fewer than usual number of cells.
21. **Hyperesthesia:** abnormally increased sensibility.
22. **Hyperalgesia:** excessive sensitivity to painful stimuli.
23. **Inflammation:** local reaction of tissues to an injury caused by chemical, physical or biological agents. The cardinal features of inflammation include swelling, redness, pain, heat (increased temperature), loss of function and fever.
24. **Infarction:** necrosis (death) of tissue secondary to sudden loss of blood supply to the affected tissue.
25. **Lesion:** pathological alteration in the structure or function of a tissue or organ.
26. **Lipoma:** cluster of fat cells forming a palpable lump. It is benign growth of mature adipocytes.
27. **Metastasis:** spread of local disease to distant parts of the body (i.e. spread of disease from one site to another).
28. **Metaplasia:** abnormal transformation of one differentiated adult tissue form to another type of adult tissue. It represents an adaptive response of tissues to injury.
29. **Malignant:** illness or growth which is resistant to treatment and tends to kill the patient.
30. **Malingering:** presenting an illness with conscious effort to deceive. It is common in females.
31. **Monoplegia:** paralysis of only one limb.
32. **Oedema:** swelling due to accumulation of fluid in the extracellular space.
33. **Paralysis:** loss of motor power (function) due to denervation or primary disease of the muscles.
34. **Paraplegia:** paralysis of both the lower limbs.
35. **Paresthesia:** perverted feeling of sensations such as pins and needles, burning, pricking, etc.
36. **Paresis:** reduction in muscle power.
37. **Prognosis:** forecasting the course and probable outcome of a disease based on the knowledge of the facts of a particular case.
38. **Pyrexia:** fever (i.e. increased body temperature).
39. **Signs:** any manifestation of disease which is objectively (physical signs) ascertained by a physician.
40. **Symptoms:** subjective complaints of the patient about his disease or disorder.
41. **Sinus:** a blind track (open at one end) lined by an epithelium.
42. **Syndrome:** a group of signs and symptoms constituting together the picture of a disease.
43. **Sarcoma:** malignant tumor of connective tissue or mesenchymal cells.
44. **Therapy:** a mode of treatment.
45. **Tumor (neoplasm):** a circumscribed, noninflammatory abnormal growth (due to uncontrollable proliferation of

cells). The benign tumors remain localized, whereas malignant tumors invade neighboring tissue and spread to other tissues and organs at a distant site, a process called metastasis.

46. **Thrombus:** a semisolid aggregate of blood cells enmeshed in fibrin and clumps of platelets within the blood vessel.
47. **Thrombosis:** formation of thrombus within a blood vessel.
48. **Ulcer:** localized breach in the surface continuity of skin or mucous membrane.

Suffixes:

(a) — **itis** = inflammation, e.g. tonsillitis (inflammation of tonsil), appendicitis (inflammation of appendix).
(b) — **ectomy** = removal from the body, e.g. tonsillectomy (removal of tonsil), appendicectomy (removal of appendix).
(c) — **otomy** = to open and then close a hollow viscus or region, e.g. laparotomy (opening and then closing abdominal cavity), hysterotomy (opening and then closing uterus).
(d) — **tomy** = act of cutting, in a surgical operation.
(e) — **ostomy** = to open a hollow organ and then leave it open for a desired period, e.g. tracheostomy (opening of trachea and then leaving it open), colostomy (opening of the colon and then leaving it open).
(f) — **oma** = a tumor, e.g. lipoma (tumor of fat cells), osteoma (bone tumor), hemangioma (tumor of blood vessels).

TERMS USED TO DESCRIBE BLOOD VESSELS

1. **Arteries:** vessels that carry oxygenated blood away from the heart.
2. **Veins:** vessels that carry deoxygenated blood towards the heart.
3. **Anastomosis:** communication between the branches of arteries and tributaries of veins.
4. **End artery:** an artery whose terminal branches do not anastomose with the branches of the arteries supplying the adjacent areas.
5. **Venae comitantes:** two veins that accompany an artery.
6. **Sinusoid:** small thin-walled blood vessels (capillaries) with irregular lumen lined by endothelial cells.
7. **Collateral circulation:** anastomotic alternate pathways (collateral channels) through which the blood can reach the field of distribution of the main artery if it is blocked.
8. **Capillaries:** microscopic vessels forming a network through which the arterioles (smallest arteries) discharge blood into smallest tributaries of veins.

TERMS USED TO DESCRIBE NERVES AND ASSOCIATED STRUCTURES

1. **Nerves:** whitish cords consisting of large number of exceedingly fine filaments called nerve fibers, bound together in bundles by fibrous tissue.
2. **Plexus:** braided structure resulting from network of nerve fibers.
3. **Ganglion:** group/collection of nerve cells outside the central nervous system.
4. **Nucleus:** group/collection of nerve cells within the central nervous system.

TERMS USED TO DESCRIBE FASCIAE

1. **Superficial fascia:** a mixture of loose areolar and adipose tissue lying deep to the dermis of the skin.
2. **Deep fascia:** dense inelastic membrane investing structures deep to the superficial fascia. It sends septa between the muscle groups.
3. **Fibrous sheath:** derived from deep fascia to form sheath around the tendons.
4. **Retinaculum:** thickening of deep fascia that retains the underlying tendons in position.

TERMS USED TO DESCRIBE MUSCLES

1. **Belly:** fleshy contractile part of the muscle.
2. **Tendon:** fibrous noncontractile, cord-like part of the muscle.
3. **Aponeurosis:** flattened tendon/flat sheet of collagen fibers extending from muscle to its attachment on bone.
4. **Raphe:** stretchable fibrous band made up of interdigitating fibers of the tendons or aponeurosis.
5. **Origin:** end of muscle which remains fixed during its contraction.
6. **Insertion:** end of muscle which moves during its contraction.
7. **Bursa:** sacs of connective tissue filled with synovial fluid, found where tendon slides over the bone.
8. **Synovial sheath of tendons:** similar to bursae in structure, consisting of double-layered synovial membrane tubes surrounding the tendons.
9. **Prime movers:** group of muscles initiating and maintaining a particular movement.
10. **Antagonists:** group of muscles which oppose the movement initiated by prime movers.
11. **Synergists:** muscles which assist prime movers.
12. **Fixators:** muscles which contract isometrically to stabilize the origin of prime movers so that it acts efficiently.

TERMS USED TO DESCRIBE LYMPH NODES AND LYMPH VESSELS

1. **Lymph nodes:** firm gland-like structures varying in size from pin head to a large bean.
2. **Lymph vessels:** fine beaded tubes containing clear fluid (lymph), found in large numbers in tissues adjacent to epithelial surfaces, *viz.*, skin, alimentary and respiratory tracts.

ANATOMICAL NOMENCLATURE

Claudius Galen (AD 130–201) and Andreas Vesalius (1514–1564), two great anatomists, wrote books on anatomy in Greek and Latin respectively. Therefore, most of the anatomical terms have Greek or Latin origin. Initially, anatomical terms used in textbooks and journals were about 30,000 in number. In 1895, the *German Anatomical Society* held its meeting at Basale and approved a list of about 5000 terms, called **Basle Nomina Anatomica** (BNA). It also laid down six strict rules, which are as follows:

1. Each part shall have only one name.
2. Each term shall be in Latin.
3. Each term shall be as short and simple as possible.
4. The terms shall be merely memory signs.
5. The related terms shall be similar, *viz.* femoral artery, femoral vein, and femoral nerve.
6. The adjectives shall be arranged as opposites, *viz.* psoas major, psoas minor, superior oblique, inferior oblique.

In 1933, the Anatomical Society of Great Britain and Ireland held its meeting at Birmingham and revised the BNA. The revised BNA was named **Birmingham Revision** (BR).

BNA was again revised by German anatomists in 1935 and was called **Jena Nomina Anatomica** (JNA). The **BR** and **JNA** restricted the Greek and Latin words to 5,000 only and allowed the terms of local contemporary language for usage.

In 1950, an International Congress of Anatomists was held at Oxford and it was agreed that further attempt should be made to establish a generally acceptable international nomenclature. In the sixth International Congress of Anatomists held at Paris in 1955, a somewhat conservative revision of BNA was done, incorporating many terms from BR and JNA and it was approved; it is known as **Nomina Anatomica.** The drafts on *Nomina histologica* and *Nomina Embryologica* were prepared by the subcommittee of the **International Anatomical Nomenclature Committee** (IANC). After a critical revision, the fourth edition of Nomina Anatomica containing *Nomina Histologica* and *Nomina Embryologica* was prepared by Roger Warwick in 1977 and published by Excerpta Medical Foundation. The author of this book had the proud privilege of having long and fruitful discussion with Roger Warwick. Now IANC is given the responsibility of bringing out the future editions as and when required.

Golden Facts to Remember

➢ Majority of anatomical terms are derived from	Greek or Latin
➢ All the terms of direction that describe the relationship of one body part to another are made in reference to	Anatomical position
➢ Sectional plane that divides the body into anterior and posterior portions	Coronal plane
➢ Sectional plane that divides the body into right and left portions is called	Sagittal plane
➢ Sectional plane that divides the body into upper and lower portions is called	Transverse/cross-sectional plane
➢ Basic procedures used for clinical examination of body are	*Observation* (visual inspection) *Palpation* (feeling with pressure) *Percussion* (detecting resonating vibrations) *Auscultation* (listening to organ sounds) *Reflex-response testing*

Continued

➢ Anatomical position	Subject stands erect and faces forward with arms at the sides and palm turned forward
➢ Adjunct motion	Voluntary independent rotation constituting a degree of freedom
➢ Conjunct motion	Obligatory coupled rotation which always accompany some other main movement
➢ *Fundamental position* is same as the anatomical position *except* that the	Palms face the sides of the body
➢ Parts of the body which are not in natural position in anatomical position	Forearm and hands
➢ Term *cephalad* refers to a position or structure close to the	Head (cephal = head)
➢ Term *caudal* refers to a position or structure closer to the	Feet (cauda = tail)
➢ Movements of supination and pronation of forearm are equivalent to	Movements of inversion and eversion of foot respectively
➢ Movement unique to human beings	Opposition of thumb
➢ Term BNA stands for	Basle Nomina Anatomica
➢ Facial feature unique to human	Prominent chin

Multiple Choice Questions

1. **Regarding anatomical position, which of the following statements is *not correct*:**
   (a) The body is erect and eyes are directed forward
   (b) The upper limbs hang by the side of the body and palms face anteriorly
   (c) The body is in fetal position
   (d) The lower limbs and feet are parallel and toes are directed forward

2. **Regarding fundamental position, select the *correct statement*:**
   (a) The body is in fetal position
   (b) The body is erect and palms face medially
   (c) The body is erect and palms face anteriorly
   (d) The arms are extended away from the body

3. **The sectional plane that divides the body into anterior and posterior portions is:**
   (a) Transverse plane
   (b) Sagittal plane
   (c) Coronal plane
   (d) Oblique plane

4. **Which of the following is not a fundamental plane:**
   (a) Coronal
   (b) Transverse
   (c) Vertical
   (d) Midsagittal

5. **Select the correct statement:**
   (a) In the supine position the person lies on the back with face directed upwards
   (b) In prone position the person lies on his back with face directed upwards
   (c) In prone position the person lies on his belly with face directed to the left side
   (d) In supine position the person lies on this back with face directed to the right side

6. **Regarding lithotomy position all are correct *except*:**
   (a) Person lies supine with buttocks at the edge of the table
   (b) Person lies prone with buttocks at the edge of the table
   (c) Person's hips and knees are semiflexed
   (d) Person's thighs are abducted and feet are in strapped position

7. **Regarding movements of hand and feet, which of the following statements is *not correct*:**
   (a) In supination the palm faces anteriorly
   (b) In pronation the palm faces posteriorly
   (c) In inversion the sole faces outwards
   (d) In eversion the sole faces outwards

8. **Regarding movements at a joint, which of the following statements is *not correct*:**
   (a) Flexion approximates the flexor surfaces of the adjoining parts
   (b) Extension approximates the extensor surfaces of the adjoining parts
   (c) In abduction limb moves close to the body
   (d) In adduction limb moves towards the body

9. **Which of the following is also called frontal plane:**
   (a) Midsagittal
   (b) Sagittal
   (c) Coronal
   (d) Transverse

Answers

1. *c*, **2.** *b*, **3.** *c*, **4.** *c*, **5.** *a*, **6.** *b*, **7.** *c*, **8.** *c*, **9.** *c*

CHAPTER

3 Architecture and Design of Human Body

Learning Objectives

After studying this chapter, the student should be able to:

- classify humans in the Animal Kingdom
- write the characteristic features of humans
- state the levels of structural organization of the human body
- identify the various regions of the human body
- outline the body cavities and their contents
- discuss the body membranes
- notify the disposition of body structures encountered during dissection
- correctly solve the review questions provided at the end of the chapter

INTRODUCTION

The human body is complex like a highly technical and sophisticated machine. Therefore, the knowledge of its organization is essential to comprehend.

Before beginning to study the organization of human body, one should know the taxonomic position of humans in the Animal Kingdom because we share many characteristics with all living animals. Like all other living animals we breathe, eat and digest food, excrete body wastes, locomote and reproduce our own kind. We are subject to disease, injury, pain, aging, mutations and death. The processes by which our bodies produce, store and utilize energy are also similar to those found in all living organisms. The fundamental patterns of development and growth of many nonhuman animals are also seen in human development.

In the scheme of classification of Animal Kingdom established by biologists to organize the structural and evolutionary relationship of living organisms, each category of classification is referred to as a **taxon**. The highest taxon is the Kingdom and the most specific category is Species. Human beings are species belonging to the **Animal Kingdom**.

Phylogeny is the origin and evolutionary development of animal species.

CLASSIFICATION OF HUMANS IN THE ANIMAL KINGDOM

Human beings are biological creatures that are classified into eight main taxonomic groupings.

The scientific classification of human beings and the characteristic features of each group are as follows:

Group	Features
Kingdom: Animalia	Eukaryotic cells that lack walls and photosynthetic pigments
Phylum: Chordata	Presence of notochord and pharyngeal pouches
Subphylum: Vertebrata	Presence of vertebral column
Class: Mammalia	Presence of mammary glands and hair
Order: Primata	Presence of well developed brain and prehensile hands
Family: Hominidae	Large cerebrum, bipedal locomotion
Genus: *Homo*	Flattened face, prominent chin and nose with inferiorly directed nostrils
Species: *sapiens*	Largest cerebrum

CHARACTERISTICS OF HUMANS

Human beings possess certain anatomical features which separate them from other animals. These are as follows:

1. **A large well developed brain:** The average adult human brain weighs between 1350 and 1400 g. This gives humans a large brain-to-body weight ratio. The human brain accounts for emotions, thought, reasoning, memory and precise coordinated movements.

2. **Bipedal locomotion:** Human beings stand and walk on two limbs and the upper limbs swing with movements of lower limbs.
3. **An opposable thumb:** The human thumb is tremendously versatile. It is opposable to fingers, hence adapted to grasp the objects.
4. **Well developed articulated speech:** Human beings have well developed articulated speech. Hence they can communicate with each other, which led to the development of culture and language.
5. **Stereoscopic vision:** The human eyes are directed forwards so that when we focus on an object, we view it from two angles. The stereoscopic vision gives us the depth of perception, a three-dimensional image.

N.B.

The human beings differ from other animals in number and arrangement of vertebrae (*vertebral formula*), the kinds and number of teeth (*dental formula*), the degree of development of facial muscles, etc.

Traits unique to human beings

- Erect posture
- Intelligence with cognitive function
- Skilled hand with opposable thumb
- Stereoscopic or binocular vision
- Prominent chin
- Fine coordination of muscles for skilled movements
- Well articulated speech

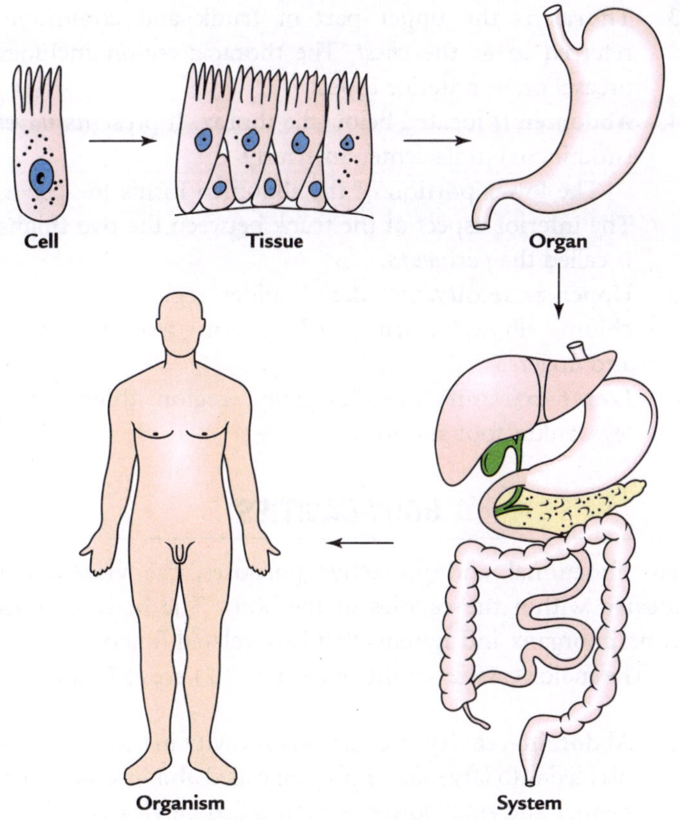

Fig. 3.1 Levels of structural organization of human body.

ORGANIZATION OF THE HUMAN BODY

Within the body there are different levels of structural organization. The five main levels of organization (Fig. 3.1) are:

1. **Cellular level:** The cell is the structural and functional unit of life. The human is a multicellular organism composed of 60–100 trillion cells. It is at cellular level that metabolism, growth, repair, etc. are carried out. The human body contains many distinct types of cells, each of which is specialized to perform specific functions. The examples of specialized cells are: (a) bone cells, (b) muscle cells, (c) fat cells, (d) blood cells and (e) nerve cells. Each of these cell types has a unique structure related to its function.
2. **Tissue level:** The tissue is a group of cells with similar structure and function including extracellular substance between them. The examples are: (a) epithelial tissue, (b) connective tissue, (c) muscle tissue and (d) nervous tissue.
3. **Organ level:** The organ is composed of two or more types of tissues that are integrated to perform a particular function. The examples of organs are: (a) heart, (b) stomach, (c) spleen, (d) eye, (e) skin, etc.
4. **System level:** A body system consists of various organs that have similar or related functions. These are 11 major systems in the body, *viz.*: (a) integumentary, (b) skeletal, (c) muscular, (d) nervous, (e) endocrine, (f) cardiovascular, (g) lymphatic, (h) respiratory, (i) digestive, (j) urinary and (k) reproductive systems.
5. **Organism level:** An organism is any living thing considered as a whole whether it is composed of one cell, *viz.* bacteria, or of trillions of cells such as human being.

The human organism is a complex of organ systems which are mutually dependent on each other, interrelated and function together.

BODY REGIONS

The human body is divided into several regions. The major body regions are: head, neck, trunk (trunk is frequently divided into thorax and abdomen), upper extremity and lower extremity:

1. **Head** is divided into (a) a *facial region*, which includes the eyes, nose and the mouth, and (b) *cranial region*, which encloses brain.
2. **Neck** is the region that extends between head and trunk and is roughly cylindrical. The neck supports the head and allows it to move.

3. **Thorax** is the upper part of trunk and commonly referred to as the *chest*. The thoracic region includes breasts on its anterior aspect.
4. **Abdomen** is located below the thorax. It presents *navel* (umbilicus) in its center anteriorly.

   The lower portion of the abdomen forms the *pelvis*. The inferior aspect of the trunk between the two thighs is called the *perineum*.
5. **Upper extremity** includes shoulder region, arm (brachium), elbow, forearm (antebrachium), wrist and hands and fingers.
6. **Lower extremity** includes gluteal region, thigh, knee, legs, ankle, foot and toes.

BODY CAVITIES

For functional and protective purposes, the viscera are located within the cavities of the body. The body cavities contain organs and systems that have related functions.

The major cavities of the body (Fig. 3.2) are as follows:

1. **Abdominal cavity:** It is the largest cavity in the body. It is divided into large upper portion called **abdominal cavity proper** and small lower portion called **pelvic cavity.**

   Abdominal cavity proper: It is oval in shape and situated in the main part of the trunk. It is bounded *superiorly* by diaphragm which separates it from thoracic cavity, *anteriorly* by muscles forming the anterior abdominal wall, *posteriorly* by lumbar vertebrae and muscles forming the posterior abdominal wall, *laterally* by lower ribs and parts of the muscles of the abdominal wall and *inferiorly* it is continuous with the pelvic cavity.

   The abdominal cavity proper contains organs and glands involved in digestion and absorption of the food:

   (a) Stomach, small intestine and most of large intestine
   (b) Liver, gallbladder, bile ducts and pancreas
   (c) Spleen
   (d) Kidneys, upper part of ureters and adrenal glands

   Pelvic cavity: It is roughly funnel shaped and extends from the lower end of the abdominal cavity. It is bounded *anteriorly* by pubic bones, *posteriorly* by sacrum and coccyx, *laterally* on either side by innominate (hip) bone, *inferiorly* by muscles of pelvic floor and *superiorly* it is continuous with the abdominal cavity.

   The pelvic cavity contains:

   (a) Terminal portion of large intestine, i.e. sigmoid colon, rectum and anus
   (b) Some loops of small intestine
   (c) Urinary bladder
   (d) Uterus
   (e) Uterine tubes
   (f) Ovaries
   (g) Prostate
   (h) Seminal vesicles
2. **Thoracic cavity:** This is situated in the upper part of the trunk. It is bounded *anteriorly* by sternum and costal cartilages of the ribs, *laterally* by 12 pairs of ribs and

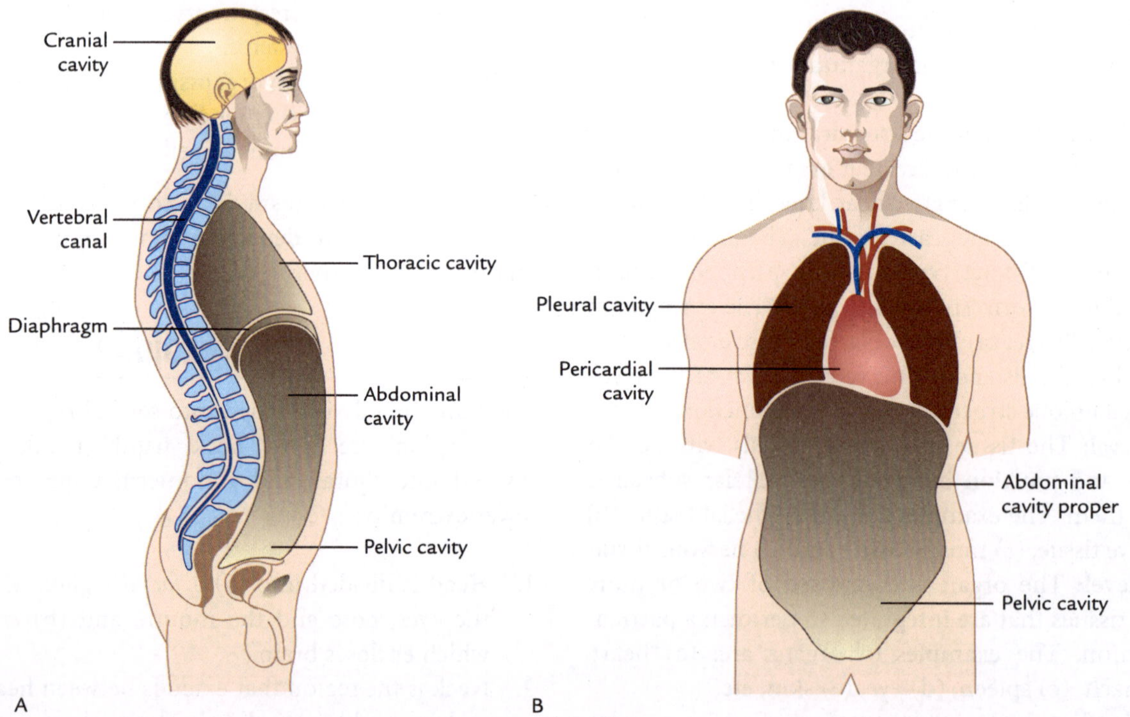

Fig. 3.2 Major cavities of the body: **A**, lateral view; **B**, anterior view.

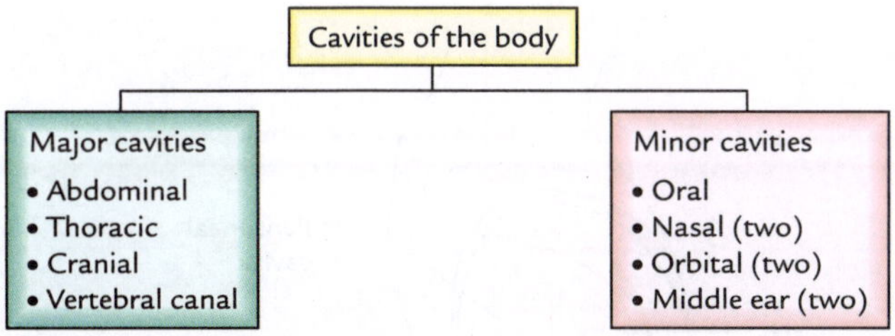

Flowchart 3.1 Body cavities.

intercostal muscles, *posteriorly* by thoracic vertebrae and intervertebral discs between the bodies of the vertebrae.

The thoracic cavity contains:

- Trachea, bronchi and lungs
- Heart, aorta, superior and inferior vena cava
- Thymus and thoracic duct
- Esophagus

3. **Cranial cavity:** It is the cavity within the skull and therefore bounded by the bones of the skull as follows: *anteriorly* by frontal bone, *posteriorly* by occipital bone, *laterally* on each side by temporal bone, *superiorly* by parietal bones and *inferiorly* by sphenoid, ethmoid and parts of frontal, temporal and occipital bones. The cranial cavity contains:
   - Brain
4. **Vertebral canal:** It is located within the vertebral column. It contains:
   - Spinal cord

The smaller/minor cavities of the body are:

1. **Oral (buccal cavity)**: it contains teeth and tongue.
2. **Two nasal cavities**: these are concerned with respiration and sense of smell.
3. **Two orbital cavities**: each of them houses eyeball and its associated muscles, nerves and vessels.
4. **Two middle ear cavities**: each of them contain ear ossicles.

The various cavities of the body are summarized in Flowchart 3.1.

BODY MEMBRANES

The membranes are sheets of epithelial cells and their supporting connective tissue layers. They cover or line the internal structures or cavities. The three main membranes are:

1. **Mucous membranes:** secrete a thick, viscid substance called **mucous** which lubricates or protects the associated organs.

   They line the various cavities and tubes that enter or exit from the body, *viz.* oral and nasal cavities, tubes of respiratory, reproductive, urinary and digestive systems.
2. **Serous membranes:** secrete a thin watery fluid called *serous fluid* which acts as a lubricant. The serous membranes cover the organs with the thoracic and abdominal cavities.

   The important serous membranes are:
   - *Pleural membrane*, covering the lungs
   - *Pericardial membranes*, covering the heart
   - *Peritoneal membranes*, covering the abdominal pelvic viscera

   The serous membranes are invaginated by the viscera and become divided into two layers: (a) visceral layer adhering to the outer surface of the organ; and (b) parietal layer lining the wall of the body cavity.

   The space between the visceral and parietal layer forms a serous cavity such as pleural cavities, pericardial cavity and peritoneal cavity (the largest serous cavity in the body).

   The pericardial cavity surrounds the heart (Fig. 3.3 A), pleural cavity surrounds the lung (Fig. 3.3 B) and peritoneal cavity surrounds the abdominal and pelvic viscera (Fig. 3.3 C).

   The space between the visceral and parietal serous membranes (serous cavity) is normally filled with a thin lubricating film of serous fluid produced by the membranes. As organs rub against the body wall or against another organ, the serous fluid and serous membranes reduce the friction.

Clinical correlation

Inflammation of serous membranes: The serous membranes sometimes become inflamed, usually as a result of infection. The inflammation of pericardium is called *pericarditis*, that of pleura is called *pleuritis* and that of peritoneum is called *peritonitis*. When inflamed, the serous membranes produce an increased amount of serous filled within serous cavities leading to clinical conditions like *pericardial effusion* (accumulation of fluid in the pericardial cavity), *pleural effusion* (accumulation of fluid in the pleural cavity) and *ascites* (accumulation of fluid in the peritoneal cavity).

The important serous membranes and serous cavities of the body are summarized in Table 3.1.

3. **Synovial membranes:** secrete clear, sticky, oily **synovial fluid** which acts as a lubricant. They line various joint cavities and surround tendons.

Table 3.1 Serous membranes and serous cavities of the body

Serous membranes	Serous cavities
Pleura	Pleural cavity
Pericardium	Pericardial cavity
Peritoneum	Peritoneal cavity

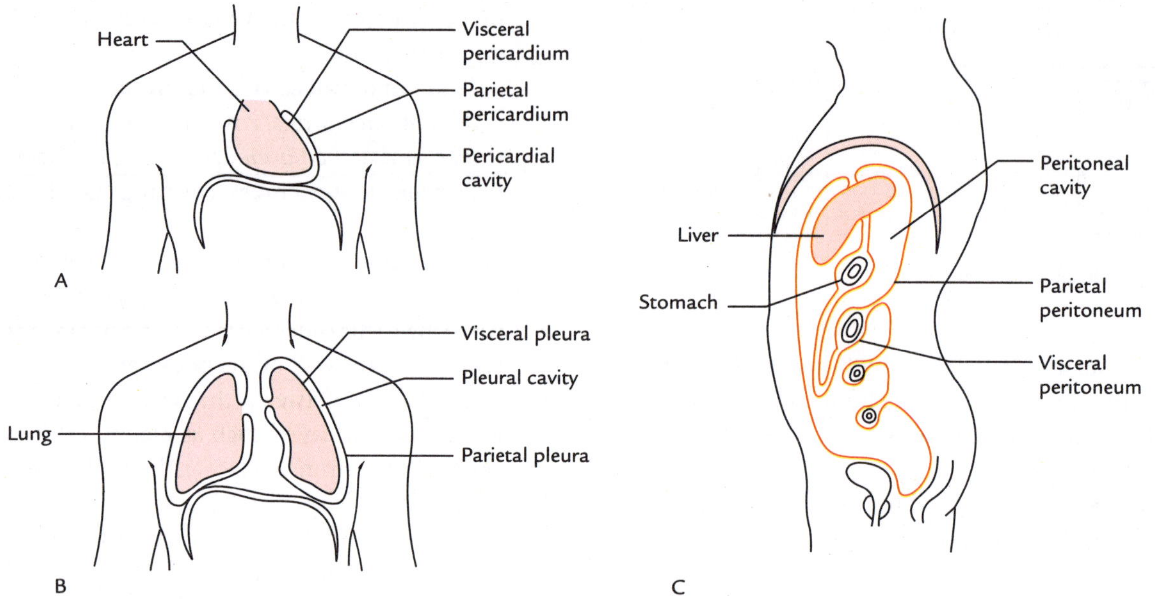

Fig. 3.3 Serous cavities surrounding the organs within thoracic and abdominal cavities: **A**, pericardial cavity surrounding the heart; **B**, pleural cavity surrounding the lungs; **C**, peritoneal cavity surrounding the abdominal organs.

BODY FLUIDS

Above 60% of body weight is formed by fluids present in the body. The body fluid is of two types:

1. **Extracellular fluid:** accounts for 22% of body weight. The extracellular fluid consists of blood, plasma, lymph, cerebrospinal fluid and fluid in the interstitial spaces of the body.

   The **interstitial fluid**, i.e. intercellular fluid (also called tissue fluid), bathes all the cells of the body except the outer layers of the skin. It is the medium through which substances pass from blood to the body cells and from cells to the blood.

   The well-being of every cell is dependent upon the composition of the intercellular fluid, which is therefore maintained at constant level by many control mechanisms in the body. This is called **homeostasis.**
2. **Intracellular fluid:** accounts for 38% of body weight. The composition of intracellular fluid is largely controlled by the cell itself, because there are selective uptake and discharge mechanisms present in the cell membrane.

GENERAL DISPOSITION OF THE BODY STRUCTURES

During dissection, following structures are encountered from superficial to deep (Fig. 3.4).

1. **Skin:** is the outermost covering of the body.
2. **Superficial fascia:** is made up of loose connective tissue and filled with variable amount of fat in different regions.
3. **Deep fascia:** is thin, tough, inelastic fibrous membrane deep to the superficial fascia and superficial to the muscles.
4. **Muscles (skeletal muscles):** are present deep to the deep fascia as red fleshy masses of different size and shape.
5. **Blood vessels and nerves:** are present between the muscles embedded in loose connective tissue. When traced distally, they give branches.
6. **Bones and joints:** bones are hard structures of different sizes and shapes deep to muscles. The junctions between the bones are called *joints*. The bones along with joints form the skeletal framework of the body.

INTRODUCTION TO THE STUDY OF ILLNESS

In order to understand the anatomical basis of specific diseases described in later chapters, it is necessary to adopt a systematic approach as outlined below:

1. **Etiology:** the cause of the disease.
2. **Pathogenesis:** the nature of disease process and its effect on normal body functioning.
3. **Complications:** the other consequences which might arise if the disease progresses.
4. **Prognosis:** the likely outcome.

Etiology: The disease is caused by one or more factors. The common factors causing the disease are:

1. **Genetic abnormalities**, inherited or acquired
2. **Infection** by microbes or parasites, *viz.* worms, bacteria or viruses

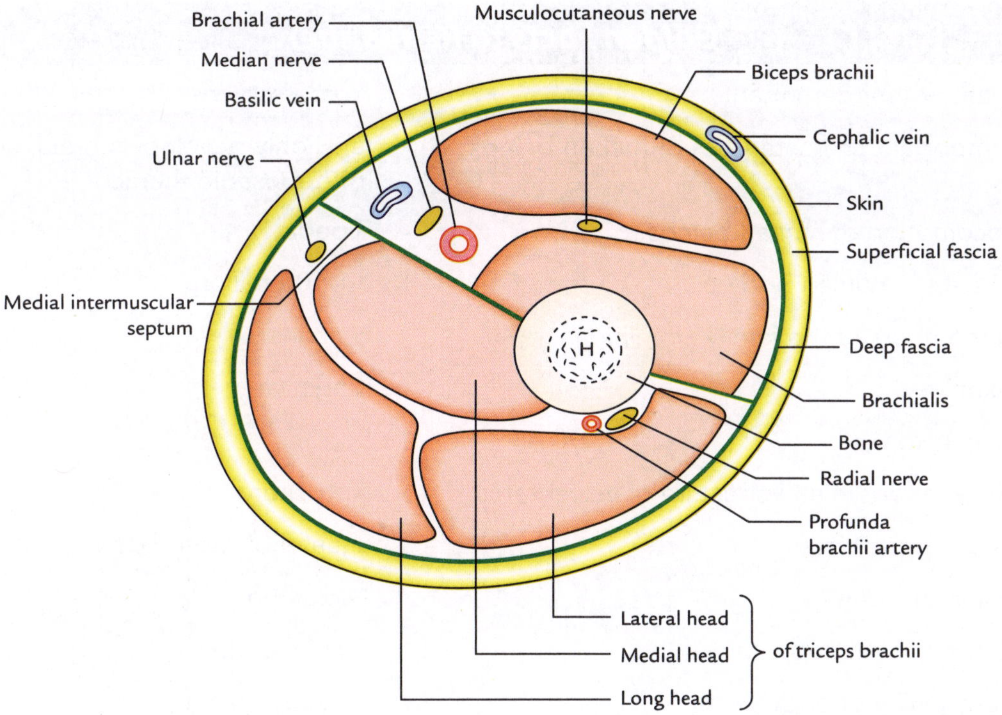

Fig. 3.4 Cross section of arm showing structures met during dissection. (H = humerus). (*Source:* Fig. 8.1, Page 93, *Textbook of Anatomy: Upper Limb and Thorax*, 2e, Vishram Singh. Copyright Elsevier 2014, All rights reserved.)

3. **Chemicals**
4. **Ionizing radiation**
5. **Physical trauma**
6. **Degeneration**, *viz.* excessive use or aging

N.B.

- If no specific cause of disease is identified, the cause is described as *idiopathic.*
- If the disease is caused by the carelessness of the doctor, the cause is described as *iatrogenic.*

Pathogenesis:

The main processes causing the illness are as follows:

1. **Inflammation,** the tissue's response to its damage is due to trauma or invasion by microbes.
2. **Tumors,** that arise when the rate of cell production exceeds that of normal cell destruction causing a mass to develop.
3. **Abnormal immune mechanisms,** sometimes the normal protective immune mechanisms of the body may cause undesirable effects.
4. **Thrombosis, embolism and infarction,** the effects and consequences of abnormal changes in the blood and/or walls of blood vessels.
5. **Degeneration,** which leads to impaired function.
6. **Metabolic abnormalities,** such as phenylketonuria cause undesirable effects.

Terminology associated with the disease

- **Acute:** a disease with sudden onset.
- **Chronic:** a long-standing disorder.
- **Congenital:** a disorder which one is born with.
- **Acquired:** a disorder which develops any time after birth.
- **Symptom:** an abnormality or disorder described by the patient.
- **Sign:** an abnormality or disorder noted by the doctor.
- **Syndrome:** a group of signs and symptoms which together constitute a disease.

Complications:

These include:

1. Spread of disease involving surrounding structures
2. Septicemia
3. Metastasis

Prognosis: It is a forecast of the probable course and outcome of a disease, e.g. the prognosis of benign tumors is generally good, whereas those of malignant tumors are poor.

Golden Facts to Remember

➢ Scientific name of modern man	*Homo-sapiens*
➢ Two most important characteristics of human beings	(a) Highly developed brain, and (b) opposable thumb
➢ Mode of locomotion of human beings	Bipedal
➢ Number of cells in human body	60–100 trillion
➢ Sole living members of the family *Hominidae*	Humans
➢ Highest taxon	Kingdom
➢ Most specific taxon*	Species
➢ Most primitive endoskeletal structure of vertebrates	Notochord
➢ Hardest tissue in the body	Enamel of tooth/bone
➢ Largest region of body	Abdomen
➢ Largest bony cavity of body	Cranial cavity
➢ Longest bony cavity of body	Vertebral canal
➢ All the chordates have three structures in common	(a) Notochord (b) Hollow neural tube (c) Pharyngeal pouches
➢ First organ of body to start functioning	Heart
➢ Largest cavity of the body	Abdominal cavity
➢ Largest serous membrane in the body	Peritoneum
➢ Largest serous cavity of the body	Peritoneal cavity
➢ Smallest level of body organization	Cell level
➢ Highest level of body organization	System level
➢ Vital functions of life are carried out at	Cellular level of body organization
➢ Cranial capacity in man	1200–1600 cm^3 (1500 cc)
➢ Oldest fossil of man discovered from South Africa	Proconsul
➢ Person who had given the scientific name of man	Carolus Linnaeus
➢ Nearest relatives of man among primates	Great Apes
➢ Organs that are similar in appearance and perform similar functions but differ in basic structure and origin	Analogous organs
➢ Organs that perform different functions but have similar structure and function	Homologous organs
➢ Family to which human beings belong	Hominidae
➢ Direct ancestor of modern living man	Cro-Magnon
➢ Animals who do not possess tail	Ape, Modern man

*In the classification scheme established by biologists to organize the structural and evolutionary relationships of organisms, each category of classification is called *'taxon'*.

Multiple Choice Questions

1. **All are correct regarding taxonomic classification of humans *except*:**
   (a) Phylum: Chordata
   (b) Class: Mammalia
   (c) Order: Primata
   (d) Family: *Homo sapiens*

2. **All are characteristics of a human being *except*:**
   (a) A large well developed brain
   (b) A well developed articulated speech
   (c) A well developed sense of smell
   (d) An opposable thumb

3. **Prehensile hands, opposable thumb, well developed brain and prominent chin are structural characteristics of grouping of animals termed:**
   (a) Primates
   (b) Humans
   (c) Mammals
   (d) Chordates

4. **Regarding serous membranes, which of the following word pairs is incorrect?**
   (a) Peritoneum/thoracic cavity
   (b) Pleura/thoracic cavity
   (c) Peritoneum/abdominal cavity
   (d) Pleura/lungs

5. **Aggregations of similar cells that perform specific functions are called:**
   (a) Organelles
   (b) Organs
   (c) Tissues
   (d) Glands

6. **The largest body cavity is:**
   (a) Cranial cavity
   (b) Thoracic cavity
   (c) Abdominal cavity
   (d) Vertebral cavity

7. **All are examples of an organ *except*:**
   (a) Heart
   (b) Skin
   (c) Muscle
   (d) Spleen

8. **All are examples of a tissue *except*:**
   (a) Epithelium
   (b) Muscle
   (c) Skin
   (d) None of the above

Answers

1. *d*, **2.** *c*, **3.** *b*, **4.** *a*, **5.** *c*, **6.** *c*, **7.** *c*, **8.** *c*

CHAPTER

4 Cells and Tissues of The Body

Learning Objectives

After studying this chapter, the student should be able to:

- describe the cell in brief and explain the structure and functions of organelles within it
- classify cells
- outline the two types of cell divisions
- describe the structure and functions of epithelium and connective tissue
- classify glands
- compare and contrast the structure and functions of exocrine and endocrine glands
- classify exocrine gland according to the mode of their secretion
- explain the capacity of regeneration in different types of tissue
- discuss the disorders of cells and tissues
- correctly solve the questions given at the end of the chapter

INTRODUCTION

The cells are the basic structural and functional units of the body (cell theory). The human body develops from a single cell called **zygote**, which results from the fusion of the ovum (female germ cell) and the spermatozoon (male germ cell).

The zygote undergoes a mitotic division (cleavage) and after several such cellular divisions, an embryonic mass consisting of 16 or more cells (blastomeres) is formed. It is called a **morula**. The fluid secreted by uterine endometrium enters in the intercellular spaces of morula and forms a fluid-filled cavity within the morula called **blastocoele**.

The appearance of a blastocoele segregates the cells into distinct groups:

1. A single layer of cells forming the outer wall—known as **trophoblast**.
2. An inner mass of cells—known as **embryoblast**.

With the establishment of these two groups of cells, the morula now becomes a **blastocyst** (Fig. 4.1). After further development, the trophoblast forms the **placenta** (fetal component) and the inner cell mass forms the **embryo**.

The inner cell mass then differentiates into three layers of cells; from superficial to deep these are:

1. Ectoderm
2. Mesoderm
3. Endoderm

These three layers are called the **primary germ layers**. *All the cells and tissues of the body are derived from these layers* (Table 4.1).

CELL

It is amazing that a single cell, the fertilized ovum (zygote), gives rise to hundreds of different kinds of cells, which compose 60–100 trillion cells that make up an adult human body. The body cells are broadly divided into two types: **somatic cells** and **germ cells**. The somatic cells are essential for growth, development, regeneration and maintenance of various tissues of the body, whereas germ cells are essential for production of gametes. The somatic cells contain 46 chromosomes arranged in 23 pairs. The cells containing two sets of chromosomes like this are called **diploid**. One set of chromosomes is derived from mother and the other is derived from father. Twenty-two pairs look alike, i.e. they are homologous. Twenty-third pair is the sex chromosomes. In the female they are both X chromosomes, while in the male there is one X and one Y chromosome.

The germ cells are essential for the production of gametes (ovum and sperms). The gametes contain 23 chromosomes, i.e. single set of chromosomes. The cells containing single set of chromosomes such as gametes are called **haploid**.

The cell division, growth, differentiation, maturation, programmed cell death (apoptosis) are the fundamental processes

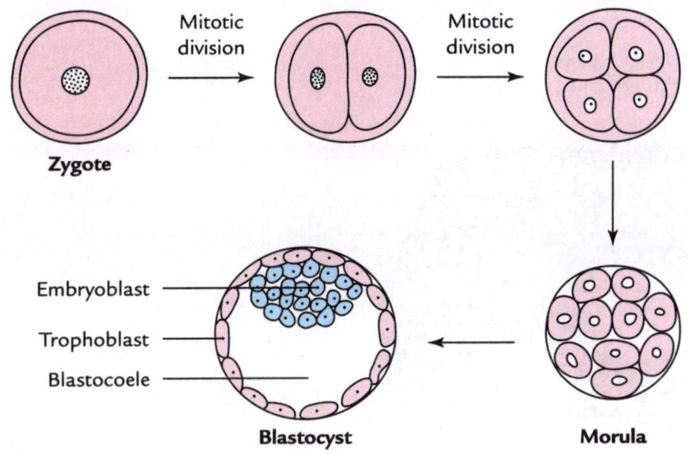

Fig. 4.1 Formation of blastocyst from zygote.

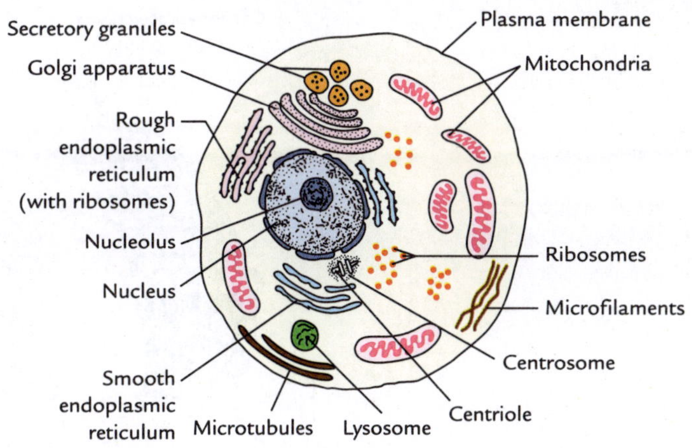

Fig. 4.2 Structure of a cell.

of the living body. Therefore, it is essential to consider the microscopic cellular anatomy:

1. The **cell membrane** separates the interior of the cell from extracellular environment.
2. The **nucleus** contains the genetic material of a cell.
3. The **cytoplasm** (watery fluid between nucleus and cell membrane) contains a number of minute structures called organelles plus deposits of carbohydrates, lipids and pigments. Most of the metabolic activities of a cell occur within the cytoplasmic organelles.

STRUCTURE

A cell consists of a **plasma membrane** enclosing nucleus and a watery fluid called **cytoplasm** (Fig. 4.2).

Plasma Membrane (Fig. 4.3 A and B)

The plasma membrane is composed of two layers of phospholipids (fatty substances) with some protein molecules embedded in it (fluid mosaic model). Some proteins traverse the entire thickness of the membrane and are called **transmembrane proteins** which contain channels for diffusion, while others penetrate only partly through it and are called **surface membrane proteins.** The phospholipid molecules have a head which is electrically charged and is hydrophilic (i.e. water loving) and a tail which has no charge and is hydrophobic (i.e. water hating). The two layers of phospholipids are arranged like a sandwich with hydrophilic heads aligned on the outer surface of the membrane and the hydrophobic tails towards the middle of the membrane (Fig. 4.3 B).

The outer surface of the cell membrane is covered by a layer of glycoprotein called **glycocalyx** or **cell-coat**. The tissue antigens, including major histocompatibility antigens (MHC), are located in the cell-coat.

The membrane proteins perform several functions:

1. They provide the cell its immunological identity.
2. They act as specific receptors for hormones and other chemical messengers.

Table 4.1 Derivatives of the three primary germ layers

Ectoderm	Mesoderm	Endoderm
Nervous system	Musculoskeletal system, i.e. muscles, bones and cartilages	Lining of gastrointestinal tract, respiratory tract, urinary bladder and urethra
Epidermis of skin including hair, nails and skin glands	Cardiovascular system (heart vessels)	Epithelium of thyroid, parathyroid, thymus, liver and pancreas
Epidermal lining of the surface of the body and orifices on the surface of the body	Dermis of skin	
Lens of eye, enamel of teeth	Dentin of teeth	
Adrenal medulla	Connective tissue, genitourinary system, adrenal cortex	

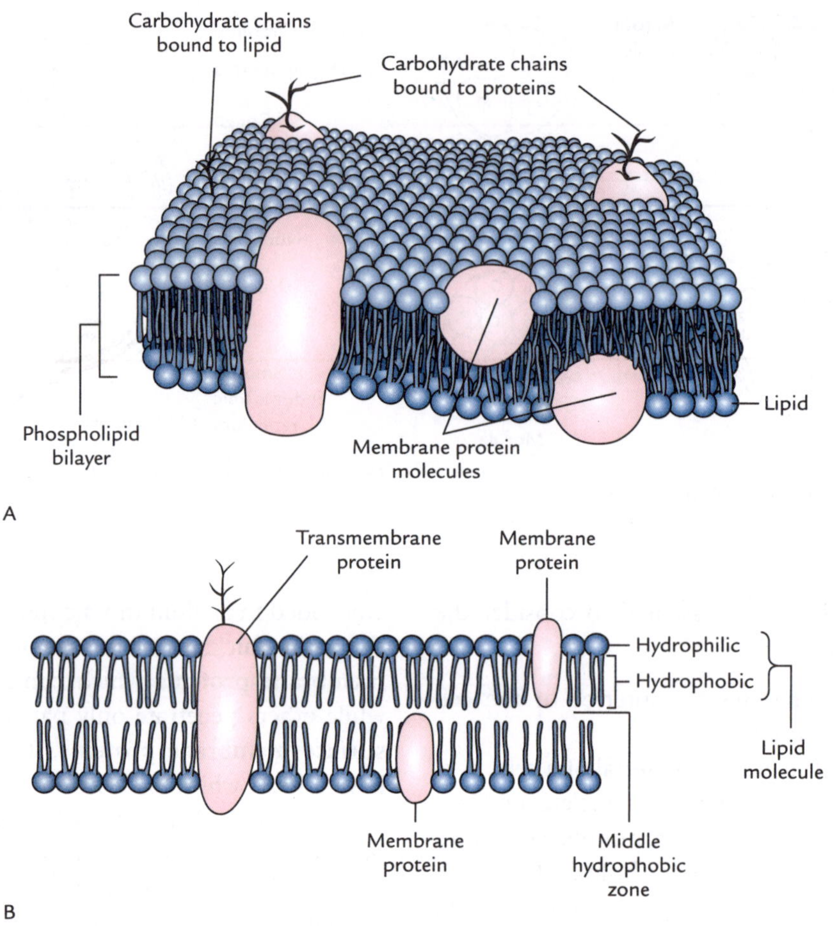

Fig. 4.3 Plasma membrane: **A**, fluid mosaic model; **B**, membrane showing two layers of phospholipids.

3. Some of them act as enzymes.
4. Some of them are involved in transportation across the membrane.

Nucleus

The nucleus is large, generally spheroid body surrounded by a membrane similar to the plasma membrane, but it has tiny pores through which some substances can pass between it and the cytoplasm. The material within nucleus is frequently called **nucleoplasm.**

The nucleus contains the genetic material of the body which directs all the activities of the cell. The genetic material is made up of **deoxyribonucleic acid (DNA)** and proteins called **histones.** These (DNA and histones) together form a fine network of threads called **chromatin.** The chromatin resembles tiny strings of beads.

During cell division the chromatin replicates and becomes more tightly coiled forming **chromosomes** (Fig. 4.4). The functional subunits of chromosomes are called **genes.** Each cell contains the total complement of genes (genome) required to synthesize all the proteins in the body but most cells synthesize only those proteins which are essential to their own specialized functions. Thus each cell uses only a part of **genome** or genetic code.

A highly refractile spherical body situated within the nucleus close to the nuclear membrane is called **nucleolus.** It is a compressed mass of a mixture of RNA granules and proteins. The RNA is liberated from the nucleolus through nuclear pores and appear in the cytoplasm.

N.B.

All cells except mature red cells contain nucleus.

Cytoplasmic Organelles

They include mitochondria, ribosomes, endoplasmic reticulum, Golgi apparatus, lysosomes, centrioles, microfilaments and microtubules.

Mitochondria

The mitochondria are sausage-shaped organelles and often described as the powerhouse of the cell. They are involved in aerobic respiration, the process by which the chemical energy in the form of **adenosine triphosphate (ATP)** is made available to the cell through a series of chemical reactions. The ATP is broken down further into free energy when required by the cell. The distribution of mitochondria varies in cells. They tend to accumulate in parts of cytoplasm where metabolic activity is more intense.

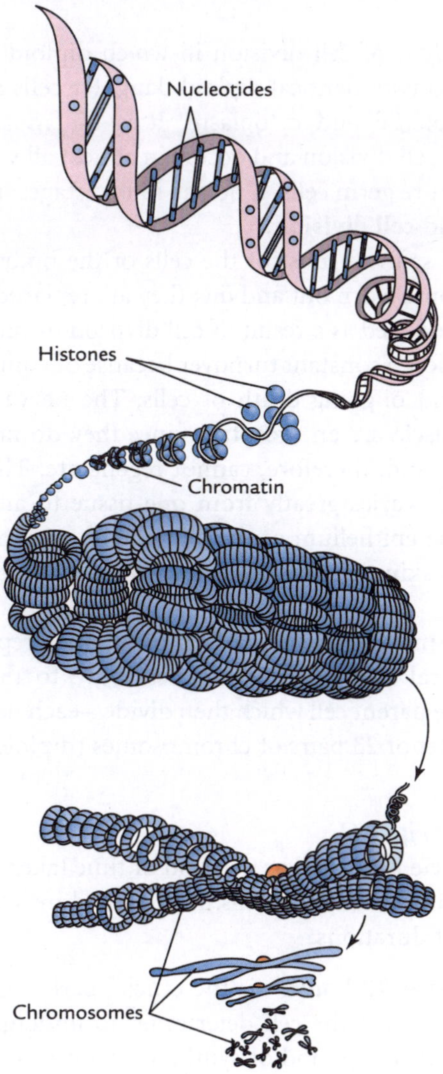

Fig. 4.4 Structural features of chromosomes during cell division.

Metabolically active cells, such as muscle cells, liver cells, have large number of mitochondria because they use energy at high rate.

Clinical correlation

Cytoplasmic inheritance: All the mitochondria in a fertilized egg (zygote) belong to the mother because head of sperm which enters the ovum during fertilization does not contain mitochondria. Thus all the mitochondrial DNA of fetus belongs to the mother. This accounts for unique form of inheritance that is passed only from mother to child. This type of inheritance is known as *cytoplasmic inheritance.* A rare cause of blindness *Leber's hereditary optic neuropathy* is believed to be inherited in this manner.

Ribosomes

These are tiny electron-dense granules (having density that prevents electrons from penetrating, therefore structures appear as dark bodies). They are composed of ribonucleic acid (RNA) and proteins. They are found in nucleus and nucleolus. They are also found on the outer surface of rough endoplasmic reticulum. The ribosomes synthesize **proteins** from amino acids.

Endoplasmic Reticulum

It is a series of interconnecting membranous canals. It is of two types: smooth and rough.

The smooth endoplasmic reticulum (SER) is devoid of ribosome granules. It synthesizes **lipids, glycogen, and steroid** hormones and is associated with the **detoxification of drugs.**

The rough endoplasmic reticulum (RER) is studded with ribosomes. It is the site of synthesis of proteins, *viz.* the **enzymes and hormones** that are exported from the parent cell to be used by other cells of the body.

Clinical correlation

Drug resistance: A person who repeatedly uses addictive drugs such as phenobarb, larpose or alcohol develops tolerance to these drugs; consequently, they require greater quantities of these drugs to achieve their effects. This is because the repeated use of drugs causes the smooth endoplasmic reticulum to proliferate in an effort to detoxify these drugs and protect the cell. With increased amount of smooth endoplasmic reticulum, the cells can handle an increased amount of drugs.

Golgi Apparatus

It is a supranuclear organelle that is composed of stacks of closely folded flattened membranous sacs. It is the site of **processing and packaging of proteins** synthesized by rough endoplasmic reticulum. The proteins move from rough endoplasmic reticulum to the Golgi apparatus where they are first processed and then packaged into small membrane-bound vesicles called **secretory granules.** These vesicles are stored and when needed, move to the plasma membrane through which proteins are exported.

Lysosomes (Lysis = Solution, Soma = Body)

These are membrane-bound vesicles which contain a large variety of hydrolytic enzymes whose main function is **intracytoplasmic digestion.** They are involved in the digestion of waste and harmful material of the cell taken into the cell from the environment. The lysosomes are present in almost all cells, but they are particularly abundant in cells exhibiting phagocytic activity, *viz.* macrophages, neutrophilic leukocytes.

Centrioles

Each cell capable of division contains two centrioles close to the nuclear membrane. The dense region of cytoplasm containing centrioles is called the **centrosome**. Each centriole presents two cylindrical bodies, placed at right angles to each other. Each cylinder consists of 27 microtubules arranged in nine bundles. Each bundle is composed of three microtubules called **triplets.** During cell division two centrioles divide to form two new centrioles. The parent centrioles migrate to the opposite sides of the cell.

The centriole synthesizes microtubules to form spindle during cell division.

Microfilaments

These are tiny strands of protein that provide structural support to the cell and maintain its characteristic shape. They are also involved in many other functions of the cell, e.g. contractile activity of muscle cells is primarily a result of the interaction between two types of microfilaments: myosin and actin.

Microtubules

These are tiny tubular structures made up of protein. They have a variety of functions such **as intracellular transport** of other organelles of the cell and movements of cell and cilia.

N.B.

All the cell organelles described above are membrane-bound organelles *except* ribosomes, centrioles, microtubules and microfilaments which are nonmembrane-bound organelles.

CELL DIVISION

There are two types of cell division: mitosis and meiosis (Fig. 4.5).

Mitosis

It is a method of cell division in which diploid parent cell gives rise to two identical diploid daughter cells in terms of genetic material and cytoplasm. It is the most common method of cell division and occurs in almost all somatic cells and immature germ cells. It occurs in two stages: **replication** of DNA and **cell division.**

The life span of most of the cells of the body is limited. Many become worn out and die; they are replaced by identical cells produced as a result of cell division or mitosis. Most tissues undergo constant turnover because of continuous cell division and ongoing death of cells. The nerve tissue and cardiac muscle are an exception since they do not multiply postnatally and, therefore, cannot regenerate. The turnover rate of cells varies greatly from one tissue to another. It is rapid in the epithelium of the alimentary canal and epidermis of the skin, whereas it is slow in the pancreas and the thyroid.

During mitosis 23 pairs of chromosomes replicate. The two identical sets of chromosomes move to the opposite poles of the parent cell which then divides–each daughter cell receives a set of 23 pairs of chromosomes (diploid number).

Cell Cycle (Fig. 4.6)

The cell cycle is defined as a period of time taken by a cell to divide into two daughter cells. It is divided into four phases of different durations:

1. **G1 phase, 12 hours**—is the crucial period of cell cycle during which the cell determines to undergo cell division. It is the period of synthesis of various metabolites required for cell division.

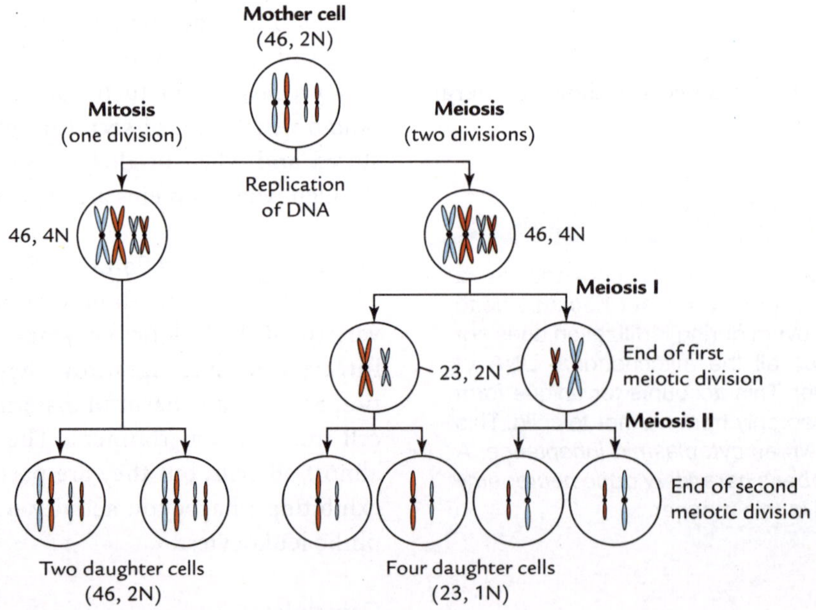

Fig. 4.5 Cell division: mitosis and meiosis.

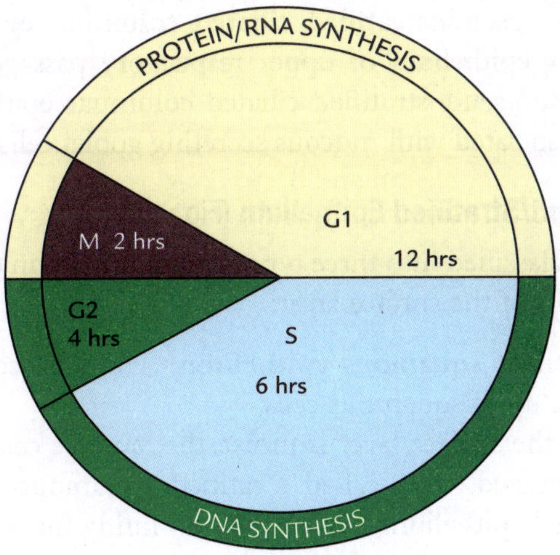

Fig. 4.6 Cell cycle.

2. **S phase (synthetic phase), 6 hours**—is the period of DNA synthesis.
3. **G2 phase, 4 hours**—is the period during which fidelity of DNA replication is checked and errors, if any, are corrected.
4. **M phase, 2 hours**—is the period during which cell actually divides.

N.B.

- The transition between G2 and M phases is regulated by the mitosis-promoting factor.
- There are regulatory mechanisms for controlled division of cells according to the need.
- The several factors that inhibit cell reproduction are collectively called *chalones*.

Meiosis (Fig. 4.5)

It is a special type of cell division that occurs only in germ cells during the production of gametes. It consists of two cell divisions (meiosis I and meiosis II). By meiotic division the diploid germ cell gives rise to four haploid gametes. During meiosis the pairs of chromosomes separate and one from each pair moves to the opposite poles of the parent cell. When it divides, each of the daughter cells has only 23 chromosomes called **haploid number.** This means that when the ovum is fertilized with spermatozoon, the resultant zygote has 46 chromosomes called **diploid number.** Thus the child has some characteristics inherited from the mother and some from the father.

The differentiating features of mitosis and meiosis are listed in Table 4.2.

TISSUES

The tissues are collections of cells performing a similar function. The term tissue includes collection of cells and intervening intercellular substance.

There are four basic types of tissues in the body:

1. Epithelial tissue
2. Connective tissue
3. Muscle tissue
4. Nervous tissue

Only epithelial and connective tissues are discussed in this chapter. The other tissues are described in detail in subsequent chapters.

EPITHELIAL TISSUE (EPITHELIUM)

The epithelium is a sheet of cells. The deep surface of this sheet rests on the basement membrane. The cells of the epithelium form continuous layer/layers. The cells are tightly packed together and there is little or no intercellular matrix between them.

Epithelium covers the body surface, lines body cavities (e.g. pleural, peritoneal), lines tubes (e.g. gastrointestinal tract, respiratory tract, genitourinary tracts, blood vessels) and forms glands (e.g. exocrine, endocrine). Epithelium has a high regeneration capacity ranging from a few days (e.g. epithelial lining, small intestine) to a month (e.g. epidermis of the skin).

Classification of Epithelium

The epithelium is classified into two main types: simple epithelium and compound (stratified) epithelium.

Table 4.2 Differences between mitosis and meiosis

Mitosis	Meiosis
Occurs in somatic cells	Occurs in germ (gametic) cells
Completes in one sequence	Completes in two sequences
Form two daughter cells (containing same number of chromosomes as in mother cell)	Form four daughter cells (containing half number of chromosomes as in mother cell)
Daughter cells are identical to mother cell	Daughter cells are not identical to mother cell
No exchange of maternal and paternal DNA occurs	Exchange of small amounts of maternal and paternal DNA occurs (to ensure genetic variability)

If the sheet is made up of a single layer of cells, it is termed as **simple epithelium** and if it is made up of multiple layers of cells, it is termed as **compound or stratified epithelium.**

Simple Epithelium (Fig. 4.7)

It is classified into three types depending upon the shape of the cells forming the epithelium:

1. **Simple squamous epithelium:** It is made of flattened cells that are bound together in a mosaic-like pattern, e.g. endothelium of heart and blood vessels, mesothelium of serous membrane, lining epithelium of alveoli of lungs.
2. **Simple cuboidal epithelium:** It is made of cube-like cells, e.g. lining of thyroid follicles, germinal epithelium of ovary.
3. **Simple columnar epithelium:** It is made up of tall columnar cells, e.g. lining epithelium of gastrointestinal tract and its glands, gallbladder, bile duct.

If the simple columnar epithelium is characterized by the presence of cilia along its free surface, it is termed as **simple ciliated columnar epithelium,** e.g. lining epithelium of central canal of spinal cord and brain vesicles.

If the simple columnar epithelium is made up of two types of columnar cells: (a) tall and thin, and (b) short and thick, the tall cells reach the surface and the short cells do not reach the surface. In such a situation nuclei of these cells lie at different levels. As a result, it gives a stratified appearance. Since the cells are almost always ciliated, this type of epithelium is termed as **pseudostratified ciliated columnar epithelium,** e.g. lining epithelium of upper respiratory passages, air sinuses. The pseudostratified ciliated columnar epithelium is always associated with mucous secreting goblet cells.

Compound/Stratified Epithelium (Fig. 4.8)

It is also classified into three types depending upon the shape of the cells of the surface layer:

1. **Stratified squamous epithelium:** The surface layer is made up of squamous cells.

   If the surface layer is moist, the surface cells are not keratinized, it is called stratified squamous nonkeratinized epithelium, e.g. epithelium lining the oral cavity, lower part of anal canal, vagina.

   If the surface layer is not moist, i.e. exposed to air, the surface cells undergo keratinization (i.e. cells are dead and the cytoplasm is replaced by keratin), it is called stratified squamous keratinized epithelium, e.g. epidermis of skin.
2. **Stratified cuboidal epithelium:** The surface layer is made up of cube-shaped cells, e.g. duct of sweat glands, seminiferous tubules.
3. **Stratified columnar epithelium:** The surface layer is made of columnar cells, e.g. large ducts of glands.

Transitional Epithelium

It is a special variety of stratified epithelium lining the urinary tract, *viz.* ureter, urinary bladder, urethra, etc. It is

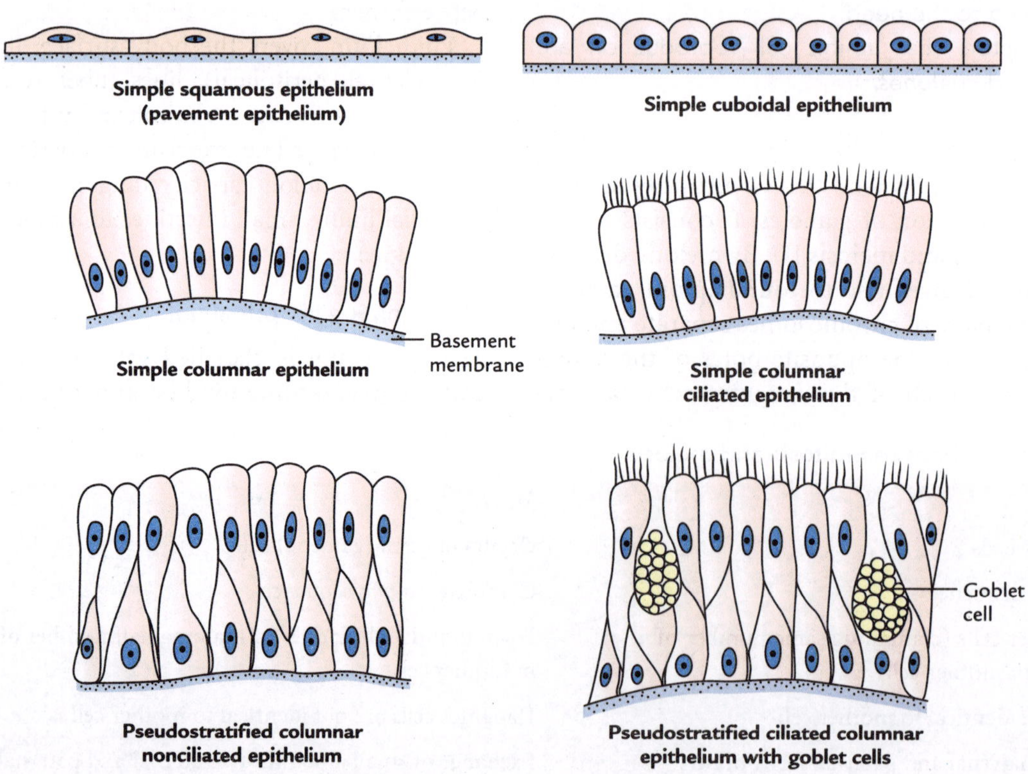

Fig. 4.7 Types of simple epithelium.

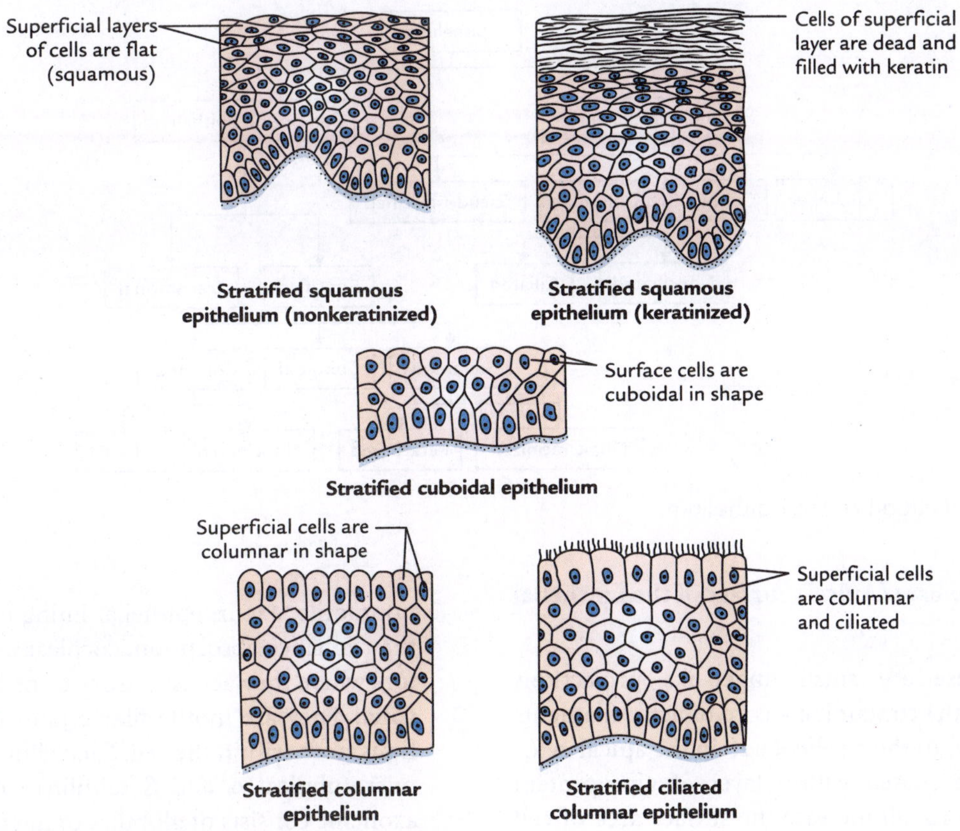

Fig. 4.8 Different types of compound/stratified epithelium.

somewhat similar to nonkeratinized stratified epithelium. But unlike the flattened surface cells of stratified epithelium, the surface cells of transitional epithelium are large and rounded with abundant cytoplasm and prominent nuclei (Fig. 4.9). The surface cells are connected by tight junctions. The transitional epithelium exhibits two types of transitions:

1. **Transition in surface of cells,** i.e. when the organ of the tube is relaxed, they are umbrella shaped but when the organ or the tube is distended, they become flattened.
2. **Transition in the number of layers of cells.** When the organ or the tube is relaxed, it is made up of 5–6 layers of cells but when stretched or distended, it is made up of only 2 or 3 layers.

The transitional epithelium is classically described to consist of three layers: superficial layer of large polyhedral cells (umbrella cells), intermediate layer of pear-shaped cells, and deeper layer of smaller (low columnar or cuboidal) cells.

The cells of all the layers are connected to the basement membrane through cell junctions. Hence, they do not get disrupted during stretching.

N.B.

The luminal surface of transitional epithelium is covered by thick osmiophilic lamella which may account for impermeability to urine.

The classification of epithelium is summarized in Flowchart 4.1.

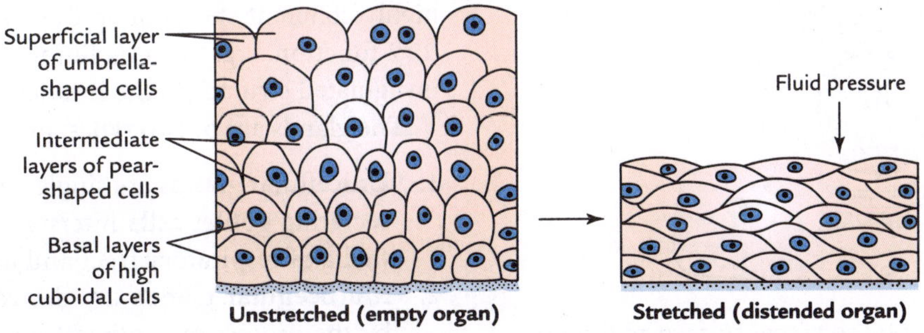

Fig. 4.9 Transitional epithelium.

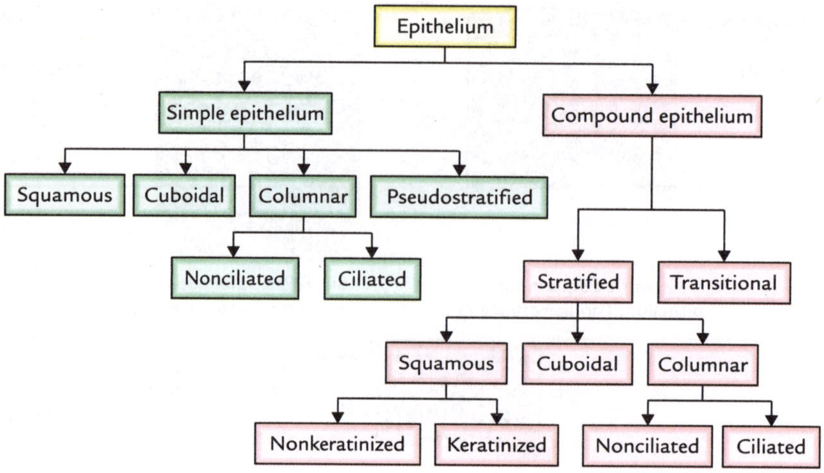

Flowchart 4.1 Classification of the epithelium.

Specialization on the Free (Apical) Surface of the Epithelial Cells (Fig. 4.10)

1. **Microvilli:** These are small finger-like projections (1–2 µm in length) containing a core of actin filaments that are anchored to the *terminal web* in the apical cytoplasm. They are coated with a layer of glycoprotein (glycocalyx). Microvilli increase the surface area of cell membrane to enhance absorption, e.g. lining epithelium of gallbladder, small intestine.
2. **Stereocilia:** These are long microvilli (about 5–10 µm in length) which lack core of actin filaments, hence nonmotile, e.g. in epithelial lining of epididymis where they enhance absorption, cochlear and vestibular receptors where they act as sensory transducers.
3. **Cilia:** They are motile filamentous cytoplasmic projections from within the cell. Each cilium contains a core of microtubules (α and ß tubulin) called **axoneme.** The axoneme consists of globules of microtubules surrounding two central microtubules (*9 + 2 arrangement*). Ciliary cells are interspersed with mucous-secreting **goblet cells.** There is always a film of mucous on the free surface of ciliary cells, e.g. epithelial lining of respiratory tract where they move the mucous towards pharynx, epithelial lining of fallopian tubes where they move the ova towards the uterine cavity. At the base of each cilium is a *basal body* that consists of 9 triplet microtubules and no central microtubules (*9 + 0 arrangement*).

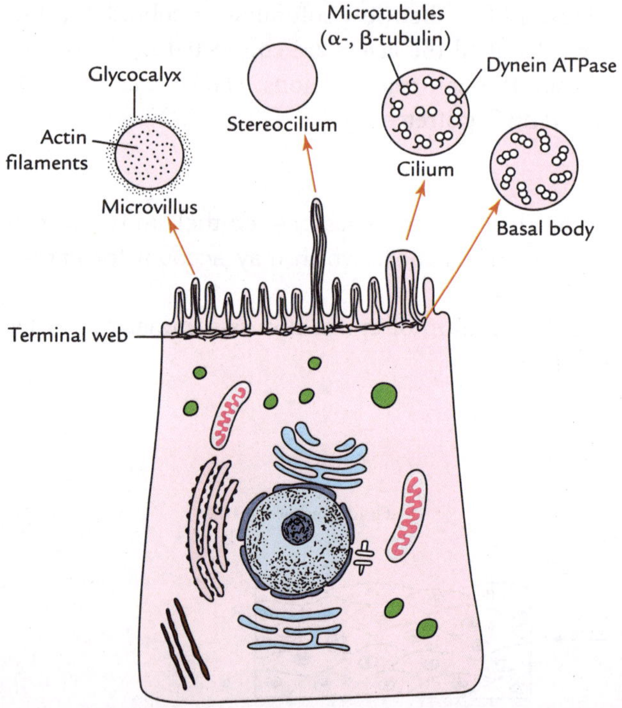

Fig. 4.10 Specializations on the apical surface of the epithelial cells.

As glands are composed of epithelial cells (these cells become specialized to produce a fluid secretion that differs in composition from blood or intercellular fluid), it is worthwhile to include a brief account of the glands in this section.

Glands

The glands are specialized epithelial cells which produce secretion. Such cells may exist in isolation among other nonsecretory cells of the epithelium, e.g. goblet cells, or may form highly coherent sheets of epithelium with a common secretory function, e.g. mucous lining of stomach and in highly invaginated structures, the multicellular glands.

The glands are of two types: unicellular and multicellular:

1. **Unicellular glands** are single-celled glands, e.g. mucous-secreting **goblet cells** interspersed in the columnar epithelia of respiratory tract and intestine.
2. **Multicellular glands** are derived from epithelial lining by the process of proliferation and evagination into the underlying connective tissue.

If the glands retain their connection with the surface epithelium, of course, by a tubular duct lined by epithelial cells, they are termed as **exocrine glands or glands with duct**. The secretions of these glands reach the surface through their ducts.

If the glands lose their connection with the surface epithelium, they are called **ductless or endocrine glands**. The secretion of these glands passes into the bloodstream.

CLASSIFICATION OF GLANDS

A. According to the branching pattern of the duct (Fig. 4.11)

1. **Simple glands**: The duct of the gland does not branch.
2. **Compound glands**: The duct of the gland branches repeatedly.

Further classification of these glands is based on the shape of the secretory portion.

1. **Tubular**: The duct is connected to the tubular secretory portion.
2. **Acinar**: The duct is connected to the sac-like secretory portion.

Simple glands: The simple glands can be tubular or acinar:

- Tubular glands are further divided into three types:
  (a) Straight tubular, e.g. intestinal glands (crypts of Lieberkuhn).
  (b) Coiled tubular, e.g. sweat glands.
  (c) Branched tubular, e.g. gastric and uterine glands.
- Acinar glands are further divided into two types:
  (a) Simple acinar, e.g. urethral and paraurethral glands in male.
  (b) Simple branched acinar, e.g. sebaceous glands.

Compound glands: The compound glands are further classified into three types according to the shape of their secretory portions:

(a) Compound tubular, e.g. bulbourethral glands of male.
(b) Compound acinar, e.g. salivary glands, exocrine pancreas.
(c) Compound tubulo-acinar, e.g. prostate gland.

B. According to the mode of secretion (Fig. 4.12)

1. **Merocrine**: The secretion is released by exocytosis through the cell membrane, e.g. most glands of the body such as salivary glands.
2. **Apocrine**: The secretion first accumulates within the cell (in the apical portion), then a portion of the cell along with the secretion is pinched off to be discharged. The pinched off portion of the cell becomes a part of secretion, e.g. mammary glands.
3. **Holocrine**: Entire secretory cell is discharged along with the secretory product. In this way the entire cell becomes a part of the secretion, e.g. sebaceous glands.

C. According to the nature of secretory product

1. **Mucous**, e.g. sublingual salivary gland.
2. **Serous**, e.g. parotid gland.
3. **Seromucous**, e.g. submandibular gland.
4. **Cellular**, e.g. testis and ovary.

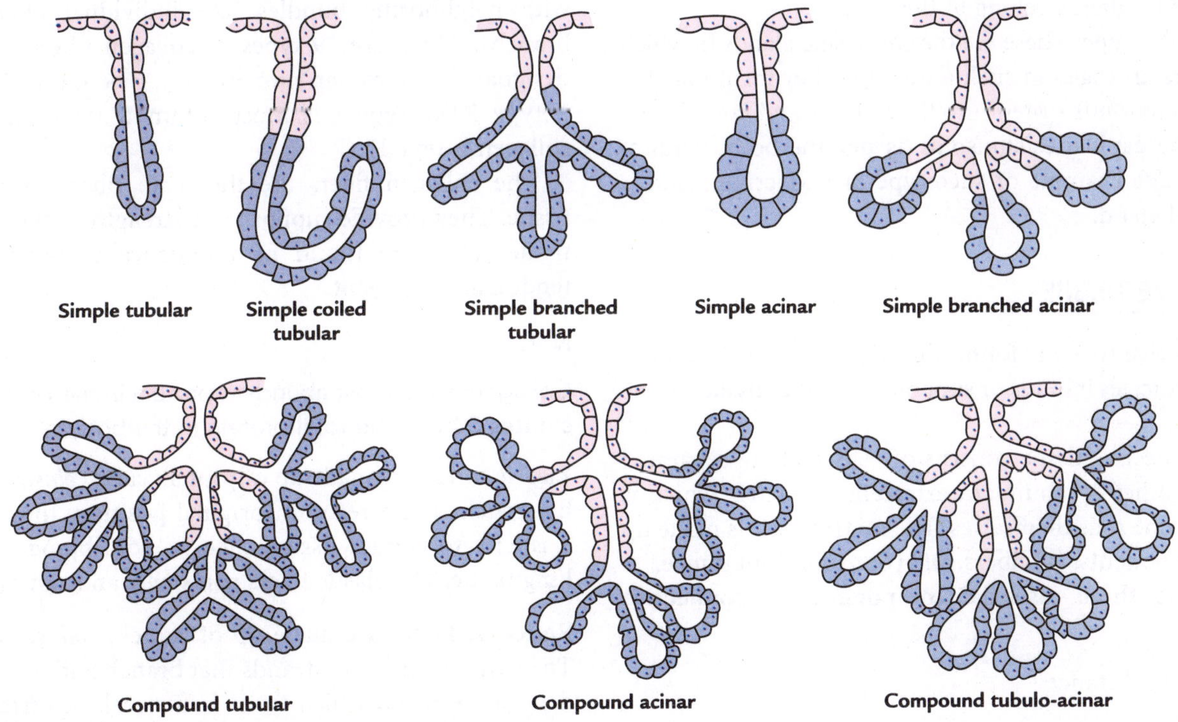

Fig. 4.11 Structural classification of exocrine glands.

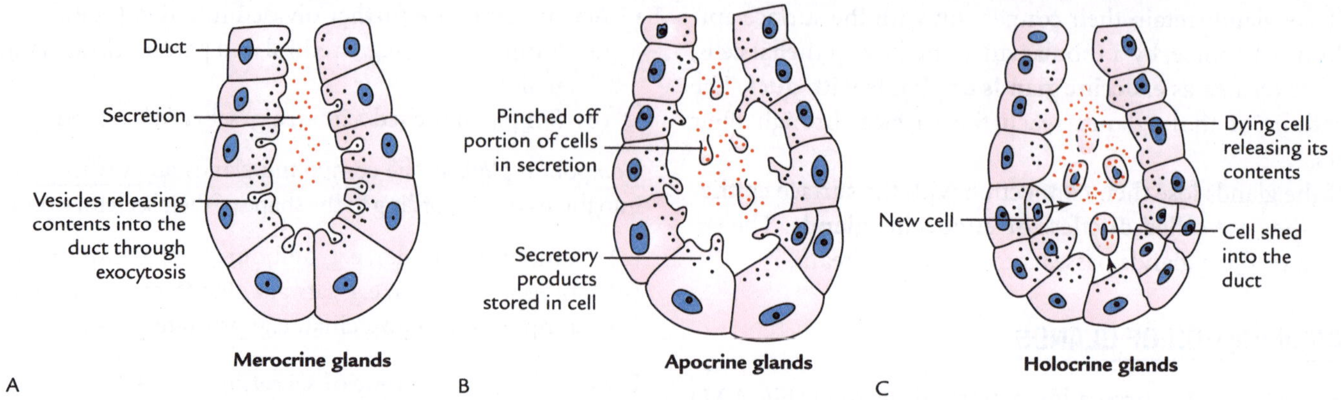

Fig. 4.12 Classification of glands according to their mode of secretion: **A**, merocrine glands empty their secretion into the duct through exocytosis; **B**, in apocrine glands, the apical portion of cell storing secretion is pinched off in the duct; **C**, in holocrine gland, the entire cell containing the secretion is shed off and the lost cell is replaced by cells deeper in the gland.

CLASSIFICATION OF ENDOCRINE GLANDS

The endocrine glands are so variable in their structure that they cannot be classified easily. However, two types of endocrine glands can be differentiated according to the grouping of cells, *viz.* cord and clump type and follicular type.

1. **Cord and clump type:** These are the endocrine glands in which cells form anastomosing cords or clumps interspersed between these cords. The clumps are dilated blood capillaries—called **sinusoids.** The secretion is directly poured out into the capillaries/sinusoids. Most of endocrine glands belong to this type.
2. **Follicular type:** These are the endocrine glands in which cells are arranged in such a way that they form follicles. The secretion is stored into the follicles and are released into the capillaries/sinusoids as per the body requirement. The example of such type of endocrine gland is thyroid gland.

CONNECTIVE TISSUE

The connective tissue is found throughout the body and as its name indicates it binds or supports the other tissues of the body.

The connective tissue consists of cells that are separated from each other by abundant extracellular matrix which is secreted by the cells themselves. The matrix itself is made up of two components: (a) fibers, and (b) ground substance.

Thus the **three essential components of connective tissue** are:

1. Ground substance
2. Fibers
3. Cells

Ground Substance: It is composed of nonfibrous protein (e.g. hyaluronic acid and chondroitin sulphate) and complex molecules of polysaccharides.

Fibers: They are of three types: collagen fibers, elastic fibers and reticular fibers (Fig. 4.13). All the three types of fibers are made up of two types of proteins, *viz.* collagen and elastin.

Collagen fibers are made up of a protein called *collagen.* They are flexible but have tremendous strength. Collagen fibers mostly occur in bundles which may branch and join with neighboring bundles (the individual fibers do not branch). There are 19 types of collagen fibers and each is designated by a roman numeral, *viz.* type I, type II, type III, ...type XIX. Type I is most common (90% of the body collagen is type I).

The collagen fibers are the main fibers of connective tissue. They provide support and strength to the connective tissue. They are found in abundance in bone, cartilage, tendon and ligament.

N.B.

Collagen is the most abundant protein in the body and constitutes 30% of the total protein in the body.

Elastic fibers are made up of protein called *elastin.* They can be stretched and recoil in original position, thus providing elasticity to certain tissues such as skin, blood vessels and lung tissue. The elastic fibers run singly and can branch.

Reticular fibers are made up of protein *collagen (type III).* They are fine delicate strands that branch and join to form a delicate network, which form framework of certain organs such as spleen, lymph node, liver, bone marrow.

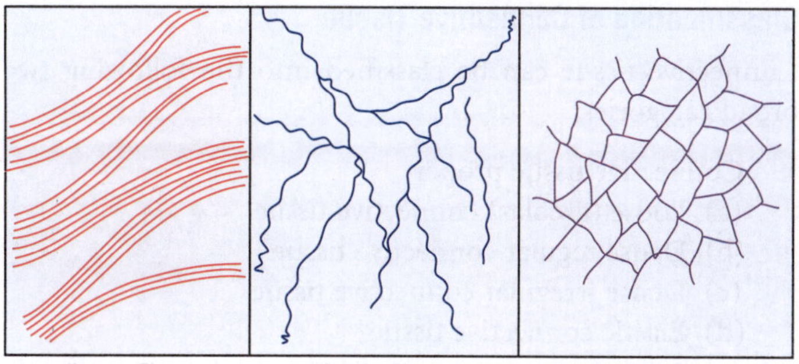

Fig. 4.13 The three types of connective tissue fibers.

Table 4.3 Types of connective tissue cells

Fixed cells	Free cells
Fibroblasts/fibrocytes	Neutrophils
Macrophages (histiocytes)	Eosinophils
Mast cells	Basophils
Adipocytes (fat cells)	Monocytes
Pigment cells (chromatophores)	B and T lymphocytes
Reticular cells	Plasma cells

N.B.

All the three types of connective tissue fibers (collagen, elastic, reticular) are synthesized by fibroblasts.

Clinical correlation

Keloid: The keloid formation is a deviation from normal wound healing whereby an excessive accumulation of collagen fibers occurs, resulting in a raised tumorous scar. Osteogenesis imperfecta is a genetic defect involving type I collagen resulting in spontaneous fractures of the bones.

Cells: The cells of the connective tissue are of two types: fixed cells and free cells (Table 4.3).

1. **Fixed cells:** These are long-lived cells and form stable population of cells that remain in the connective tissue (Fig. 4.14).

Fibroblasts/fibrocytes: They are the most abundant connective tissue cells present in almost all the types of connective tissues. They are large and irregular cells. They have an ovoid nucleus with prominent nucleolus. Fibroblasts are involved in the synthesis and secretion of ground substance and all types of connective tissue fibers (e.g. collagen, elastin and reticular). The fibroblasts and fibrocytes are the same cells with a functional difference:

1. **Fibroblast** is the active form that produces matrix.
2. **Fibrocyte** is the inactive form of fibroblast which retains the capability to revert in 'blast' form. They are smaller and thinner than fibroblasts, hence morphologically different.

Fibroblasts play a key role in wound healing by synthesizing collagen fibers. The fibrocytes perform only the maintenance levels of activity. In cases of need such as wound healing, the fibrocytes revert to the active fibroblastic form. The collagen formation is impaired in vitamin C deficiency.

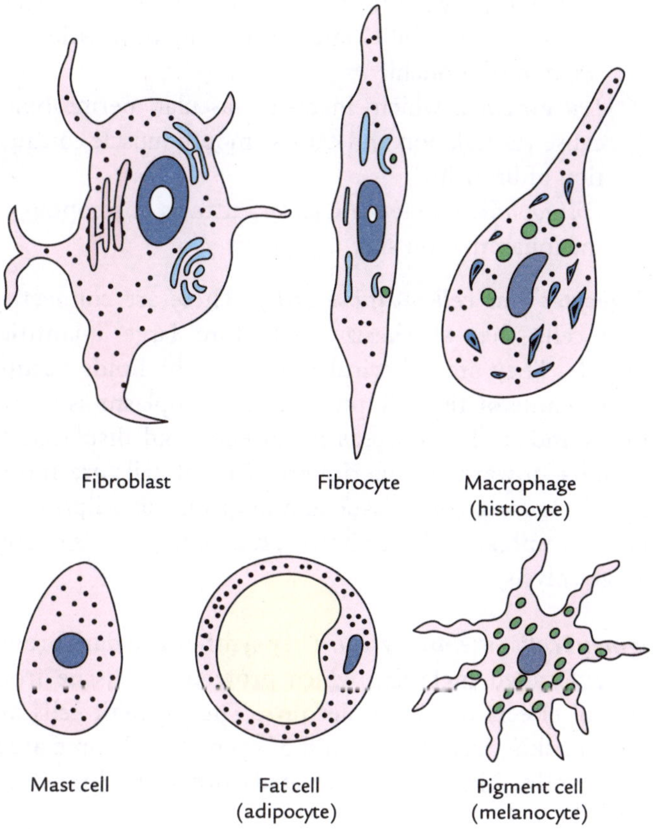

Fig. 4.14 Types of fixed connective tissue cells.

N.B.

The fibroblasts act as stem cells for other cellular components of the connective tissue.

Macrophages (histiocytes): They are irregular shaped cells with short branching projections. They are derived from monocytes within the circulating blood. Once monocytes enter the tissue they mature and are called **macrophages**. The macrophages are present in almost all the tissues. Macrophages have phagocytic function.

Mast cells: These are small oval cells with centrally placed nucleus and contain many granules in their cytoplasm. They arise from the stem cells in the bone marrow. Mast cells have a function in **immediate (type I) hypersensitivity reactions** (**anaphylactic reaction**). The surface of mast cells possesses receptors for immunoglobulins (antibodies) produced by plasma cells upon first exposure to an allergen (e.g. plant pollen, snake venom, foreign serum) which sensitizes the mast cells.

Mast cells secrete the following substances upon second exposure to the same allergen causing a classical '**wheal and flare reaction in the skin**':

- *Heparin*—an anticoagulant.
- *Histamine*, which dilates small blood vessels to increase vascular permeability and causes smooth muscle contraction of bronchi.
- *Leukotrienes*, which increase vascular permeability, cause vasodilation and causes smooth muscle contraction of bronchi.
- *Eosinophilic chemotactic factor*, attracts eosinophils to the inflammation site.

Adipocytes (fat cells/adipose cells): These are connective tissue cells that synthesize and store large quantities of lipids. They are spherical in shape. The lipids occupy almost whole of the cell, pushing the cytoplasm as a thin rim around it. The nucleus is flattened and displaced to one side—towards the periphery. The fat cells are found singly in loose areolar tissue and in groups in adipose tissue. They uptake and metabolize glucose to provide energy (via glycolysis).

Pigment cells (melanocytes): They synthesize a dark brown pigment called **melanin,** which protects the tissue from harmful effects of ultraviolet rays. The pigment cells are found in skin, iris and choroid of eyeball, and some areas of the brain. They are star shaped with many branching processes.

The cytoplasm contains melanin granules in membrane-bound organelles called **melanosomes.**

Reticular cells: The reticular cells are found in the reticular connective tissues. They are branched flattened cells with poorly staining nuclei and cytoplasm. They resemble fibroblasts and produce reticular fibers to which cells are attached.

2. **Free cells:** The **free cells** are short-lived wandering cells that are continually replaced from cells of blood, i.e. they enter the connective tissue from blood usually during inflammation. They are described in detail in chapter Cardiovascular System.

Classification of Connective Tissue

Connective tissue can be classified into the following two broad categories:

1. Connective tissue proper
   (a) Loose (areolar) connective tissue
   (b) Dense regular connective tissue
   (c) Dense irregular connective tissue
   (d) Elastic connective tissue
   (e) Adipose connective tissue
   (f) Reticular connective tissue
2. Specialized connective tissue
   (a) Bone
   (b) Cartilage
   (c) Blood

Loose connective tissue (Fig. 4.15): It is the most widely distributed connective tissue of the body. It consists of loosely woven network of all three types of fibers (collagen, elastic, reticular) and contain almost all kinds of connective tissue cells, predominantly fibroblasts. The fibers and cells are dispersed in semifluid ground substance. Much of the body fluid is found within loose connective tissue. Loose connective tissue is packing and binding tissue that surrounds muscles, nerves and vessels, and binds skin to the underlying deep fascia. It permits the skin to move when a part of the body is rubbed.

Dense regular connective tissue (Fig. 4.16): It consists predominantly of densely packed bundles of collagen fibers. The bundles of collagen fibers lie parallel to the direction of force placed on this tissue. The fibroblasts are present in rows between bundles of collagen fibers. Dense connective tissue is silvery white in appearance and forms tendons, aponeuroses, ligaments.

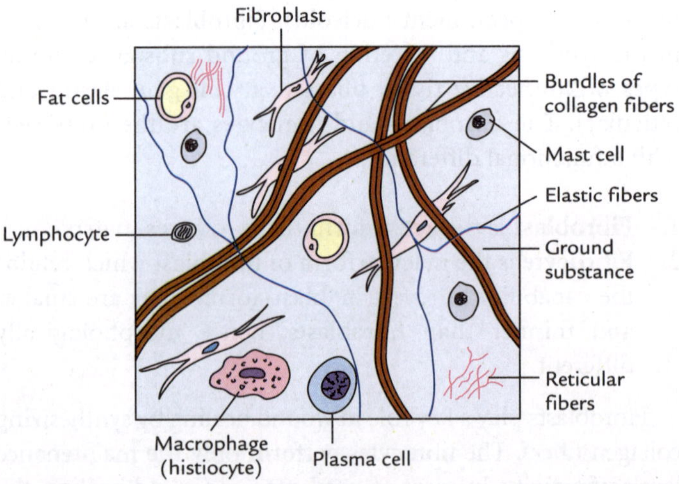

Fig. 4.15 Loose connective tissue.

Dense irregular connective tissue (Fig. 4.17): It consists of densely packed bundles of collagen fibers that are interwoven to provide tensile strength in any direction. The dense irregular connective tissue forms, dermis of skin, periosteum, fibrous capsule of joints, collagenous matrix of bone called osteoid.

Elastic connective tissue: It consists predominantly of elastic fibers that are yellowish and irregularly arranged. They can be stretched to 1.5 times their original length and will snap back to their original form. Elastic connective tissue is found in the walls of elastic arteries (e.g. aorta and large arteries), vocal cords of larynx, ligamentum nuchae on the back of neck, ligamenta flava between arches of vertebrae, etc.

Adipose connective tissue: It consists of large aggregations of **adipose cells** or adipocytes. Adipose cells store droplets of fat within their cytoplasm, causing them to swell, thus forcing their nuclei to one side, and the cytoplasm is present as a thin rim around it. The fat functions not only as food reserve but protects and supports various organs. The adipose tissue is present in abundance in superficial fascia deep to the skin, around kidneys, blood vessels around heart, in breasts of sexually mature females, etc.

Reticular connective tissue: It consists of network of reticular fibers and reticular cells. Reticular tissue also contains macrophages (phagocytic cells). The reticular connective tissue forms stroma or reticular framework of certain organs (e.g. spleen, lymph node, liver, bone marrow) and reticular lamina of basement membrane.

N.B.

Mucoid tissue: It consists of copious matrix having fine meshwork of collagen fibres with fibroblasts, e.g. Wharton's jelly of umbilical cord and vitreous humor of the eyeball.

The specialized types of connective tissue are described in separate chapters.

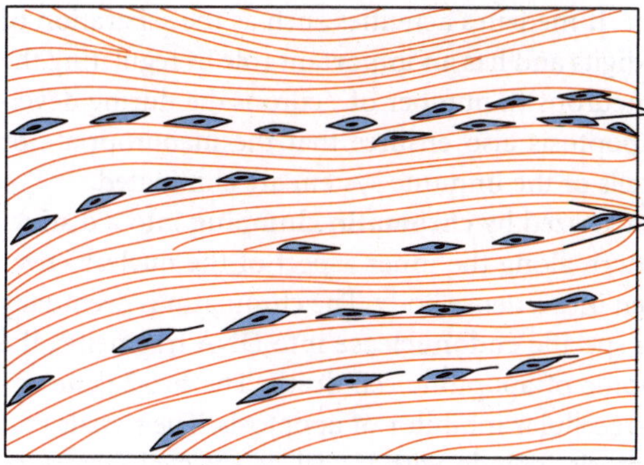

Fig. 4.16 Dense regular connective tissue (white fibrous connective tissue, e.g. tendons, ligaments).

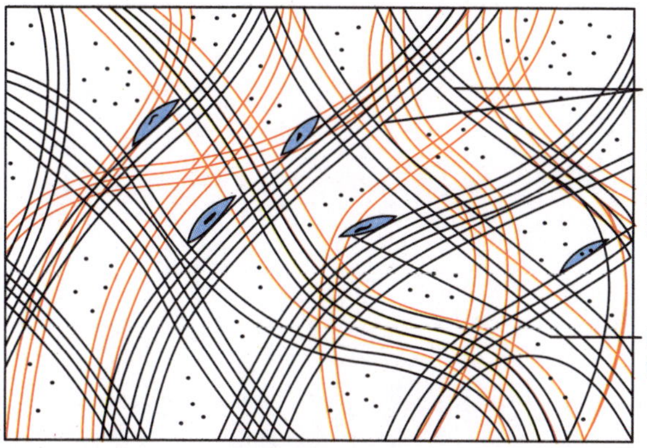

Fig. 4.17 Dense irregular connective tissue (e.g. reticular layer of dermis, fibrous capsules of joints and organs, periosteum and perichondrium).

MUSCLE TISSUE

The muscle tissue is made up of specialized contractile cells called muscle cells/muscle fibers. The muscle tissue is of three types:

1. Skeletal muscle
2. Smooth muscle
3. Cardiac muscle

Muscle tissue is described in detail in chapter Muscular System.

NERVOUS TISSUE

The nervous tissue is made up of the following two types of cells:

1. **Neurons:** These are **excitable cells**. They initiate, receive, conduct and transmit information.
2. **Neuroglia:** These **are nonexcitable cells**. They provide structural and functional support to neurons.

The nervous tissue is described in detail in chapter Nervous System.

TISSUE REGENERATION

The tissue regeneration occurs by replication of original cells (by mitosis). The rate of regeneration depends on the normal rate of physiological turnover of particular types of cells. Those with rapid turnover regenerate very fast. According to the rate of physiological turnover, the cells are divided into the following three types:

1. **Labile cells.** These are cells in which replication is a continuous process. They include cells of:
   (a) Epithelium of skin, mucous membrane, secretory glands, ducts, lining of uterus
   (b) Bone marrow
   (c) Blood
   (d) Spleen and lymphoid tissue
2. **Stable cells.** These are cells which are capable of replication but do so infrequently. They include:
   (a) Liver, kidney and pancreatic cells
   (b) Fibroblasts
   (c) Smooth muscle cells
   (d) Osteoblasts and osteoclasts of bone
3. **Permanent cells.** These cells are incapable of replicating after the normal growth is complete. They include:
   (a) Nerve cells (neurons)
   (b) Skeletal and cardiac muscles

CELL DIFFERENTIATION

The cells are differentiated into different types with particular structural and functional characteristics in an early stage of development, *viz.* epithelial cells develop different characteristics from lymphocytes.

In postnatal life when cells replicate to produce daughter cells, if daughter cells have same appearance, functions and genetic make-up as the parent cells they are easily recognized and are called **well differentiated cells**. On the other hand, if daughter cells cannot be recognized due to change in their appearance, function and genetic make-up, they are called **poorly differentiated cells**.

Clinical correlation

Tumor or neoplasm: It is a mass of tissue when the cells replicate faster than normal in an uncoordinated manner, and continue to do so even after the initial stimulus is ceased. Remember that normally cells divide in an orderly manner.

The tumors are of two types: benign and malignant. The *benign tumors* grow slowly and are not likely to spread and become worse. On the other hand, *malignant tumors* grow fast. They are likely to spread and cause harm.

The differentiating features of benign and malignant tumors are presented in Table 4.4.

Table 4.4 Differences between benign and malignant tumors

	Benign tumor	Malignant tumor
Growth	Slow	Rapid
Cell differentiation	Well differentiated	Poorly differentiated
Encapsulation	Usually encapsulated	Nonencapsulated
Spread	Does not spread	Spreads — by local infiltration — via lymph — via blood
Recurrence	Rare	Common

APOPTOSIS

Apoptosis is programmed cell death (i.e. regulated cell suicide). It is a central mechanism controlling multicellular development. It mediates activities such as the separation of developing digits and has an important role in regulating the number of neurons (a number of neurons die during development). Apoptosis also ensures that the inappropriate or inefficient cells of the immune system are eliminated.

It is characterized by **chromatin clumping** into a distinct crescent pattern along the inner aspect of the nuclear envelope and then into a dense body. The chromatin is eventually cleaved by a specific **endonuclease** into DNA fragments, the pathognomonic of apoptotic cell death. The **bcl-2 gene** encodes an intracellular inhibitor of apoptosis. The signals that trigger apoptosis include withdrawal of survival factors or exposure to inappropriate proliferative stimuli.

Golden Facts to Remember

➢ Largest cell in the body	Ovum (130 µm)
➢ Least differentiated cell in the body	Zygote
➢ Most differentiated cells in the body	Neurons, myocytes of cardiac muscle
➢ Largest membrane-bound structure within the cell	Nucleus
➢ All the cells in the body possess nucleus *except*	Mature erythrocytes
➢ Longest cell in the body	Neuron (sensory neurons of S1 spinal nerve)
➢ Longest period of cell cycle	G1 phase (12 hours)
➢ Most common type of cell division	Mitosis
➢ Powerhouse of cell	Mitochondria
➢ Unicellular glands	Goblet cells
➢ Most widely distributed connective tissue in the body	Loose connective tissue
➢ Most abundant connective tissue cells	Fibroblasts
➢ Most abundant protein in the body	Collagen
➢ Most numerous connective tissue cells	Fibroblasts
➢ Most common connective tissue fibers	Collagen fibers
➢ First connective tissue fibers to appear during development	Reticular fibers
➢ First person to observe the cell wall in dead cells of cork	Robert Hooke (1635–1703)
➢ Term 'cell' was coined by	Robert Hooke (1635–1703)
➢ First person to describe free-living cells	Antonie van Leeuwenhoek (1632–1723)
➢ Building blocks of every organism	Cells
➢ The famous 'cell theory' was formulated by	Separately by MJ Schleiden (1804–1881) and Theodor Schwann (1810–1882)
➢ Term 'nucleus' was coined by	Robert Brown (1773–1858)
➢ First person to describe nucleolus	MJ Schleiden
➢ Most important feature of prokaryotic cells	Absence of nuclear envelope
➢ Most important feature of eukaryotic cells	Nucleus is surrounded by a nuclear envelope (nuclear membrane)
➢ The term 'tissue' was coined by	Bichat (1771–1802)
➢ The term 'histology' was coined by	Mayer (1819)
➢ A separate branch of science for study of tissues was proposed by	Marcello Malpighi (1628–1694)

Multiple Choice Questions

1. **All of the following structures are derived from ectoderm *except*:**
   (a) Lens of eye
   (b) Enamel of tooth
   (c) Dermis of skin
   (d) Adrenal medulla

2. **All of the following structures are derived from mesoderm *except*:**
   (a) Muscles
   (b) Bones
   (c) Thyroid
   (d) Dentin of teeth

3. **Lumen of all of the following structures is lined by transitional epithelium *except*:**
   (a) Urinary bladder
   (b) Ureter
   (c) Urethra
   (d) Esophagus

4. **Connective tissue, muscle and dermis of skin are derived from:**
   (a) Ectoderm
   (b) Mesoderm
   (c) Endoderm
   (d) None of the above

5. **Exocrine glands are considered merocrine in nature, if:**
   (a) The secretion is discharged along with pinched off apical portion of the cell
   (b) The secretion is released by exocytosis through cell membrane
   (c) The entire cell is discharged along with secretary product
   (d) The secretion is not discharged

6. **Most abundant protein in the body is:**
   (a) Collagen
   (b) Elastin
   (c) Reticulin
   (d) Globulin

7. **All of the following are fixed cells of connective tissue *except*:**
   (a) Fibrocytes
   (b) Mast cells
   (c) Adipocytes
   (d) Monocytes

8. **All of the following are free cells of connective tissue *except*:**
   (a) Neutrophils
   (b) Eosinophils
   (c) Basophils
   (d) Macrophages

9. **Which of the following cell is called histiocyte:**
   (a) Fibroblast
   (b) Monocyte
   (c) Macrophage
   (d) Plasma cell

Answers

1. *c*, **2.** *c*, **3.** *d*, **4.** *b*, **5.** *b*, **6.** *a*, **7.** *d*, **8.** *d*, **9.** *c*

CHAPTER 5

Skin, Superficial Fascia and Deep Fascia

Learning Objectives

After studying this chapter, the student should be able to:
- describe the structure and functions of the skin
- compare and contrast the thin and thick skin types
- enumerate the types of surface irregularities of skin and discuss the types of papillary ridges in 'fingerprints'
- list the epidermal derivatives and discuss the structure and function of each of them
- compare and contrast the structure and function of eccrine and apocrine sweat glands
- present the anatomical basis of clubbing, acne, sebaceous cyst
- classify the types of burns and discuss the characteristic features of each type
- estimate the surface area of skin applying the 'rule of nine' and discuss its importance in treatment of burns
- outline the stages involved in wound healing
- discuss the structure and functions of superficial and deep fasciae
- correctly solve the review questions given at the end of the chapter

SKIN

The skin is the outer covering of the body. It provides the dynamic interphase between the body and the external environment.

The skin is considered as an organ since it consists of several kinds of tissues that are structurally arranged to function together.

It is the largest organ of the body, covering over 7600 sq cm (3000 sq inch) area in an average adult and accounts for approximately 7% of the person's body weight.

The general appearance and condition of the skin is clinically important because it provides clues to certain body functions and dysfunctions. Thus skin reflects our general health. A healthy skin indicates a healthy body.

STRUCTURE OF SKIN

The skin consists of two principal layers: the epidermis and the dermis (Fig. 5.1).

The surface epithelium of skin is **epidermis**. It is of the keratinized stratified squamous variety. The various appendages of skin, *viz.* sweat glands, sebaceous glands, hair and nails are specialized derivatives of this epidermis. The deeper **dermis** consists mainly of bundles of collagen fibers together with some elastic tissue, blood vessels, lymphatics and nerve fibers.

Epidermis

The epidermis is a superficial avascular layer of stratified squamous keratinized epithelium derived from surface ectoderm of the body. It varies in thickness from 0.007 to 0.12 mm.

It consists of four main types of cells:

(a) Keratinocytes (90%)
(b) Melanocytes (8%)
(c) Langerhans cells
(d) Merkel cells

The *keratinocytes* are arranged in four or five layers. They produce keratin, a protein that protects the skin from heat, microbes and chemicals.

The *melanocytes* produce melanin pigment that imparts color to skin and absorbs ultraviolet light to protect the skin from cancer to certain extent.

The *Langerhans cells* arise from bone marrow and migrate to epidermis. They participate in immune response and protect the skin against viral and other infections.

The *Merkel cells* are located in the deeper part of epidermis and come in contact with sensory neuron. They act as receptors for touch sensations.

Layers of Epidermis

Depending on the skin type—thick or thin—skin is made up of either four or five layers (Fig. 5.2).

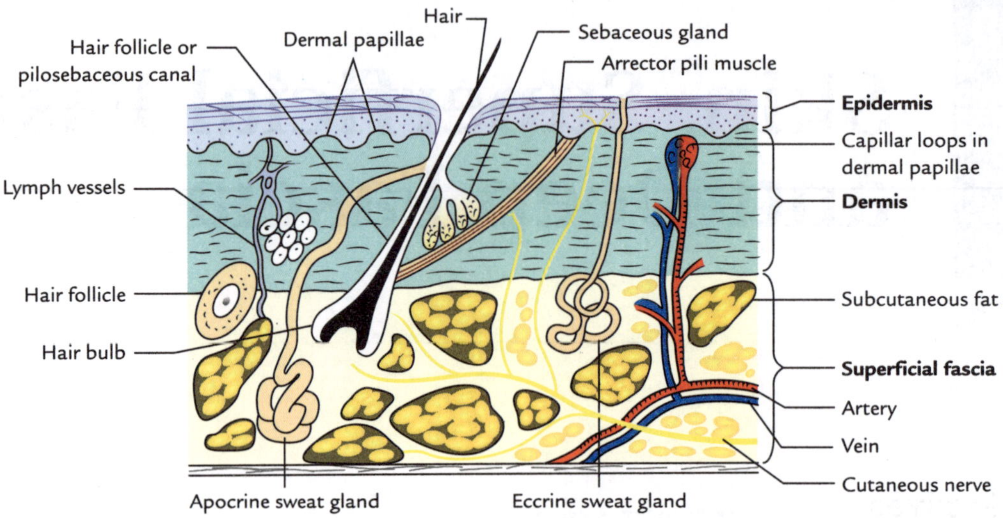

Fig. 5.1 Structure of the skin.

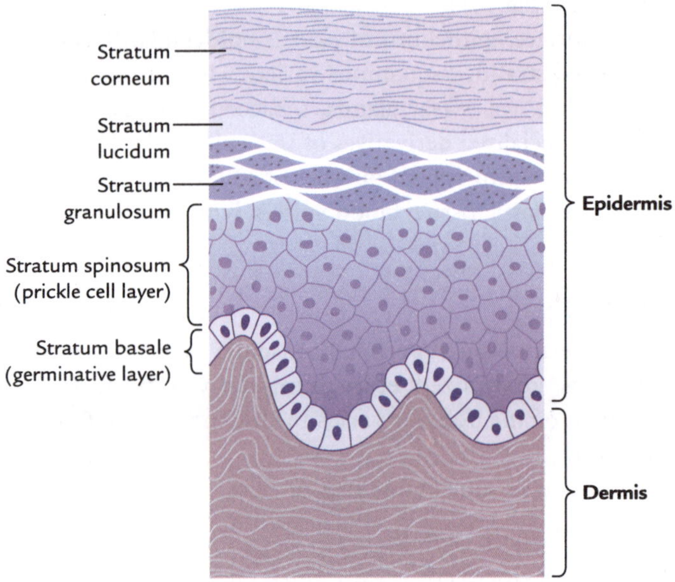

Fig. 5.2 Structural features of the epidermis.

From deep to superficial the name and characteristics of various layers of thick skin are as follows:

1. **Stratum basale/stratum germinatum (syn. basal layer, malpighian layer):** It consists of a single layer of cuboidal or columnar cells. A thin basement membrane is situated between stratum basale and dermis. The cells of this layer constantly divide by mitotic activity. The newly formed cells move towards the superficial layer to renew the epidermis. It usually takes about 6–8 weeks for the cells to move from stratum basale to the surface of the skin. This layer also contains melanocytes which synthesize and produce melanin pigments which protect the skin from harmful effects of ultraviolet rays of sunlight.
2. **Stratum spinosum (spiny layer):** It consists of several layers of polygonal cells, each with a centrally located large oval nucleus. The cells are held together by desmosomes. Fixation during histological preparation causes shrinkage of cell membrane, giving the cell a spiny appearance, i.e. cells present spine-like processes, hence the name stratum spinosum or **prickle cell layer.**
3. **Stratum granulosum (granular layer):** It consists of three or four rows of flattened cells with pyknotic nuclei showing signs of degeneration. The cytoplasm contains **keratohyalin granules** which are made up of histidine-rich protein called filaggrin.
4. **Stratum lucidum (clear layer):** It is a thin clear homogeneous glassy layer. The nucleus, organelles and membrane of cells are not visible under a microscope. It is a highly refractile layer of epidermis. It is found only in thick glabrous skin such as soles of feet and palms of hands.
5. **Stratum corneum:** It is the most superficial layer of the skin. It consists of many (25–30) layers of fully keratinized flattened scalelike dead cells. These cells are filled with a protein called **keratin.** This layer is cornified and is the real protective layer of the skin. When desmosomes between the cells of the outermost layers become weak, the surface cells desquamate.

Dermis

The dermis is the deep vascular layer of the skin derived from mesoderm. It is thicker than epidermis and consists of collagen (type I) and elastic fibers. In addition, it contains glands, nerves, lymphatics and blood vessels. The smooth muscles of the dermis are associated with hair follicles as '**arrectores pili muscles**'.

Layers of Dermis

The dermis is usually divided into two layers:

1. A superficial papillary layer
2. Deep reticular layer

Papillary layer: This layer is in contact with epidermis and accounts for about one-fifth of the entire thickness of the dermis. It forms numerous conical blunt projections called **dermal papillae** extending into the epidermis.

The dermal papillae fit into the reciprocal depressions on the undersurface of the epidermis (epidermal ridges) and serve to interlock the dermis and the epidermis.

Reticular layer: It is chiefly composed of collagen fibers arranged mostly in parallel bundles. The direction of these bundles produces **cleavage lines** or **Langer's lines**. The cleavage lines are horizontal in the trunk and neck, and longitudinal in the limbs.

This layer is quite distensible, as is evident in pregnant women and obese individuals, but if stretched too much, the white fibers rupture and their repair causes scar formation. These scars are seen as white streaks called **stretch marks** or **linea albicans.** The linea albicans are frequently found in lower part of abdomen, buttock, thigh and breasts of multiparous females.

Clinical correlation

Making of leather: The strong resilient reticular layer of dermis in domestic animals is used in making leather. In tanning process (i.e. treatment with chemicals), the epidermis with its hair and papillary layer of the dermis are separated from the reticular layer. The reticular layer is then softened and treated with protective chemicals to make it usable in various forms such as leather jackets, purses, etc.

COLOR OF SKIN

The color of the skin is imparted by combination of the following three pigments:

1. Melanin
2. Carotene
3. Hemoglobin

Melanin is a black-brown pigment produced by melanocytes, which are derived from neural crest cells and migrate to epidermis.

The amount of melanin leads to variation in color of skin from pale to tan to black. Melanocytes are plenty in the epidermis of penis, nipple and areolae of the breast.

Carotene is a yellow-orange pigment. It is an exogenous pigment taken up from the food. It is present in stratum corneum and fat cells of the dermis and superficial fascia.

The **purple hemoglobin** and **red oxyhemoglobin** present in cutaneous blood vessels is responsible for the pink color of the skin.

N.B.

All races have the same number of melanocytes, but the amount of melanin produced and distribution of melanocytes and melatonin determines whether the color of the individual will be black, brown or white.

Clinical correlation

- **Albinism:** It is a clinical condition in which skin, hair, and eyelashes of an individual are white. It occurs due to failure of development of melanin pigment. It is important to remember that the skin of the genetically determined albinos has normal number of melanocytes in the dermis but lacks the enzyme tyrosinase that converts the amino acid tyrosine to melanin.
- **Vitiligo:** It presents as white spots in the skin and occurs due to partial or complete loss of melanocytes at that site.

TYPES OF SKIN

The skin varies in thickness. It is thickest in palms and soles, which are exposed to wear and tear. In these areas it is 6 mm thick. Skin is thinnest on the eyelids, external genitalia and tympanum (eardrum), where it is approximately 0.5 mm thick. The average thickness of skin is 1.0–2.0 mm.

On the basis of thickness, the skin is classified into the following two types (Fig. 5.3):

1. Thin–hairy skin
2. Thick–hairless skin

Thin skin is present all over the body except in palms and soles. In thin skin the epidermis is thin.

Thick skin is present only in the palms and soles. In thick skin the stratum corneum is very thick, an adaptation to resist trauma in the skin of the palms and soles. There is an additional layer of stratum lucidum underneath the stratum corneum. It is a homogeneous layer where the cells are not clearly seen. The hair follicles and sebaceous glands are totally absent in thick skin. At the same time sweat glands are seen in abundance.

The differences between the thin and thick skin are provided in Table 5.1 (see also Fig. 5.3).

N.B.

Thick skin is composed of five layers, whereas thin skin is composed of four layers (stratum lucidum is absent).

SURFACE IRREGULARITIES (ALSO CALLED SURFACE PATTERNS) OF SKIN

The surface of the skin presents three types of irregularities:

1. Tension lines
2. Flexor lines
3. Papillary (friction) ridges

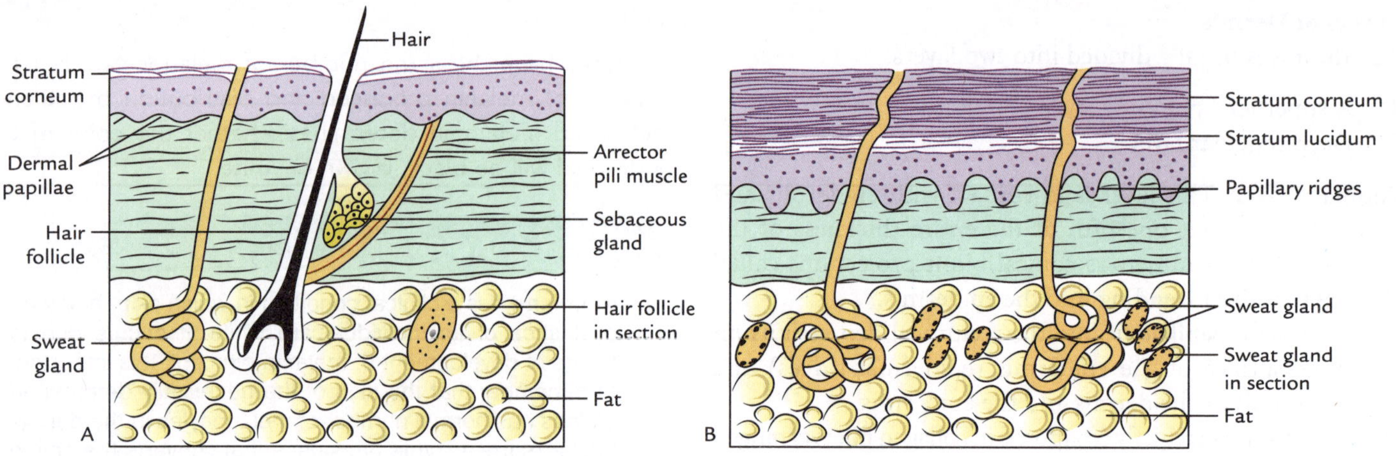

Fig. 5.3 Features of skin: **A,** thin skin; **B,** thick skin.

Table 5.1 Differences between the thin and thick skin

	Thin skin	Thick skin
Epidermis	Thin (0.10–0.15 mm) Stratum corneum thin Stratum lucidum absent	Thick (0.6–4.5 mm) Stratum corneum thick Stratum lucidum present
Friction ridges	Absent	Present
Hair follicles	Present (hairy)	Absent (nonhairy)
Sebaceous glands	Present	Absent
Sweat glands	Few	More
Sensory nerve endings	Few	More
Distribution	Present all over the body except for palms and soles	Present in palms, soles and palmar surfaces of fingers

Tension lines (synonym cleavage lines, Langer's lines), as mentioned earlier, are caused by the patterns of arrangement and pull of collagen fibers within the dermis. These are in the form of linear furrows invisible to naked eye. They are horizontal in trunk and neck and longitudinal in the limbs (Fig. 5.4).

Clinical correlation

The tension lines are of special interest to surgeons: incisions made parallel to these lines heal more rapidly and produce a hairline scar as minimum number of fibers are cut and pull is along the longitudinal axis of the incision, whereas incisions made across these lines heal poorly and produce wide ugly scar because most of the fibers are cut and the pull is at right angles to the long axis of the incision.

Flexor lines and flexor creases are acquired permanent lines and creases in the skin. The flexor creases are well marked in the palms and soles and are produced by habitual movements. The skin along these lines is thin and firmly bound to the deep fascia. The lines are prominent on the flexure aspects of the joints.

Wrinkle lines are caused by contraction of underlying muscles and are usually perpendicular to the lines of the muscle pull.

The furrows or lines on the forehead and face are produced due to continuous contraction of the muscles of facial expression. Hence on the face, they are known as **lines of expression.**

Papillary ridges (friction ridges) are present on the finger and the toe pads and on the palms and soles. They form narrow ridges separated by parallel grooves arranged in curved arrays. They correspond to the dermal ridges.

The designs formed by these lines have basic similarities, but they are not identical in any two individuals. Because they are precise and easy to reproduce, **fingerprints** are customarily used for identifying individuals. The study of these ridges is termed as **dermatoglyphics.** There are four basic dermatoglyphic patterns in the digits: (a) arches, (b) whorls,

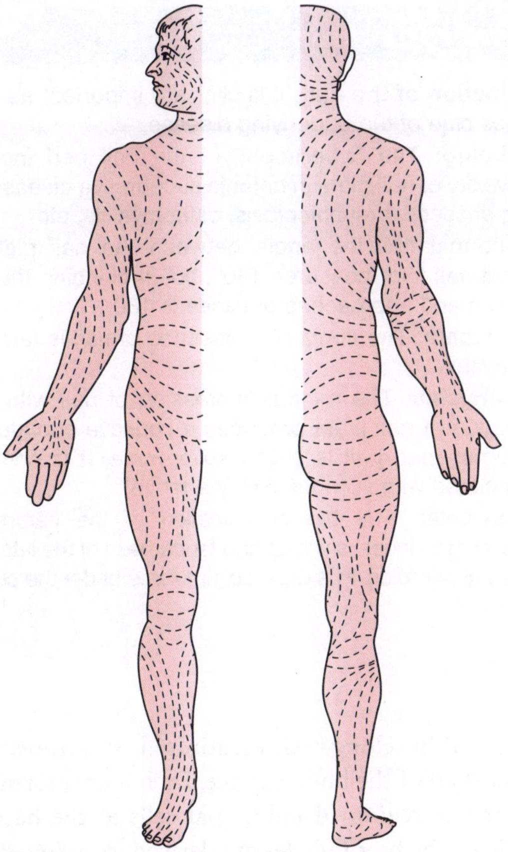

Fig. 5.4 Tension lines of the skin: **A**, front; **B**, back.

(c) loops and (d) composite. There may be a combination of the above three patterns (Fig. 5.5). These patterns are determined genetically.

Clinical correlation

Finger prints: The science known as dermatoglyphics deals with the classification and identification of fingerprints. Every individual's print is unique, including those of identical twins. So fingerprints are used for medicolegal purpose to identify criminals. Further, in certain diseases, particularly mental disorders, there is deviation from normal patterns.

APPENDAGES OF SKIN (ACCESSORY STRUCTURES OF SKIN)

The appendages of skin are epidermal (i.e. ectodermal) derivatives. These include: nails, hair, sweat glands and sebaceous glands.

Nails (Fig. 5.6)

These are hardened plates of keratinized epithelial cells of stratum corneum (i.e. nails consist of hard keratin) found on the dorsal surface of the tips of fingers and toes and are accordingly termed as finger and toe nails.

Both finger and toe nails serve to protect the digits. The fingernails also help in grasping and picking small objects and are also used for scratching.

The nails are found only in primates, whereas most other mammals have claws or hooves.

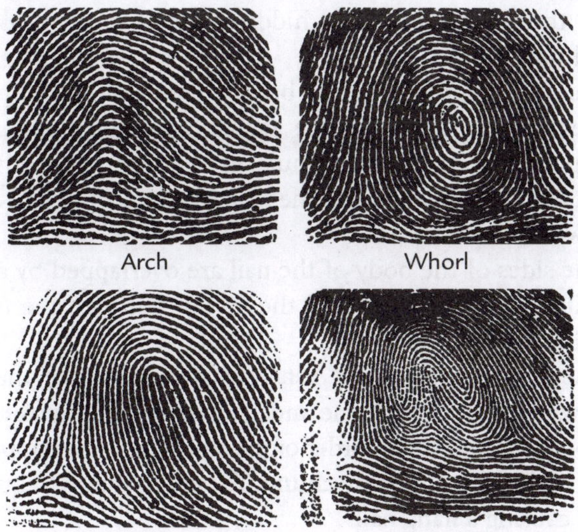

Fig. 5.5 Four types of fingerprints. (*Source:* Fig. 7.3, Page 77, *Textbook of Clinical Embryology*, Vishram Singh. Copyright Elsevier 2012, All rights reserved.)

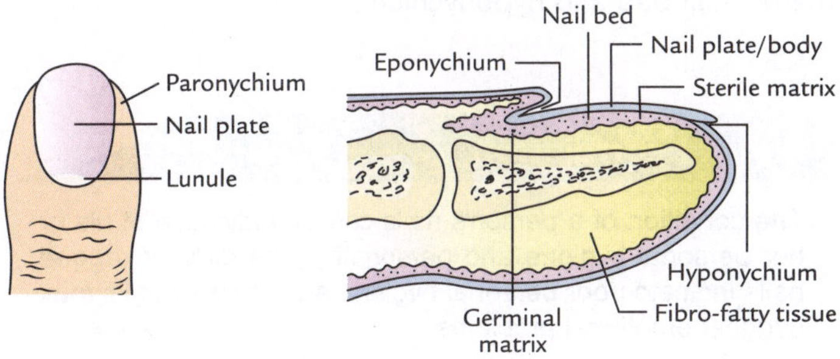

Fig. 5.6 Structure of a nail.

Parts of the Nail

Each nail consists of the following parts:

1. Root }
2. Body } Nail plate
3. Free border
4. Hidden border

The nail plate rests on the nail bed, which is actually made of stratum basale and stratum spinosum of the epidermis. The large exposed part of the nail plate is called **nail body** while the smaller proximal hidden part of the nail plate is called **nail root.**

The proximal part of the body presents a white opaque crescent called **lunule.*** The tissue (corneum) under the transparent body (except lunule) is very vascular. This accounts for the pink color of the nail. In anemia the nails look pale white.

The sides of the body of the nail are overlapped by a fold of skin called **nail folds** and the furrow between the two is called the **nail groove.**

The **free border** is the distal exposed border of the nail plate which is attached to the undersurface by **hyponychium.**** The proximal attached border of the nail plate is overlapped by a fold of the skin, the **eponychium.** The eponychium frequently splits, causing a hang nail.

The nail bed beneath the root and lunule is thick and is called **germinal matrix.** The rest of the nail bed is thin and is called **sterile matrix.** The nail matrix is the source of nail plate.

N.B.

The *nail apparatus* consists of nail plate, nail folds, nail matrix, nail bed and hyponychium.

Clinical correlation

The condition of a person's nails can be indicative of his or her personal hygiene and personality. The dirty or ragged nails indicate poor personal hygiene and chewed nails may suggest emotional problems.

Growth of Nails

Like hair, nails grow from the base. The nail grows by proliferation of germinal matrix and transformation of the superficial cells of the matrix into the nail cells. The hard transparent nail cells are then pushed forward over the thin sterile matrix. The nails grow continuously throughout life and do not have resting phase.

The fingernails grow at an average rate of about 1 mm per week. The growth rate of toenails is somewhat slower. It takes about 3–4 months for the whole nail to grow. For this reason in fungal diseases of the nails the course of treatment should last for not less than this period.

N.B.

The growth of nail is fastest (0.1 mm per day) in the middle finger (longest finger) of the hand.

Clinical correlation

Examination of the nail: It is clinically important as it often provides clue of the underlying disease.

- **Clubbing:** The hypertrophy of the nail bed increases convexity of nail plate in chronic suppurative diseases, *viz.* lung abscess, bronchiectasis, osteomyelitis, etc.

  In normal nail the angle between the nail plate and proximal nail fold measures 160°, but in clubbing the angle increases and approaches or exceeds 180°.
- **Anonychia:** The congenital absence of nail is termed as anonychia.
- **Koilonychia:** The central depression of nail with lateral elevation of nail plate produces a concave curvature, i.e. spoon-shaped nail is called *koilonychia*. It is commonly associated with iron-deficiency anemia.
- **Paronychia:** It is the inflammation of the paronychium producing redness, swelling and tenderness of the lateral and proximal nail folds. Pus often accumulates under the cuticle.

Hair

These are thin elongated keratinized structures present over almost all of the body surface. Each hair is formed from hair matrix, a region of epidermal cells at the base of the hair follicle. The hair follicles are derived from invaginations of epidermal epithelium. Hair is found everywhere on the body except on palms, soles, lips, glans penis, clitoris and labia minora.

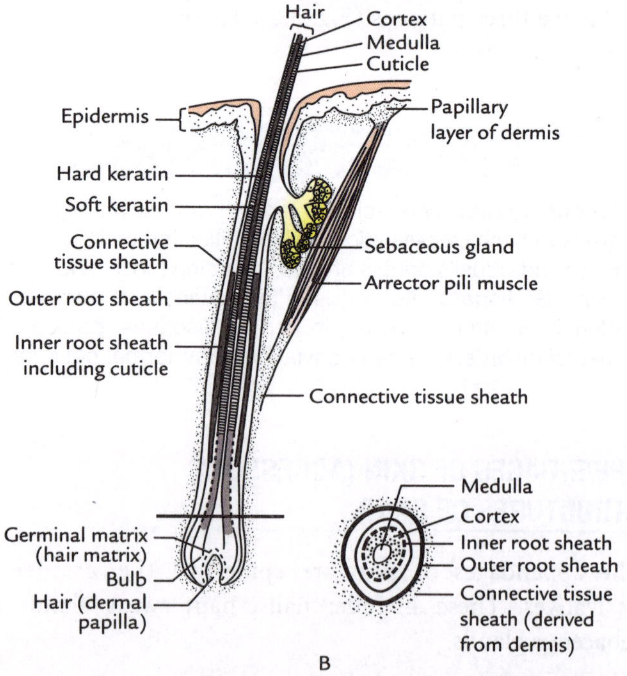

Fig. 5.7 Detailed structure of the hair follicle: **A**, longitudinal section of hair in a follicle; **B**, transverse section of hair in the follicle.

*Lunule: L. *Lunula* = small moon
**Hyponychium: Gk. *Hypo* = under; *onyx* = nail

The presence of hair is a characteristic of all mammals. The humans are relatively hairless, with only the scalp, the face, the pubis and the axilla being densely haired. For this reason anthropologists have referred to humans as **naked animals**. The primary function of hair is protection.

Parts of Hair

Each hair consists of three parts:

1. Shaft
2. Root
3. Bulb

Shaft of hair—projects above the surface of the skin. It is the dead portion of hair consisting of keratinous material and is diagonally placed.

Root of hair—is embedded within the skin. It is surrounded by hair follicle (a sheath of epidermis and dermis). The hair follicle, in fact, is a tubular invagination of the epidermis and dermis.

Bulb of hair—is the enlarged base of the root of the hair within the hair follicle. Each hair develops from stratum basale cells within the bulb of the hair. The bulb of the hair is invaginated by highly vascular connective tissue, the **dermal papilla,** which provides nutrition to the developing hair.

Clinical correlation

In a healthy person, hair grows at a rate of 1 mm every 3 days. The life span of a hair varies from 3 to 4 months for eyelashes to 3 to 4 years for scalp hair. Each hair lost is replaced by a new hair that grows from the bulb of hair and pushes the old hair out. Baldness results when hair are lost and not replaced by new hair. Baldness may occur due to a disease but is generally inherited and most frequently occurs in males because of genetic influences combined with male sex hormone testosterone. No treatment is effective in reversing genetic baldness; however, flaps of the skin containing healthy follicles from hairy parts of the body can be grafted.

Arrector pili muscles: These are thin slips of smooth muscle attached to the hair follicles. Arrector pili muscle makes an obtuse angle with the skin surface. A sebaceous gland is often enclosed between the arrector pili and hair follicle.

The arrector pili muscles are involuntary and respond to thermal or psychological stimuli. The contraction of the arrector pili muscles has two effects: when they contract (a) the hair are pulled in more vertical position (*stand on end appearance*) causing goose bumps ('*goose skin*'), and (b) squeezes out sebum into the hair follicles. The 'goose flesh' appearance of skin is a common feature on exposure to cold or emotional stimuli.

N.B.

- The *pilosebaceous apparatus* (unit) consists of hair follicle, sebaceous gland and arrector pilorum muscle.
- *Arrector pili muscles are absent* in facial and axillary hairs, eye brows, eye lashes, hairs of nostrils and hairs of external auditory meatuses.

Structure of Hair (Fig. 5.7)

The hair consists of three layers as seen in its cross-section. From deep to superficial these are:

1. Medulla
2. Cortex
3. Cuticle

Medulla consists of moderately keratinized and loosely arranged cells. They are separated by many air spaces (also called air cells).

Cortex consists of heavily keratinized and compactly grouped cells.

Cuticle consists of a single layer of cells with serrate edges. They provide hair a scaly appearance under dissection microscope.

A hair is surrounded by three sheaths:

1. Internal root sheath
2. External root sheath
3. Connective tissue sheath

The **internal root sheath** completely surrounds the initial part of the shaft. Its cells degenerate and disappear above the sebaceous glands.

The **external root sheath** is continuous with epidermal cells and near the surface it shows all the layers of epidermis.

The **connective tissue sheath** is derived from dermis.

Color of Hair

The color of hair is determined by the amount of melanin produced by melanocytes in the germinal matrix of the hair follicle. The varying amounts of melanin produce hair color, ranging from **blonde-** to-**brunette**-to-**black**.

Clinical correlation

Greying of hair: In old age hair become grey or white. It is due to lack of production of melanin due to progressive decrease of tyrosinase and increase in the number of air spaces in the cells of medullary shaft that generally accompany aging.

Texture of Hair

The texture of hair is determined by its cross-sectional shape. **Straight hair** is round in cross-section, **wavy hair** is oval and **kinky hair** is flat.

Types of Hair

The humans have three types of hair:

1. Lanugo
2. Angora or terminal
3. Definitive or vellus

Lanugo are fine silky hair which cover the fetus. They develop during the third trimester of development and are usually not evident on the baby's body at birth unless the baby is born prematurely.

Angora or terminal hair are long, coarse and pigmented. They grow continuously in length. The examples are: hair of scalp and face of male, hair in axillary and pubic regions, eyelashes and eyebrows.

Definitive or vellus hair are the most common type. They grow to certain length and then cease to grow. They are short, fine and usually unpigmented.

Sweat (Sudoriferous) Glands

The sweat glands are long coiled tubular glands. Each sweat gland consists of two parts: a secretory portion and an excretory duct.

The **secretory portion** is located in the deep dermis in the form of a twisted coil. The **excretory duct** is long and extends from secretory position to the surface of the skin. The sweat glands are most numerous in the palms, soles, axilla, pubic region and forehead.

Types of Sweat Glands

The sweat glands are of two types:

1. Eccrine
2. Apocrine

The **eccrine sweat glands** are widely distributed all over the body, especially on the forehead, palms and soles. These glands are fully formed before birth.

The eccrine glands help in regulation of the body temperature by evaporation of sweat and also help in excretion of the body salt. In response to thermal and emotional stimuli, these glands are capable of producing 8–10 L of sweat per day. The eccrine sweat glands are stimulated by cholinergic fibers of sympathetic nerves.

The eccrine (or epicrine) glands are distributed throughout the body except for lip margins, eardrums, nail beds, inner surface of the prepuce and glans penis.

The **apocrine sweat glands** are much larger sweat glands and their ducts open in the apical part of the hair follicles. They are found in axillary and pubic regions, areolae of breasts, labia minora and perianal region. Their secretion is viscous containing protein and lipid. It is poured into the hair follicles. The apocrine sweat glands are stimulated by adrenergic fibers of sympathetic nerves.

N.B.

- In apocrine sweat glands secretion is by exocytosis (merocrine), hence the term apocrine is a misnomer.
- As a rule, postganglionic sympathetic neurons use norepinephrine as their neurotransmitter; however, there is exception to the rule in regulation of the body temperature.

The apocrine sweat glands differ from eccrine sweat glands in the following three ways:

1. They secrete a viscous product containing protein and lipids via merocrine secretion.
2. They discharge their secretion into the apical part of the hair follicle, i.e. pilosebaceous canal of a hair follicle (rather than directly onto the surface).
3. They are under endocrine control (androgens and estrogens).

The apocrine glands are not functional until puberty and their odoriferous secretion is thought to attract opposite sex.

N.B.

- In animals the apocrine glands secrete *pheromones* which influence heterosexual drive, important for courtship and social behavior.
- In humans the secretion of the apocrine sweat glands is initially odourless but later due to bacterial decomposition produces a characteristic *adult body odor* in 'blacks' and 'whites'.

  For this reason people use different kind of exogenous sexual attractions such as perfumes, scents while attending functions and parties.

The main differences between the eccrine and apocrine sweat glands are presented in the Table 5.2.

N.B.

- The *ceruminous glands* present in the external auditory meatus are modified apocrine sweat glands. They discharge waxy secretion called *cerumen* which provides a sticky barrier for foreign bodies and protects the tympanic membrane from damage. Accumulation of cerumen in external auditory meatus (earwax) may prevent sound waves from reaching the tympanic membrane.
- The modified apocrine glands of eyelashes are called *glands of Moll.*

The mammary glands or breasts are modified sweat glands, located in the superficial fascia in the region of the chest. They secrete milk during lactation. The mammary glands reach their greatest development during child-bearing years.

The breast consists of 15–20 pyramidal lobes/acini of glandular tissue which are drained by lactiferous ducts onto the nipple.

Table 5.2 Differences between eccrine (merocrine) and apocrine sweat glands

	Eccrine sweat glands	Apocrine swe at glands
Nature of secretion	Watery, containing sodium chloride, potassium, urea and ammonia	Viscid, containing proteins and lipids
Site of discharge of secretion	On the skin surface on sweat pores	Into the pilosebaceous canal around the hair shaft
Distribution	Widely distributed throughout the body	Found in axilla, mons pubis and anal regions
Function	Regulate body temperature	Provide characteristic body odor (malodorous body scent)
Age of activity	Active throughout life	Active at puberty
Neurogenic control	*Cholinergic* postganglionic sympathetic neurons	*Adrenergic* postganglionic sympathetic neurons
Endocrine control	Absent	Present (androgens and estrogens)

The glandular tissue of each lobe is surrounded by fat or adipose tissue. Adipose tissue within the breast contributes largely to the contour and size of the breast. Proliferation of the glandular tissue during pregnancy is due to estrogen and progesterone. The secretory activation of glandular tissue is due to prolactin.

The suspensory ligaments (of Cooper) which are connective tissue septa attach the breast to the skin and to the underlying deep fascia (pectoral fascia). They provide support and maintain posture of the breast.

Clinical correlation

Gynaecomastia: The lobes of mammary glands are only slightly developed in male or remain rudimentary. If they develop, the condition is called as *gynecomastia*.

Sebaceous Glands (Oil Glands)

They are associated with hair follicles as they develop from the follicular epithelium of the hair. Each hair follicle is provided with one to six sebaceous glands. They are simple branched glands that are connected to the hair follicle. They secrete an oily material, the sebum, onto the shaft of the hair. The sebum which mainly consists of lipids is dispersed along the shaft of the hair to the surface of the skin. It lubricates and waterproofs the surface of the skin and also prevents the hair from being brittle. They are widely distributed all over the skin of the body except palms and soles.

N.B.

Sebaceous glands mostly open into the hair follicles. However, in certain areas of the body sebaceous glands open directly onto the surface of the skin, e.g.:

- *On nose*, where the opening of the ducts when occluded with debris appear as 'black heads'.
- In *genital* and *perianal* regions.
- In *areola* around the nipple, where they form *Montgomery's tubercles*.
- In the *eyelids*, where they are called *tarsal glands*.

Clinical correlation

- **Acne at puberty:** Under the influence of the sex hormones, the sebaceous glands grow in size and increase their production of sebum. If the drainage of sebum is blocked, the sebaceous glands become infected and produce acne. The acne are small elevations of skin (pimples). They may contain pus (pustule) and are usually confined to the face particularly in teenaged males.
- **Sebaceous cysts:** The mouth of sebaceous glands opens into the hair follicle. If the mouth of a sebaceous gland becomes blocked, the gland becomes distended by its own secretion producing *sebaceous cyst*.
  Most sebaceous cysts are found in the hairy part of the body. The scalp, scrotum, neck, shoulder and back are the common sites, but they can occur wherever there are sebaceous glands. Most sebaceous cysts are tense and consequently spherical.
- **Sebaceous horn:** If the sebum of a sebaceous cyst exudes slowly, it may dry and harden into a conical spike called sebaceous horn.

FUNCTIONS OF SKIN

The skin is a dynamic organ. It not only protects the body from pathogens and external injury, but it also plays a major role in maintaining body homeostasis.

The major functions of the skin include:

1. Protection
2. Hydroregulation (i.e. prevents the loss of body fluids)
3. Thermoregulation
4. Sensory reception (i.e. acts as a sensory organ)
5. Absorption of lipid-soluble substances and ultraviolet rays

6. Synthesis of vitamin D
7. Excretion of waste material
8. Communication of emotions

Protection: Skin acts as a protective barrier between the external environment and internal tissues of the body. It protects the body from pathogens and external injury.
Hydroregulation: Skin being (virtually) waterproof, it prevents dehydration (loss of body fluids) in hot weather and absorption of water when immersed in water. The waterproofing is provided by cornified layer of the skin.
Thermoregulation: Skin plays a crucial role in regulation of body temperature. It maintains the normal body temperature, i.e. at 37°C, by effects of sweating and shivering. The excess heat is lost from the body by three ways, all involving the skin: (a) through the excretion and evaporation of sweat, (b) through radiation from dilated blood vessels, and (c) through convection of heat directly through skin. The heat is conserved by the fat and the hair.
Sensory reception: Skin is an important sensory organ for perceiving sensations like pain, touch, temperature and pressure. This is because skin contains a large number of sensory nerve endings called **cutaneous receptors.**
Absorption: Skin being a protective barrier, it has limited capacity of absorption. Lipid-soluble substances such as vitamins A, D, E and K are absorbed slowly. Some gases, *viz.* O_2 and CO_2, may pass through skin into blood, small amounts of ultraviolet light are absorbed readily and certain toxins and pesticides enter the body through the skin.
Synthesis: Vitamin D is synthesized in skin with the help of ultraviolet rays of the sun. In addition, keratin and melatonin are also synthesized in the skin. The melanin and keratin remain in the skin while vitamin D is used elsewhere in the body.
Excretion: The skin also acts as an excretory organ. The excess of water, salts and waste products such as ammonia and urea are excreted through the skin by sweating.
Communication of emotions: Skin can also communicate emotions, e.g. in anger a person's face becomes red and in anxiety the palms become cold and damp or the person may start sweating.

BLOOD SUPPLY TO THE SKIN

The epidermis of the skin is avascular. The blood vessels within the dermis supply the glands and hair follicles within the dermis and metabolically active stratum basale of the epidermis.

A special feature of the blood supply to the skin is the presence of numerous arteriovenous anastomoses which regulate blood flow through the capillary bed and thus help in maintaining the body temperature.

Clinical correlation

Bed sores: Proper circulation of blood in skin is essential for a healthy skin. When a person lies in one position on bed for a long period, the dermal flow of blood is reduced at sites where the body presses against the bed. As a result cell necrosis occurs at these sites, leading to ulceration. The ulcers thus produced are called *bed sores* or *decubitus ulcers*.

NERVE SUPPLY TO THE SKIN

The nerves supplying to the skin are:

1. Motor nerves
2. Sensory nerves

Motor nerves: These are autonomic nerve fibers which activate glands and control blood flow.
Sensory nerves: These are somatic nerve fibers which innervate the skin in the form of large number of sensory nerve endings which carry different types of sensations from the skin.

Sensory nerve endings in the skin (Fig. 5.8)

(a) *Free nerve endings* enter the epidermis and carry pain and temperature sensations.
(b) *Merkel's discs or endings* terminate on the Merkel cells of stratum basale and functions as **mechanoreceptors.**
(c) *Meissner's corpuscles* are present in the dermal papillae and function as **mechanoreceptors** to detect fine touch.
(d) *Pacinian corpuscles* are present in the dermis and function as **mechanoreceptors** to detect deep pressure and vibrations.
(e) *Ruffini's endings* are present deep within the dermis and function as **heat receptors** to detect heat.
(f) *Bulbs of Krause* are located in the superficial part of the dermis and function as **thermoreceptors** to detect cold.

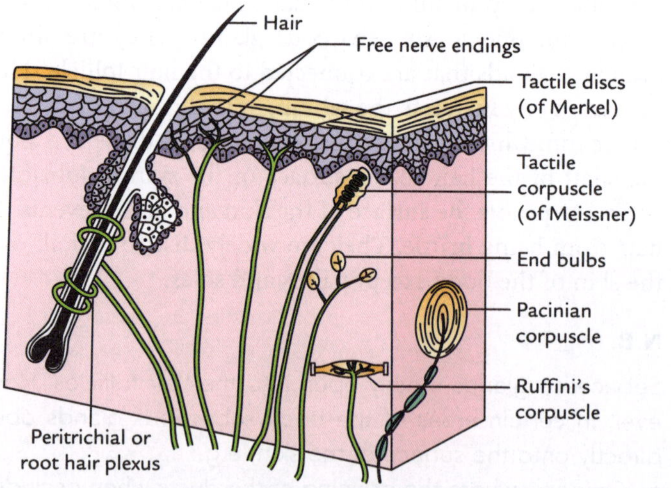

Fig. 5.8 Sensory nerve endings in the skin. (*Source:* Fig. 4.1, Page 29, *Textbook of Clinical Neuroanatomy*, Vishram Singh. Copyright Elsevier 2010, All rights reserved.)

(g) *Root hair plexuses* are the plexuses of nerve fibers around roots of hair follicles and function as **tactile receptors** to detect movement.

All the cutaneous receptors are located in the dermis except free nerve endings and Merkel's discs which are located in the epidermis.

WOUND HEALING

The healing of wound occurs in three steps or stages:

1. Inflammation
2. Proliferation
3. Maturation

Inflammation: The cut surfaces become inflamed, blood clots and cell debris fills the gap between them in the first few hours. The phagocytes and fibroblasts migrate into the blood clot:

(a) Phagocytes remove the blood clot and cell debris.
(b) Fibroblasts secrete collagen fibers which bind the cut surfaces.

Proliferation: The epithelial cells proliferate across the clot. The epidermis meets and grows upwards until the full thickness is restored. **Granulation tissue** consisting of new capillary buds, phagocytes and fibroblasts develop. The fibroblasts continue to secrete collagen fibers as the clot and any bacteria are removed by phagocytosis. The clot above the new tissue becomes the **scab** and separates after 3–10 days.
Maturation: The granulation tissue is replaced by fibrous scar tissue.

N.B.

The healing is described to be of two types: (a) primary healing (healing by first intention), and (b) secondary healing (healing by second intention). The primary healing follows minimal destruction of tissue when the damaged edges of wound are in close opposition. The secondary healing follows destruction of a large amount of tissue or when the edges of a wound cannot be brought in opposition. The stages of healing are same in both types.

SKIN BURNS

The skin burns are generally caused by heat, electricity or chemicals. The skin burns are classified as **first degree, second degree** or **third degree** based on their severity.

First degree burn

- Destroys only epidermis
- Presenting symptoms are: redness, pain and edema (swelling).
- Shedding of surface layer a few days later
- Heals in 3–6 days.

Second degree burn

- Involves epidermis and part of dermis
- Blisters appear
- Heals completely within few weeks

Third degree burn

- Destroys both epidermis and dermis completely and frequently some of the underlying muscle
- Skin appears waxy or charged
- Are insensitive to touch
- Wounds develop
- Heals by forming scar tissue
- Requires skin grafting to promote healing.

N.B.

Major burns include: (a) third degree burns involving 10% of the body surface, or (b) second degree burns involving over 25% of the body surface.

Estimation of Surface Area of Skin

The total surface area of the skin covering the entire body is 1.5–2.0 sq m. The estimation of the percentage of surface area damaged in case of burns is important in treating the patient with intravenous fluid which replaces the fluids lost from tissue damage.

(a) **Rule of nine**: This rule is a quick means of estimating the surface area affected by burn.
According to this rule, the total surface area of the body is divided into regions, each of which accounts for 9% (or a multiple of 9%) of the total skin surface (Table 5.3; Fig. 5.9).
(b) **Hand area rule**: A rough estimation of surface area affected by burn can be calculated by '*hand area rule*'. According to this rule, the area of patient's hand is approximately 1% of the total body surface.

Regeneration of the skin

The skin has high capacity of regeneration and repair. For this reason, the skin grafting is a common procedure in plastic surgery especially after burns. If a patch of epidermis gets removed, the repair and regeneration takes place by a proliferative activity of the stratum germinativum; however, there is no regeneration of hair follicles. If the dermis remains intact, the pattern of papillary ridges (fingerprints) is reproduced as earlier. If the dermis is damaged, the papillary ridges regenerate but do not conform to the original pattern.

SUPERFICIAL FASCIA

It is a subcutaneous layer of loose areolar tissue which unites dermis of skin to the underlying deep fascia (Fig. 5.10). It allows mobility of the dermis on the underlying structures.

Table 5.3 The surface area of skin in percentage for various regions of the body

Region of the body	% of the surface area of the skin
1. Head and neck (both anterior and posterior surfaces)	9 (4½ + 4½)
2. Right upper limb (both anterior and posterior surfaces)	9 (4½ + 4½)
3. Left upper limb (both anterior and posterior surfaces)	9 (4½ + 4½)
4. Anterior surface of the trunk	18 (9 × 2)
5. Posterior surface of the trunk including buttocks	18 (9 × 2)
6. Right lower limb (both anterior and posterior surfaces)	18 (9 + 9)
7. Left lower limb (both anterior and posterior surfaces)	18 (9 + 9)
8. Perineum	1
Total	100

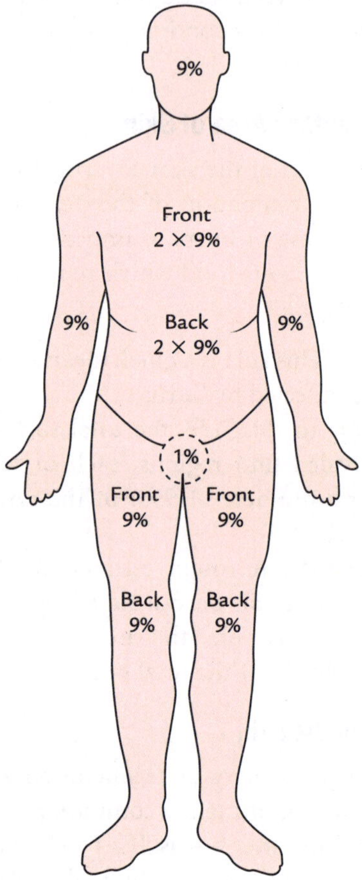

Fig. 5.9 Rule of nine—to determine the surface of the skin affected by burns.

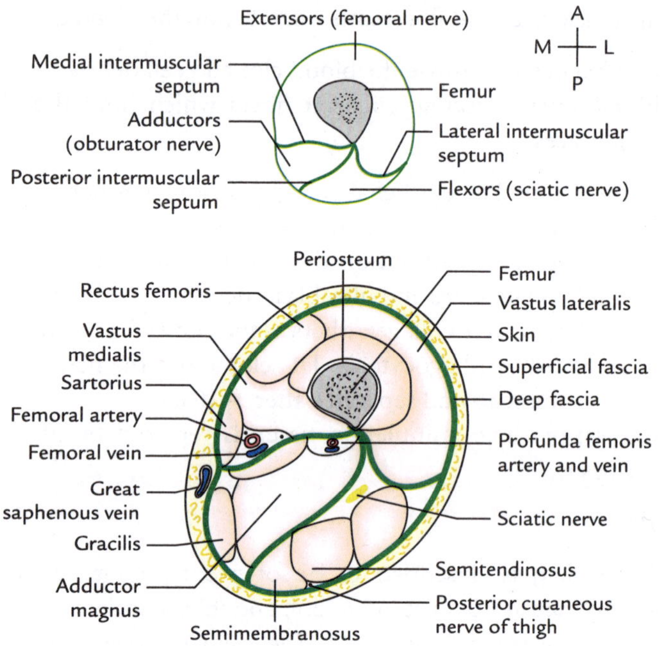

Fig. 5.10 Transverse section through the middle of the right thigh to show the three intermuscular septa and three osteofascial compartments as seen from above.

It is heavily infiltrated with fat. The amount of fat varies in different parts of the body. The superficial fascia almost everywhere in the body contains fat *except* in the:

1. Eyelids
2. External ear/pinna
3. Penis
4. Scrotum
5. Flexion creases of the digits

The amount of fat in superficial fascia is more in females and children. The fat being a bad conductor of heat, the females and children feel less cold. Further, it is the main factor responsible for the smooth external contours of the females.

Special fat deposits at certain sites in women form their secondary sexual characteristics. These sites are:

1. Gluteal and lumbar region
2. Front of thigh
3. Anterior abdominal wall below the navel (umbilicus)
4. Breasts

5. Post-deltoid region
6. Cervical thoracic region

The superficial fascia acts as a distributing layer, in which the blood vessels, lymphatics and nerves can travel before entering the dermis.

N.B.

- The subcutaneous fascia in the lower animal contains a thin sheet of muscle called *panniculus carnosus*. Its fibers are inserted into the skin. The twitch of its fibers prompts the insects to go away or fly off.
  In humans the panniculus carnosus is represented by:
  — muscles of facial expression (skeletal muscles)
  — platysma in the neck (skeletal muscle)
  — subareolar muscle of the breast (smooth muscle)
  — palmaris brevis (skeletal muscle)
  — dartos in the scrotal wall (smooth muscle)
  — corrugator cutis ani (smooth muscle)

FUNCTIONS OF SUPERFICIAL FASCIA

The functions of superficial fascia are as follows:

1. Forms an insulating layer deep to skin
2. Responsible for smooth external contours of females and children
3. Allows mobility of the skin on the underlying structures
4. Provides easy passage to nerve, vessels and lymphatics
5. Acts as cushion at certain sites (due to excessive accumulation of fat, e.g. buttocks)

Clinical correlation

- **Subcutaneous injections:** Subcutaneous injections are painful due to presence of pain receptors in it. Drugs administered by this route are absorbed slowly because subcutaneous tissue has poor blood supply. Only small doses (0.5–1 ml) of water-soluble drugs are given subcutaneously. For example, insulin injections in diabetic persons are given subcutaneously in small doses for slow release over a long duration.
- **Sites of subcutaneous injections:** The ideal sites of subcutaneous injections are:
  (a) Posterior aspect of arm
  (b) Anterior aspect of forearm
  (c) Anterior abdominal wall
  (d) Anterior aspect of thigh

DEEP FASCIA

The deep fascia is a tough, inelastic membrane of fibrous tissue which encloses the body deep to subcutaneous tissue, like a tight sleeve (Fig. 5.10). It keeps the soft tissues in place and maintains the shape of the body. The deep fascia is best marked in the limbs and neck. In the limbs, it sends septa (intermuscular septa) between the groups of muscles to attach with the periosteum of the bone. These septae enable a group of muscles to contract individually and slide freely over the adjacent muscle groups.

In the neck, it forms three layers:

1. **General investing layer,** which encloses the structures of the neck like a collar
2. **Pretracheal fascia,** which passes in front of the trachea
3. **Prevertebral fascia,** in front of the cervical part of the vertebral column. Thus the neck is divided into two compartments: visceral compartment and musculoskeletal compartment.

Axiom: Wherever the deep fascia encounters the bone, it does not cross, rather attaches itself to it for the simple reason that both are derived from the mesoderm.

MODIFICATIONS OF DEEP FASCIA

The modifications of deep fascia are as follows:

1. **Retinacula:** At certain sites deep fascia thickens to form thick bands to retain the tendon of long muscles in place and prevent their bowstringing during action of these muscles. These bands are called **retinacula,** *viz.* flexor and extensor retinacula around wrist and ankle joints.
2. **Aponeurosis:** In palms and soles it thickens to form palmar and plantar aponeurosis to protect the underlying structures. In true sense, an aponeurosis is a thick, wide sheet of fibrous tissue that provides attachment to muscles. The palmar and plantar aponeurosis represent the degenerated tendons of palmaris longus and plantaris muscles, respectively.
3. **Fibrous sheaths:** At certain sites, deep fascia condenses to form a sheath around neurovascular bundles, *viz.*
   (a) *Carotid sheath* enclosing common carotid artery, internal jugular vein and vagus nerve
   (b) *Axillary sheath* enclosing axillary artery and axillary vein (deep fascia is dense around the artery and rather loose around the veins to allow the veins to distend)
4. **Fibrous capsules:** At some sites it splits to enclose certain glands to form their capsule, *viz.* parotid gland, submandibular gland, thyroid gland, etc.
5. **Interosseous membranes:** In the forearm and leg the deep fascia is modified to form interosseous membranes.
6. **Intermuscular septa:** In the limbs, deep fascia sends fibrous septa from its deep surface to help form the compartments of the muscles.
7. **Fibrous flexor sheaths:** On the flexor surfaces of fingers and toes, the deep fascia thickens to form the fibrous flexor sheath around the long flexor tendons. These sheaths prevent the tendons from bowing out of position.

8. **Ligaments:** The ligaments of joints are considered as localized thickened bands of the deep fascia.
9. **Fascial sheath:** It forms sheath around certain muscles *viz.* psoas sheath.

Clinical correlation

- Since deep fascia defines fascial planes between the muscles, these planes form potential pathways for infection to spread.
- Pus tends to force its way along the lines of least resistance provided by the planes of the deep fascia.
- Pus can track down through the fascial sleeves formed by deep fascia around the blood vessels and muscles, e.g. pus from root of neck can track down into the arm through axillary sheath.
- Pus from tubercular thoracic spine can track down in the inguinal region through psoas sheath
- Surgeons can operate along the fascial planes with minimal injury to the adjoining structures.
- Deep fascia is least marked, i.e. scarcely demonstrable in the region of anterior abdominal wall and is considered to be absent.

SITES WHERE DEEP FASCIA IS ABSENT

The deep fascia is absent at the following sites:

1. Face
2. Breast
3. Anterior abdominal wall
4. Penis and scrotum
5. Ischiorectal fossa

NERVE SUPPLY OF DEEP FASCIA

The deep fascia is very sensitive. Its nerve supply is derived from:

1. Nerves supplying overlapping skin.
2. Nerves supplying enclosed muscles.

FUNCTIONS OF THE DEEP FASCIA

The functions of deep fascia are as follows:

1. Keeps the underlying structures in position and preserves the characteristic surface contour, *viz.* limbs, neck.
2. Provides extra surface for muscular attachments
3. Facilitates venous and lymphatic drainage
4. Binds bones, *viz.* interosseous membranes
5. Retains the long tendons in place to prevent their bowstringing and also serves as pulleys during their actions.

Golden Facts to Remember

➢ Largest organ in the body (area-wise)	Skin
➢ Largest sensory organ in the body	Skin
➢ Thickest skin in the body	Palms of hands, soles of feet
➢ Thinnest skin in the body	Glans penis, eyelids, eardrum
➢ Commonest site of skin cancer	Face
➢ Commonest congenital disorder of skin	Mole
➢ Mole (melanocyte nevi)	Melanocyte clustered in high densities
➢ Most common skin cancer	Basal-cell carcinoma
➢ Largest modified gland of skin	Mammary gland (modified sweat gland) in female
➢ Fingerprints were first used in criminal investigation by	Henry Faulds in 1880
➢ Exoskeleton in humans is represented by	Hair and nails
➢ Largest sensory receptors of skin	Pacinian corpuscles
➢ Longest coarse hair in the body	Hair on scalp

➢ Smallest coarse hair in the body	Eyelashes of lower eyelid
➢ Naked apes	Humans
➢ Most common type of hair in the body	Definitive or vellus hair
➢ Sites with maximum number of sweat glands	Forehead, palms, soles
➢ Site with maximum number of sebaceous gland	Scalp
➢ Nails with fastest growth	Nails of middle finger of hand
➢ Sites with abundant fat in superficial fascia	Breasts, buttocks, flanks, anterior abdominal wall (below umbilicus)
➢ Sites where fat is absent in superficial fascia	Eyelids, penis, scrotum
➢ Most common tumor arising from subcutaneous tissue	Lipoma
➢ Ideal sites for subcutaneous injections	Posterior aspect of arm, anterior aspect of forearm, anterior abdominal wall, anterior aspect of thigh
➢ Toughest deep fascia in the body	Temporal fascia, fascia lata
➢ Sites where deep fascia is absent	Face, external genitalia
➢ Thinnest deep fascia in the body	Fascia of Gallaudet (deep fascia on the anterior abdominal wall)

Multiple Choice Questions

1. **All of the following statements are true regarding skin *except* that it:**
   (a) Forms the dynamic interphase between the body and the external environment
   (b) Is the largest organ in the body
   (c) Develops from both ectoderm and mesoderm
   (d) Forms about 27% of body weight in adult

2. **Epidermal layer not present in thin skin is:**
   (a) Stratum granulosum
   (b) Stratum spinosum
   (c) Stratum lucidum
   (d) Stratum corneum

3. **All of the following contribute to skin color *except*:**
   (a) Dermal papillae
   (b) Melanin
   (c) Carotene
   (d) Hemoglobin

4. **Regarding cleavage (Langer) lines, all of the following statements are true *except*:**
   (a) They are caused by the pull of elastic and collagen fibers in the dermis
   (b) Their direction is vertical in chest and abdomen
   (c) Incisions made parallel to these lines heal quickly and produce hairline scar
   (d) Incision made across these lines heal poorly and produce wide thick scar

5. **Not true about apocrine sweat glands, all of the following statements are true *except* that they:**
   (a) Are not functional until puberty
   (b) Are found in axillary and pubic regions
   (c) Discharge their secretion always on the skin surface
   (d) Discharge their secretion into the pilosebaceous canal/hair follicle

6. **Regarding dermis, all of the following statements are true *except*:**
   (a) It develops from surface ectoderm
   (b) It consists of superficial papillary layer and deep reticular layer
   (c) Reticular layer is used for making leather from domestic animals
   (d) It contains sweat glands, sebaceous glands, hair follicles and arrector pili muscles

7. **In which kind of burn is healing slow and leads to scarring:**
   (a) First degree burn
   (b) Second degree burn
   (c) Third degree burn
   (d) None of the above

8. **Fat is absent in superficial fascia of:**
   (a) Eyelids
   (b) Penis
   (c) Anterior abdominal wall below umbilicus
   (d) External ear/pinna

9. **All of the following muscles are present in the superficial fascia *except*:**
   (a) Muscles of facial expression
   (b) Platysma
   (c) Pectoralis major
   (d) Corrugator cutis ani

10. **All of the following are modifications of deep fascia *except*:**
    (a) Axillary sheath
    (b) Pretracheal fascia
    (c) Retinacula
    (d) Platysma

Answers

1. *d*, **2.** *c*, **3.** *a*, **4.** *b*, **5.** *c*, **6.** *a*, **7.** *c*, **8.** *c*, **9.** *c*, **10.** *d*

CHAPTER 6

Skeleton

Learning Objectives

After studying this chapter, the student should be able to:

- enumerate the types of skeleton and list the bones in each type
- list the functions of the bone
- enumerate the different type of cells of bone
- classify the bones according to their shape and give an example of each
- describe the sesamoid bones and list their characteristic features
- outline the parts of a growing long bone and discuss its arterial supply
- describe intramembranous ossification
- describe intracartilaginous ossification
- compare and contrast the structure of compact and spongy bones
- classify different types of cartilages and give an example of each
- describe the growth of the bone
- discuss remodeling of bone and its clinical significance
- correctly solve the review questions given at the end of the chapter

INTRODUCTION

The skeleton of the body is composed of bones and cartilages. Both bones and cartilages are made up of specialized connective tissue called skeletal (**sclerous**) **tissue**, which can bear weight without bending and has considerable tensile strength. The skeletal tissue consists of same components (e.g. cells, matrix) as that of general connective tissue, but physically differs from it as its matrix is solidified.

The functions of skeletal system are as follows:

1. Forms a rigid framework of the body.
2. Provides protection to the viscera (*viz.* brain, heart, lungs, etc.) of the body from external injury.
3. Provides leverage for the body movements.

TYPES OF THE SKELETON

For the convenience of study, the skeleton is divided into two types (Fig. 6.1):

1. Axial skeleton
2. Appendicular skeleton

AXIAL SKELETON

The axial skeleton consists of bones and cartilages that lie close to the central axis of the body. It includes skull, auditory ossicles, hyoid bone, vertebral column, and rib cage:

1. **Skull:** It consists of two sets of bones—the cranial bones that form the cranium or brain case and the facial bones.
2. **Auditory ossicles:** These are the three small bones present in each middle ear cavity.
3. **Hyoid bone:** It is located above the larynx and below the lower jaw.
4. **Vertebral column (back bone):** This consists of 33 vertebrae, 7 cervical, 12 thoracic, 5 lumbar, 5 sacral and 4 coccygeal; however, sacral vertebrae fuse to form **sacrum** and coccygeal vertebrae fuse to form **coccyx**, thus vertebral column consists of 26 individual or movable bones (vertebrae).
5. **Rib cage:** It forms the bony and cartilaginous framework of the thorax. The bone forming the rib cage includes 12 pairs of ribs with associated costal cartilages and sternum (breast bone).

APPENDICULAR SKELETON

The appendicular skeleton is bilaterally symmetrical and comprises the bones of the upper and lower extremities (or limbs) and bony girdles which anchor these extremities with the axial skeleton. Thus, it includes bones of pectoral girdle, upper limb, pelvic girdle and lower limb (Fig. 6.1).

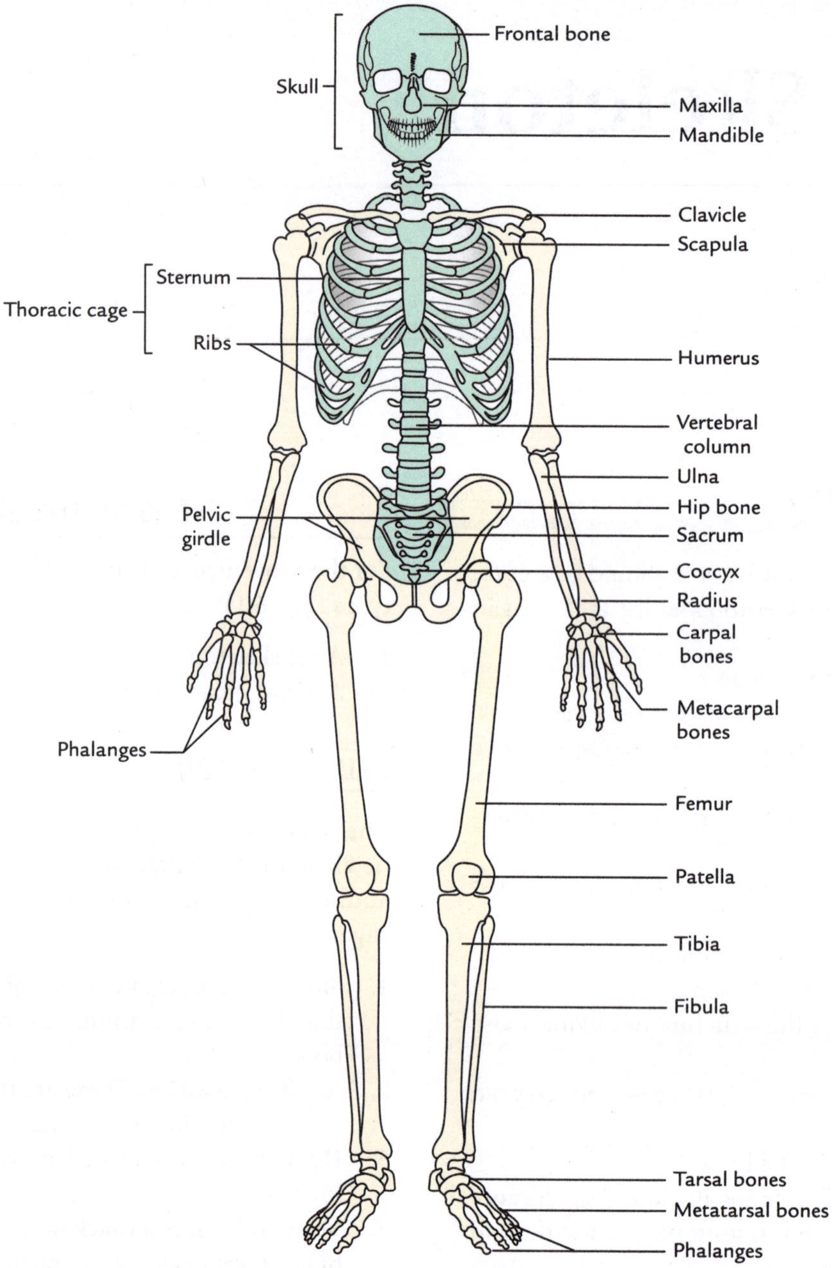

Fig. 6.1 Axial (green color) and appendicular (light brown color) skeleton.

1. **Pectoral girdle:** It consists of paired scapulae and clavicles. It is not a complete girdle as it is attached only anteriorly.
2. **Bones of upper limb:** Each upper limb contains the humerus within the arm (brachium); the radius and ulna within the forearm (antebrachium); the carpal bones, the metacarpal bones and the phalanges within the hand.
3. **Pelvic girdle:** It consists of two hip bones. It is a complete girdle as it is united anteriorly with symphysis pubis and posteriorly with the sacrum of vertebral column.
4. **Bones of lower limb:** Each lower limb contains the femur within the thigh; the tibia and fibula within the leg; the tarsal bones, the metatarsal bones and the phalanges within the foot.

The bones forming axial and appendicular skeleton are listed in Table 6.1 and shown in Figure 6.1.

BONES

The bones are the hard structures, which form the rigid framework of the body.

Structurally, bone is a highly vascular mineralized connective tissue consisting of cells and dense intercellular organic matrix impregnated with inorganic salts. The organic material mainly consists of collagen fibers and forms one-third of the bone. It provides resilience to the bone. The inorganic material mainly consists of calcium phosphate and traces of other salts. It

Table 6.1 Number of bones present in axial and appendicular skeleton

	Number of bones
	Axial skeleton
Skull	
Cranial bones	8
Facial bones	14
Hyoid	1
Ear ossicles (3 in each ear)	6
Vertebral bones	26
Rib cage	
Sternum	1
Ribs	24
Total	80
	Appendicular skeleton
Pectoral (shoulder) girdles	
Clavicle	2
Scapula	2
Upper limbs	
Humerus	2
Ulna	2
Radius	2
Carpals	16
Metacarpals	10
Phalanges	28
Pelvic (hip) girdle	
Hip bone	2
Lower limbs	
Femur	2
Fibula	2
Tibia	2
Patella	2
Tarsals	14
Metatarsals	10
Phalanges	28
Total	**126**
Total bones of axial skeleton	80
Total bones of appendicular skeleton	126
Total bones of the body	**206**

provides hardness and rigidity to the bone and makes it radiopaque in x-ray films.

The bone is not an inert material as often thought of by some students but it is a living structure. It is supplied by blood vessels, lymph vessels and nerves. It has the power of regeneration and repair. In fact, bones have greater regenerative power than any other tissues of the body, *except* blood.

The bones are subject to diseases like any other tissue of the body.

Clinical correlation

Bone health: The bones undergo atrophy, i.e. become thinner and weaker if not used, e.g. bones of a paralyzed limb atrophy; on the other hand, they hypertrophy, i.e. become thicker and stronger if subjected to support an increased weight. Therefore, regular exercise is essential to maintain the health of the bones.

N.B.

- The skeletal system of adult human is composed of approximately 206 bones.
- At birth, the skeleton consists of approximately 270 bones (in adult the number of bones decreases due to gradual fusion of separate bones).

FUNCTIONS OF BONES

The following are the functions of bones:

1. Form rigid framework of the body to give it a shape and support.
2. Provide surface for attachment of muscles, tendons, ligaments, etc.
3. Serve as levers for muscles to bring about a movement.
4. Protect certain viscera, e.g. brain, spinal cord, heart, lungs, liver, bladder, etc.
5. Contain marrow which is factory of blood cells, e.g. white blood cells, red blood cells and platelets.
6. Storehouse of calcium and phosphorus, about 95% of the phosphorus within the body is deposited in the bones and the teeth.
7. Some bones around the nose contain large cavities filled with air (paranasal air sinuses which affect the timber of the voice).

MICROSCOPIC STRUCTURE OF BONES

The bone is a specialized connective tissue and consists of the following three components:

1. Cells
2. Ground substance
3. Fibers

The ground substance and fibers together form the intercellular substance or matrix which gets mineralized.

Cells: The bone cells are of three types: osteoblasts, osteocytes and osteoclasts.

Osteoblasts

1. The osteoblasts are derived from pluripotent **osteoprogenitor cells** located in mesenchyme, periosteum and endosteum.
2. They secrete **osteoid**, which is unmineralized matrix, consisting of proteoglycans, glycoproteins and type I collagen fibers.
   (a) For mineralization to occur, the osteoblasts secrete **osteocalcin** and **alkaline phosphatase** which release calcium and phosphate radicals from substances containing them.
   (b) In addition, osteoblasts release **matrix vesicles** (membrane bound vesicles), which concentrate calcium and phosphate, and are the **most important factors necessary for mineralization to occur.**
3. They undergo mitosis.
4. They are the precursor cells of the osteocytes.

N.B.

The blood alkaline phosphatase level can be monitored clinically to assess osteogenesis during bone repair.

Osteocytes

1. The osteocytes are derived from osteoblasts. Once an osteoblast becomes surrounded by matrix, it becomes an **osteocyte.**
2. The osteocytes are flattened cells with numerous cytoplasmic processes. They are located in spaces within matrix called **lacunae** and **canaliculi**, respectively. The cytoplasmic processes of neighboring cells communicate by **gap junctions.**
3. The osteocytes unlike osteoblasts do not undergo mitosis.
4. The canaliculi radiate from each lacuna and permit diffusion of nutritive material (Fig. 6.2). Thus, cells remain alive in calcified matrix and maintain the bone by their balanced osteogenic and osteoclastic activity. They secrete alkaline phosphatase to maintain calcification. When bone cells die, the matrix is decalcified.

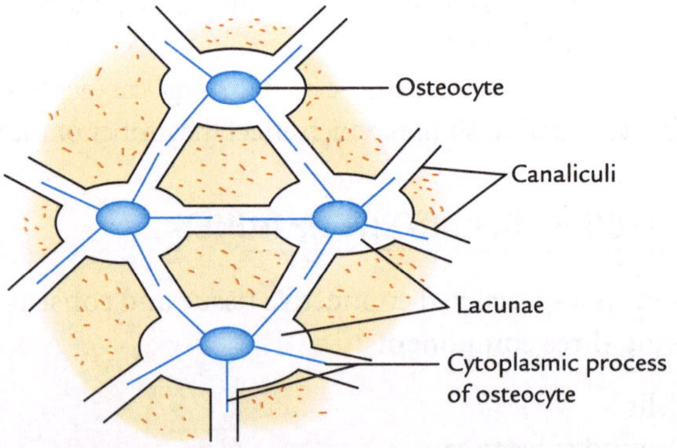

Fig. 6.2 Osteocytes, lacunae and canaliculi.

Osteoclasts

1. The osteoclasts are derived from the fusion of uncommitted cells of red bone marrow that are related to a type of white blood cell called **monocyte** similar to the formation of *giant cells* by the fusion of macrophages.
2. They are large cells with multiple nuclei.
3. They help in resorption of the bone and play an important role in bone remodeling.
4. They reside in shallow depressions of the bone called **Howship's lacunae.**
5. They do not undergo mitosis.

Ground substance: It consists of the following components:

1. **Proteoglycans** containing a side chain of glycosaminoglycans (GAGs), specifically *chondroitin sulfate* and *keratan sulfate.*
2. **Glycoproteins,** such as *osteonectin* and *osteocalcin* (a calcium binding protein).
3. **A mineral component** that includes *hydroxyapatite* (calcium phosphate crystals), *citrate ions* and *bicarbonate ions.* Mineral component mainly consists of hydroxyapatite crystals of calcium phosphate ($Ca_{10}[PO_4]_6[OH]_2$), and contributes to the hardness/rigidity of bone.
4. **Water (tissue fluid),** which contributes to a low degree of bone hydration (7%).

Fibers: They are type I collagen fibers and provide tensile strength to the bone.

CLASSIFICATION OF BONES

The bones are usually classified in three ways:

(a) According to the shape
(b) According to the structure (structural classification)
(c) According to the development (developmental classification)

A. Classification according to the shape

Depending on the size, shape, etc., the bones are classified into the following types (Fig. 6.3):

1. Long bones
2. Short bones
3. Flat bones
4. Irregular bones
5. Pneumatic bones
6. Sesamoid bones
7. Accessory bones

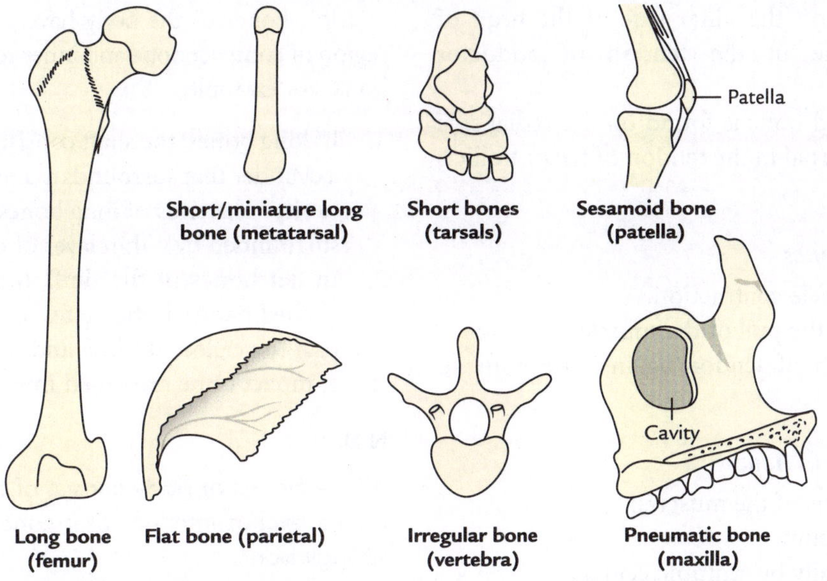

Fig. 6.3 Types of bones—depending on their shapes.

Long bones are those in which length exceeds the breadth and thickness. The long bones are of two types: typical and miniature/short.

(a) **Typical long bones.** They have the following features:
1. Consists of three parts: one elongated tubular shaft (diaphysis) and two expanded ends (epiphyses).
2. Contain medullar cavity filled with bone marrow.
3. Ossify in the cartilage.
4. Lie vertically in the body.
5. Are weight bearing.
6. Are found in limbs and act as levers for muscles.

The examples of typical long bones are humerus, radius, ulna, femur, tibia and fibula.

N.B.

The *clavicle* is the only long bone which lies horizontally, ossify mainly in membrane and does not contain medullary cavity.

(b) **Miniature/short long bones:** These are much shorter in length as compared to typical long bones with epiphysis present at one end only.

The examples of miniature long bones are metacarpals, metatarsals and phalanges. *All the metacarpals and metatarsals have epiphysis at their distal end except first metacarpal and first metatarsal which have epiphysis at their proximal end.*

Short bones are small in size and usually cuboidal in shape, presenting six surfaces. These bones are found in wrist (carpal bones) and foot (tarsal bones).

N.B.

All the short bones ossify in cartilage after birth except talus, calcaneus and cuboid which start ossifying before birth.

Flat bones are flat and shallow plate-like bones. They form boundaries of certain body cavities, e.g. cranium, thoracic cavity. The examples of flat bones include: (a) bones forming cranial vault (frontal, parietal, occipital, etc.), and (b) bones forming thoracic cage (scapulae, ribs, sternum, etc.).

Irregular bones are highly irregular in shape, *viz.* hip bone, vertebrae, bones forming base of the skull.

Pneumatic bones are a variety of irregular bones which contain air-filled cavity or cavities within them. These bones are mainly located around the nasal cavity, *viz.* maxilla, frontal, sphenoid and ethmoid bones. The air-filled cavities in these bones are called **paranasal air sinuses.**

The paranasal air sinuses not only make the skull light but also add resonance to the voice. They also act as air conditioning chambers for the inspired air.

Sesamoid bones (Arab. *sesame* = seed) are seed-like bony nodules which develop in certain muscle tendons where they rub against convex bony surfaces during the movements of the joint. The rubbing surface of the sesamoid bone is covered with an articular cartilage.

Sites of Sesamoid Bones

1. *Patella* in the tendon of quadriceps femoris in front of the knee joint.
2. *Fabella* in the lateral head of gastrocnemius behind the knee joint.
3. Two sesamoid bones below the head of the first metatarsal bone in the tendon of flexor hallucis brevis.
4. One sesamoid bone in the tendon of peroneus longus where it binds around the cuboid bone.
5. *Pisiform* in the tendon of the flexor carpi ulnaris.

6. One sesamoid bone on the ulnar side of the head of 1st metacarpal bone in the tendon of adductor pollicis.
7. Sometimes a sesamoid bone is found on the radial side of head of 1st metacarpal in the tendon of flexor pollicis brevis.

Functions of Sesamoid Bones

1. Act as pulleys for muscle contraction.
2. Alter the direction of the pull of the muscle.
3. Minimize the friction of tendon against the bone to prevent its attrition.

Characteristics of Sesamoid Bones

1. Develop in the tendons of the muscles.
2. Are devoid of periosteum.
3. Ossify after birth usually by multiple centers.
4. Lack haversian system.

N.B.

- *Patella* is the *largest sesamoid bone* in the body and the cartilage covering, its articular surface is the *thickest articular cartilage* in the body.
- *Sesamoid bones* are not classified as true bones as they are not covered by periosteum.

Accessory Bones

These are bones that are not generally present in the body. If present they do not cause any harm, sometimes clinicians confuse it with a fractured bone. Accessory bones may be formed due to:

1. Appearance of extra ossification centers in skull sutures, *viz.* **sutural or wormian bones.**
2. Nonfusion of an epiphysis. The examples are:
   (a) *Os trigonium:* the posterior tubercle of the talus that fails to fuse with the rest of the bone.
   (b) *Os vesalianum:* the styloid process of the 5th metatarsal that fails to fuse with the rest of the bone.
   (c) *Patella cubiti*: occasionally, the center of ossification for the olecranon process of ulna fails to fuse to the proximal end of the shaft.

N.B.

Heterotopic bones sometimes formed in soft tissues where they are not normally found, e.g., *rider's bone* in the tendon of adductor longus muscle of the thigh.

B. Structural Classification

Macroscopically (i.e. as seen on naked eye examination of a section of a long/flat bone), the architecture of bone may be compact (dense) or cancellous (spongy).

Most bones of the body have a basic structure of an outer region of compact bone and inner region of spongy (cancellous) bone. For example:

1. In long bones, the shaft consists of compact bone forming a cylinder that surrounds a central cavity called **medullary cavity**. The ends of long bones consist of cancellous bone surrounded by a thin layer of compact bone.
2. In flat bones of the skull, the cancellous bone is sandwiched between the plates of compact bone. The spongy part is called **diploe** and outer and inner plates of compact bone are called inner and outer **tables.**

N.B.

All the bones of body consist of both compact and spongy bones *except* inferior nasal concha which consists of only spongy bone.

Compact (Dense) Bone

The texture of compact bone is dense, ivory-like with no visible spaces on naked eye examination. The compact bone consists of (a) lamellae of collagenous sheets, and (b) haversian systems or osteons (Fig. 6.4).

Lamellae

The compact bone consists of three types of bony lamellae:

1. **Concentric lamellae** which surround the haversian canal.
2. **Interstitial lamellae**—lie between the osteons. The **interstitial lamellae** are remnants of old outer circumferential lamellae or old haversian systems.
3. **Circumferential lamellae** which are flat plates that extend around the bone.

Haversian System (Osteon)

Each haversian system consists of a **haversian canal** (or central canal), surrounded by **concentric lamellae of bone.**

Haversian canal runs parallel to the long axis of the bone and contains blood vessels, nerves and loose connective tissue.

The concentric lamellae, 4–20 in number, form rings around haversian canal. The osteocytes are located between the lamellar rings in lacunae.

The lacunae communicate with one another in between and across the lamellae, and with the central canal by numerous radiating **canaliculi.**

Haversian canals are lined by endosteum and communicate with each other, with the medullary cavity and with the surface of bone by numerous **Volkmann's canals**. The Volkmann's canals run perpendicular to the long axis of the bone.

The blood vessels from the periosteum or endosteum enter the bone through Volkmann's canals.

The haversian canals receive blood vessels from Volkmann's canals.

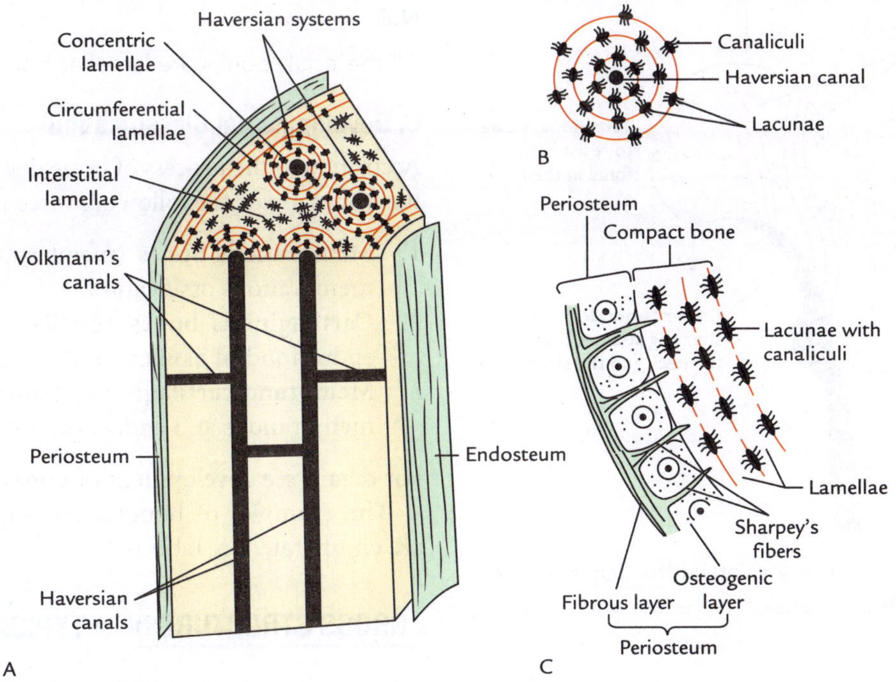

Fig. 6.4 Structure of compact bone: **A**, haversian systems and lamellae; **B**, an osteon; **C**, periosteum and outer circumferential lamellae of a compact bone.

The osteocytes receive nutrients and eliminate waste products through the canal system.

Cancellous (Spongy) Bone

The cancellous bone is a meshwork of bony spicules. It consists of interconnecting rods and plates of bone called **trabeculae**, enclosing large spaces filled with **red bone marrow.** The trabeculae:

(a) consist of superimposed lamellae and do not form **haversian system** because they get nutrition from the blood vessels of tissues around them;
(b) have a layer of osteoblasts on their surfaces.
(c) are oriented along the lines of stress.

The differences between the compact and spongy bone are given in Table 6.2.

Wolff's Law (Trajectory theory of Wolff, 1892): According to this law, the bone formation (osteogenesis) is directly proportional to stress and strain. The tensile force favors bone formation, whereas compressive force favors bone resorption. This theory, however, no longer holds good because now it is noticed that both tensile and compressive forces can stimulate bone formation in appropriate conditions.

The **architecture of cancellous bone** is often interpreted in terms of Wolff's law. Thus, the arrangement of bony lamellae is governed by the lines of maximal stress (Fig. 6.5):

1. **Pressure lamellae** are arranged parallel to the line of weight transmission.
2. **Tension lamellae** are arranged at right angles to the pressure lamellae.

Table 6.2 Difference between compact and spongy bone

	Compact bone	Spongy bone
Density	Dense like an ivory	Porous like a sponge
Haversian systems	Present	Absent
Arrangement of bony lamellae	Regular	Irregular
Location in bone	Outer region	Inner region
Bone marrow	Absent	Present
Amount in the body by weight	75%	25%

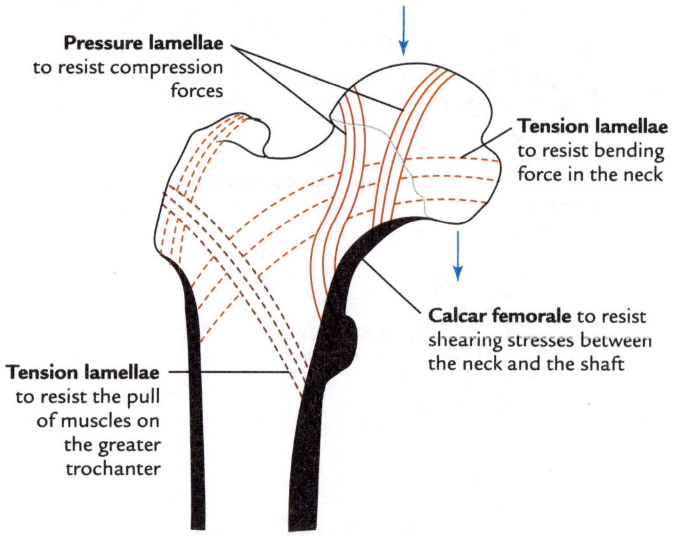

Fig. 6.5 Diagrammatic sagittal section of the upper end of femur showing pressure and tension lamellae, and calcar femorale.

N.B.

The compact arrangement of pressure lamellae form *bony buttresses to provide additional support, viz. calcar femorale (Fig. 6.5).*

Clinical correlation

The trabeculae are oriented along the line of stress within a bone. If the direction of weight-bearing stress is changed slightly, for example, because of a fracture that heals improperly, the trabecular pattern realigns with new lines of stress. For this reason, patient often complains of pain at the fracture site in later life.

Microscopically, bones are of two types:

1. Woven
2. Lamellar

This classification is based on the manner in which the different components of the matrix are arranged.

Woven bone: The collagen fascicles and bone crystals within a woven bone are arranged randomly forming a network resembling the warp and weft of a woven fabric and hence the name 'woven bone'. The examples of woven bone are **young fetal bones** (most immature bone), **callus** at fracture repair sites.

Lamellar bone: In lamellar bone, the mineralized matrix is arranged in thin layers (lamellae). The lamellae are arranged in two different patterns:

1. In number of concentric cylindrical units (haversian system), e.g. compact bone.
2. In number of branching and anastomosing curved plates, e.g. spongy bone.

N.B.

All the adult bones are lamellar bones.

C. Developmental Classification

According to the process of bone development (ossification), the bones are of the following three types:

1. **Membranous bones** (membrane bones), developed by membranous ossification.
2. **Cartilaginous bones** (cartilage bones), developed by endochondral ossification.
3. **Membrano-cartilaginous bones**, developed by both membranous and endochondral ossification.

For details see development of bones on page 77.

The examples of bones according to their development are enumerated in Table 6.3.

GROSS STRUCTURE OF A TYPICAL LONG BONE

A typical long bone consists of three parts: a shaft (or body) and two ends (Fig. 6.6).

1. The **shaft** is an elongated part between the two expanded ends. It is made of an outer thick shell of compact bone (cortex) enclosing a cavity called **medullary cavity,** thus providing maximum strength with minimal material and weight.

   The medullary cavity is filled with yellow bone marrow (remember that at birth it is filled with red bone marrow and is involved in active hemopoiesis).
2. The **ends** are knobby (expanded) and largely made up of cancellous bone covered by a thin shell of a compact bone. The ends of long bone are covered by an articular hyaline cartilage and take part in the formation of joints.

Table 6.3 Examples of bones according to their development

Types of bones	Examples
Membranous	Bones of cranial vault Facial bones
Cartilaginous	Bones of limbs Bones of base of skull Bones of vertebral column (vertebrae) Bones of thoracic cage (ribs, sternum)
Membrano-cartilaginous	Mandible Clavicle Occipital bone Temporal bone Sphenoid bone

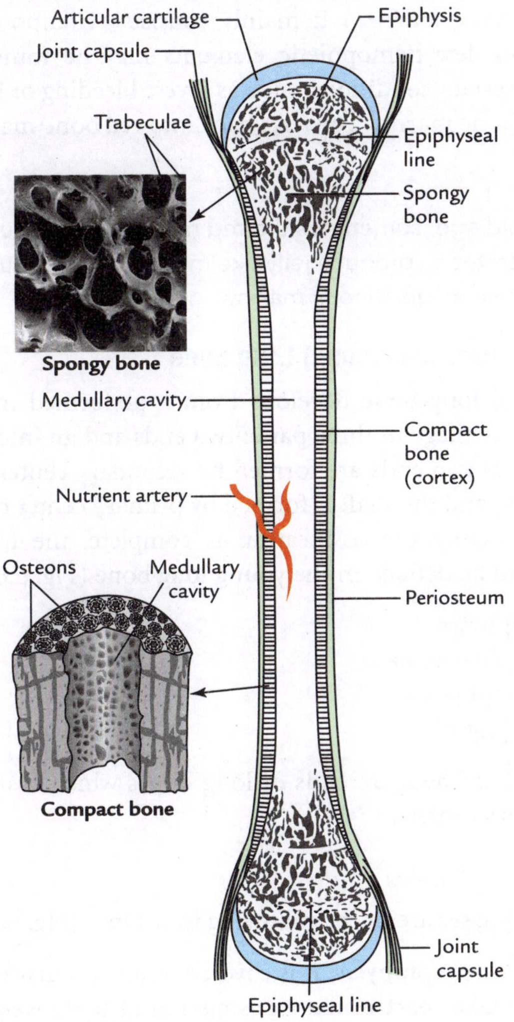

Fig. 6.6 Gross structure of a typical long bone. The insets show details of spongy (above) and compact (below) bones.

Periosteum and Endosteum

The outer surfaces of all the bones are covered by a thick fibrous membrane called *periosteum*, whereas their inner surfaces are lined by a thin fibrous membrane called *endosteum*. Both periosteum and endosteum contain osteoprogenitor cells, osteoblasts and osteoclasts which are essential for formation, remodeling and repair of bone.

The **periosteum** (Figs 6.4 and 6.6) is a thick fibrous membrane covering the entire surface of bone *except* at the areas covered by an articular cartilage. At the articular margin, the periosteum is continuous with the joint capsule.

It is made up of two layers:

1. Outer dense fibrous layer.
2. Inner cellular layer which is osteogenic in nature.

The periosteum is united to the underlying bone by extrinsic collagen fibers, the **Sharpey's fibers**. These are coarse collagenous fibers from inner layer which extends inward to penetrate the bone matrix (outer cortical bone tissue) like spikes of a shoe, thus bolting the periosteum to the bone.

Functions of Periosteum

1. Protects and maintains the shape of the bone.
2. Nourishes the outer part of the underlying cortex by abundant periosteal arteries.
3. Provides attachment to ligaments, tendons, muscles and intermuscular septa.
4. Provides regenerative capability to the bone.

The **endosteum** is cellular membrane that lines the medullary cavity of the shaft. The osteoblasts and osteoprogenitor cells within the endosteum play an important role in bone remodeling and repair.

Nutrient foramen is usually present near the middle of shaft for the entry of nutrient artery.

Clinical correlation

The periosteum is important in the repair of fractures.

It has unique capability of forming new bone, hence bone stripped of its periosteum will not survive.

The periosteum is very sensitive to pain, particularly to tearing and tension. Therefore, drilling into the bone without anesthesia is very painful. For the same reason, during intramuscular injection, if needle penetrates periosteum, severe pain is felt by the patient.

Bone Marrow

The bone marrow is a soft, loose, vascular tissue consisting of delicate network of reticular fibers and various types of cells. It is the main site of hemopoiesis.

It is present in the medullary cavity of the long bones and in the cavities of the spongy bone.

Types of Bone Marrow

Two types of bone marrow are described according to their appearance on gross examination.

1. Red bone marrow
2. Yellow bone marrow

Red bone marrow: It is vascular and appears red in color due to the presence of red blood cells. It consists of network of fine reticular fibers containing blood forming cells, showing all stages of development: immature (nucleated) and mature (non-nucleated) red blood cells, myeloblasts, myelocytes, granulocytes, megakaryocytes, etc. At birth it is present in all the bones at all sites, and is an important site of hemopoiesis, but as the age advances the marrow in the medullary cavity of long bones is gradually replaced by yellow marrow. Hence in the adults, the red marrow is found in the cancellous bone. The sites (Fig. 6.7) are as follows:

(a) Ends of long bones
(b) Sternum
(c) Ribs
(d) Skull bones
(e) Iliac crests of hip bones
(f) Vertebrae

Clinical correlation

- **Bone marrow aspiration:** It is often performed by the clinicians for diagnostic purpose. The sites commonly used for bone marrow aspiration are: sternum, anterior and posterior iliac spines of hip bones, ribs, lumbar spinous processes and upper end of tibia.
- In the adult, the *common sites of bone marrow aspiration* are manubrium of sternum and spinous processes of lumbar vertebrae.
- In the children, the common sites of bone marrow aspiration are iliac crests of hip bones.

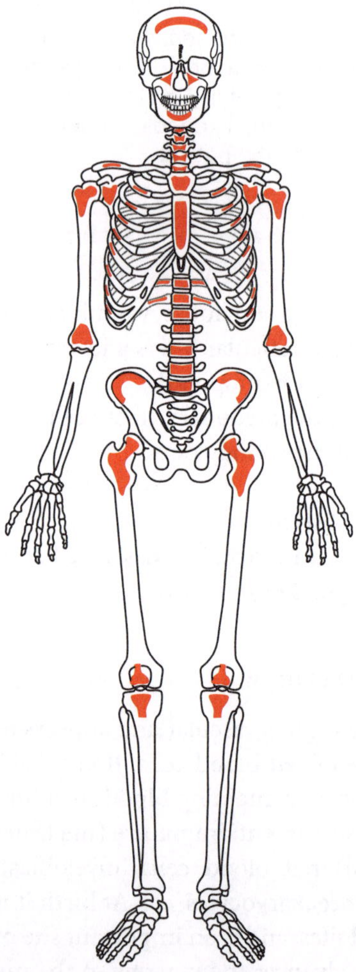

Fig. 6.7 Sites of red bone marrow.

Yellow bone marrow: It mainly consists of adipose tissue. However, few hemopoietic elements may be found in it. Under certain conditions, such as severe bleeding or hypoxia, yellow bone marrow converts back into red bone marrow.

N.B.

In the old age, sometimes the red marrow in the skull bones degenerates to produce jelly-like material (gelatinous mass). It is known as *gelatinous marrow*.

Parts of Growing (Young) Long Bone

A typical long bone develops from a preformed model of hyaline cartilage in three parts: two ends and an intervening shaft. The two ends are formed by secondary centers of ossification and the shaft is formed by primary center of ossification. Before the ossification is complete, the following parts can be defined in the young long bone (Fig. 6.8):

1. Epiphyses
2. Epiphyseal plates
3. Metaphyses
4. Diaphysis

Epiphyses: These are ends of long bones which ossify from secondary centers.

Types of Epiphyses

The epiphyses are of the following four types (Fig. 6.9):

1. **Pressure epiphysis:** It is covered by an articular cartilage and takes part in the transmission of body weight, e.g. head of femur, humerus, lower end of radius, etc.

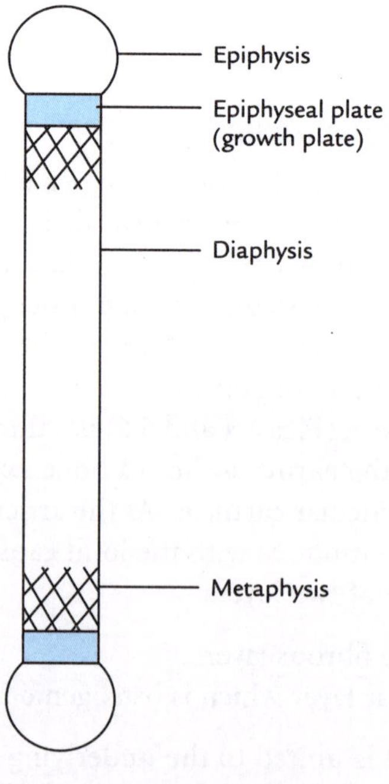

Fig. 6.8 Parts of a growing long bone.

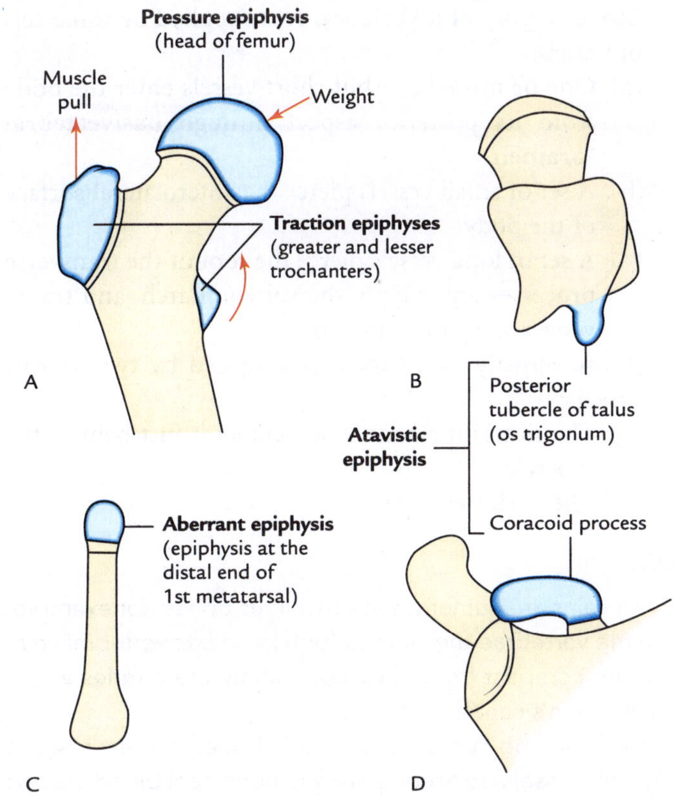

Fig. 6.9 Types of epiphyses: **A**, pressure and traction epiphyses; **B** and **D**, atavistic epiphyses; **C**, aberrant epiphysis.

2. **Traction epiphysis:**
   (a) It is produced by a pull of the muscle or muscles, e.g. greater and lesser trochanters of femur, greater and lesser tubercles of humerus, etc.
   (b) It is always nonarticular and provides attachment to the muscle or muscles.
   (c) It always ossifies later than the pressure epiphysis.
3. **Atavistic epiphysis:** It is an independent bone in lower mammals, which in man gets fused to the nearest bone to receive nutrition from the host bone. It grows like a parasite, e.g. coracoid process of scapula, posterior tubercle of talus which is also known as *os trigonum*.
4. **Aberrant epiphysis:** It is an epiphysis which appears at unusual end of a short long bone, e.g. epiphysis at the head of first metacarpal. Remember, normally epiphysis appears at the base of the first metacarpal bone.

Epiphyseal (Growth) Plate: It is a plate of hyaline cartilage which intervenes between the epiphysis and diaphysis of a growing long bone. The proliferation of cells in the epiphyseal cartilage is responsible for growth in length of a long bone (for details see page 85). After the fusion of epiphysis with diaphysis, the bone can no longer grow in length. The epiphyseal plate/cartilage is nourished by both epiphyseal and metaphyseal arteries.

N.B.

The fusion between epiphysis and diaphysis occurs 2 or 3 years earlier in females, hence they are shorter in length than males.

Metaphysis: The end of diaphysis toward the epiphyseal cartilage is called metaphysis. It is the most actively growing area of a long bone. Before fusion of epiphysis, the metaphysis is profusely supplied by blood from nutrient, periosteal and juxta-epiphyseal arteries. These are end arteries and form hair-pin-like bends. Therefore, metaphysis is the common site of osteomyelitis in children for bacteria and emboli are easily trapped in the hair-pin bends leading to infarction. After the epiphyseal fusion the communications are established between the epiphyseal and metaphyseal arteries, as a result metaphysis contains no more end arteries. For this reason, osteomyelitis in this region is rare in adults.
Diaphysis: It is the elongated part of bone between the metaphyses. It develops from primary ossification center.

BLOOD SUPPLY OF BONES

1. **Blood Supply of a Long Bone:** The long bone is supplied by the following four sets of arteries: nutrient artery, periosteal arteries, metaphyseal arteries and epiphyseal arteries (Fig. 6.10).
   (a) *Nutrient artery*: It enters the middle of the shaft through a nutrient foramen, runs obliquely through the cortex and then divides into ascending and descending branches in the medullary cavity. Each branch then subdivides into a number of smaller parallel vessels which enter the metaphysis and form

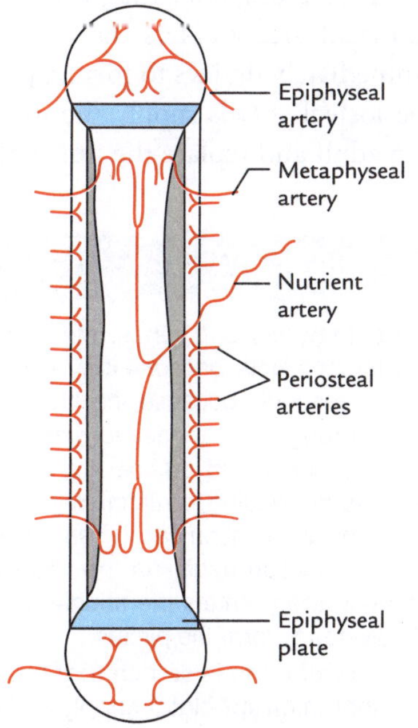

Fig. 6.10 Blood supply to a growing long bone.

hair-pin loops. These loops anastomose with epiphyseal, metaphyseal (juxta epiphyseal) and periosteal arteries. Therefore, the metaphysis is the most vascular zone of the long bone.

The nutrient artery supplies the medullary cavity containing bone marrow and inner two-third of the outer shell of compact bone of diaphysis and metaphysis.

N.B.

- Oblique direction of nutrient foramen in shaft is opposite to the growing end of the long bone.
- Before entering the nutrient foramen the nutrient artery is tortuous, so that it is not affected during the movements of the bone.
- The nutrient artery of tibia is the largest nutrient artery of the body.

(b) *Periosteal arteries*: They are numerous and ramify beneath the periosteum. They enter the bone through Volkmann's canals to supply the outer one-third of the cortex. The periosteal vessels are especially numerous beneath the muscular and ligamentous attachments.

(c) *Metaphyseal (juxta-epiphyseal) arteries*: They are derived from neighboring arteries and enter the metaphysis directly along the attachment of joint capsule.

(d) *Epiphyseal arteries*: They are derived from arterial anastomosis around the joint (*circulus vasculosus*). They enter the epiphysis either directly or after piercing the epiphyseal cartilage.

2. **Blood Supply to Short Long Bones:** To an extent it is similar to that of a long bone *except* that:
   (a) The nutrient artery enters the middle of the shaft and immediately divides to form a plexus.
   (b) The periosteal vessels supply the major part of the bone in adult and replace the nutrient vessels.

Clinical correlation

- **Osteomyelitis:** In typical long bones, infection occurs in the metaphyseal regions firstly because they are richly supplied with blood and secondly because the blood supply in the metaphyses is through end arteries forming 'hair-pin bends'. Therefore, the bacteria and emboli are easily trapped in these hair-pin bends, leading to infarction (necrosis) of bone, resulting in a clinical condition called *osteomyelitis*. In short long bones, the infection begins in the middle of the shaft because nutrient artery enters the middle of the shaft and immediately divides to form the plexus.
- The blood supply of bone is so rich that the passing of a metal pin cannot interrupt blood supply sufficiently to kill the bone.

3. **Blood Supply of a Vertebra:** It is supplied by three sets of vessels:
   (a) One or more large but short vessels enter the body from its posterior aspect through **basivertebral foramen**.
   (b) A set of small vessels pierce the anterolateral surface of the body.
   (c) A set of long vessels pierce the root of the transverse processes and supply the vertebral arch, and transverse and spinous processes.
4. **Blood Supply of a Rib:** It is supplied by two sets of vessels:
   (a) The nutrient artery which enters it just behind the tubercle.
   (b) The periosteal arteries.

N.B.

- The veins are numerous in cancellous bones; for example, in the vertebrae they join to form large *basivertebral vein*. In the compact bone they accompany the arteries in the Volkmann's canals.
- There are no lymphatics in the bone, however some lymph vessels do accompany the periosteal blood vessels and drain in the regional lymph nodes.

FRACTURE OF BONE

The fracture is a break in the continuity of the bone. It is the most common type of bone injury. Fracture mostly occurs due to trauma (**traumatic fractures**), however, they may occur spontaneously due to disease that weakens the bone (**spontaneous** or **pathological fractures**).

A fracture may be simple or compound.

1. **Simple or closed fracture**: the fractured bone is not exposed to the exterior through skin.
2. **Compound fracture**: the fractured bone is exposed to the exterior through an opening in the skin.

When a bone fractures, the treatment involves realigning the broken ends and then immobilizing them until the fracture is healed (repaired).

Repair of a Fractured Bone

It involves the following steps:

1. When bone is fractured, the blood collects and coagulates to form **fracture hematoma** in and around the fracture site.
2. Two or three days later, new blood capillaries and uncommitted cells from the surrounding tissue invade the hematoma.
3. After 1 week, some of the uncommitted cells differentiate into fibroblasts, which produce a fibrous network

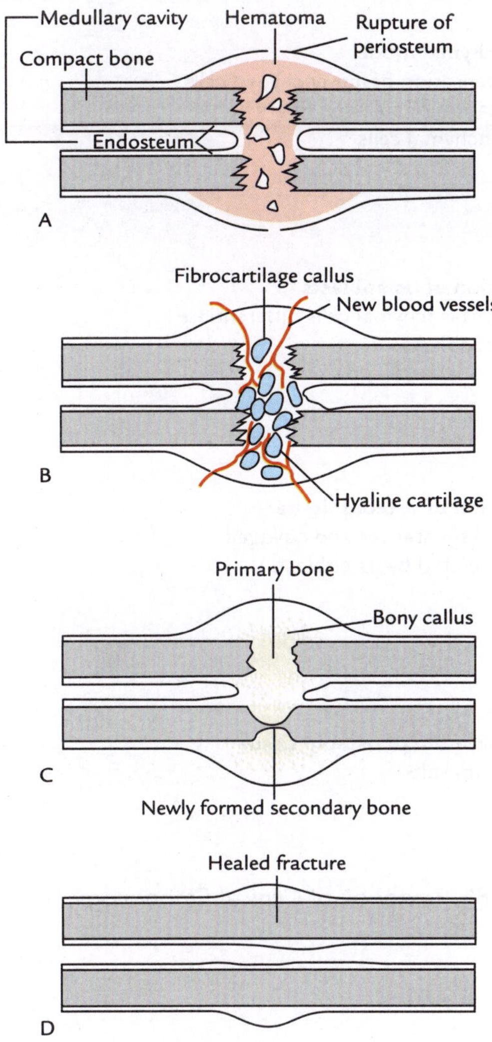

Fig. 6.11 Repair of a fractured bone: **A**, bone fracture with formation of hematoma; **B**, formation of fibrocartilage callus; **C**, formation of bony callus; **D**, healed fracture.

between fractured ends. The other cells differentiate into chondroblasts, which produce islets of fibrocartilage in the fibrous network forming a **fibrocartilage callus (temporary callus)**.

4. The **osteoprogenitor cells** in the periosteum and endosteum around the fracture site proliferate and differentiate into the bone-forming cells, the **osteoblasts**, which invade the temporary callus and lay down the woven-bone (primary bone tissue or osteoid) which unites the extremities of the fractured bone. It is called **bony callus**.
5. The primary bone tissue of the callus is gradually replaced by a secondary bone (mature bone).
6. Remodeling takes place and restores the original bone structure.

Figure 6.11 depicts repair of a fractured bone.

DEVELOPMENT AND GROWTH OF BONES

Development

All the bones develop from a mesenchyme by a process called ossification.

Ossification

As stated above it is the process of bone formation.

Types of Ossification

There are two types of ossifications:

1. Intramembranous ossification.
2. Intracartilaginous (endochondral) ossification.

In intramembrane ossification mesenchymal models of bones undergo ossification, while in intracartilaginous ossification, cartilaginous models of bones undergo ossification. The details are as under:

Intramembranous ossification: It involves the following steps:

Step 1: Mesenchymal tissue condenses to form a membranous sheet model. Osteoprogenitor cells located in this sheet differentiate into osteoblasts. The sites where the osteoblasts first appear are called ossification centers.

Step 2: Osteoblasts secrete organic substance (ground substance and collagen fibers) in the intercellular spaces to form osteoid tissue or bone matrix.

Step 3: Under the influence of alkaline phosphatase secreted by osteoblasts, the osteoid tissue is mineralized with calcium salts to become bone. The osteoblast now becomes trapped in mineralized matrix and are called *osteocytes*.

The intramembranous ossification is shown in Figure 6.12. Bones formed by the intramembranous ossification include flat bones of skull, viz. frontal, parietal, occipital, clavicle, etc.

> **Clinical correlation**
>
> **Cleidocranial dysostosis**: It is a congenital condition presenting the following features:
> (a) Complete or partial absence of clavicles.
> (b) Defective development of cranial vault with large fontanelles and delayed closing of the sutures. This condition occurs due to defective intramembranous ossification.

Intracartilaginous (endochondral) ossification: The intracartilaginous ossification is more complicated, but clinically more important because all the long bones of limbs (and many others) are ossified by this process.

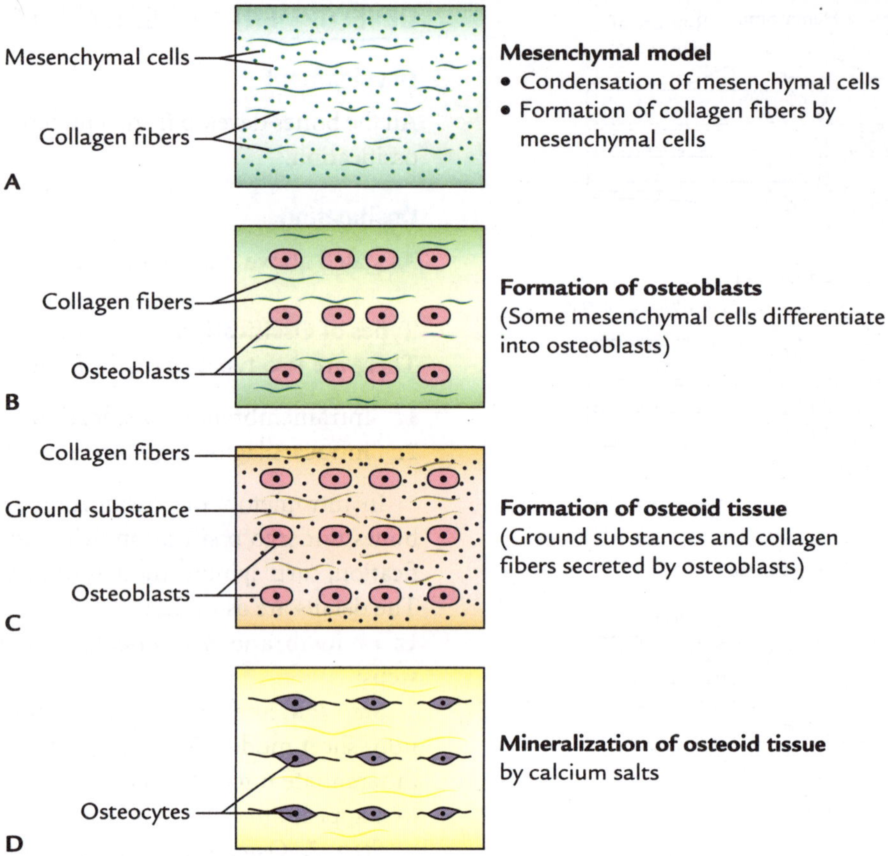

Fig. 6.12 Steps of intramembranous ossification. (*Source:* Fig. 8.1, Page 85, *Textbook of Clinical Embryology*, Vishram Singh. Copyright Elsevier 2012, All rights reserved.)

It involves the following steps (Fig. 6.13):

Step 1: The cartilage cells (chondroblasts) of cartilaginous model enlarge and matrix surrounding them is calcified under the influence of alkaline phosphatase secreted by cartilage cells.

Step 2: The cartilage cells die and disappear leaving behind empty spaces called *primary areolae.*

Step 3: The cells on the surface of periosteum differentiates into osteoblasts which enter at the site of ossification along with blood vessels (*periosteal bud*).

Step 4: The most of calcified matrix is absorbed forming large empty spaces called *secondary areolae*, leaving behind only thin bars of calcified matrix.

Step 5: The new bone (osteoid) is laid down on the surface of calcified bars of matrix.

Step 6: The mineralization of osteoid.

OSSIFICATION OF A LONG BONE

The following is a simplified account of intracartilaginous ossification of a long bone (Fig. 6.14).

Step 1: First the bone is laid down as a hyaline cartilaginous model surrounded by perichondrium.

Step 2: A **primary centre of ossification** then appears in the center of the shaft and this spreads toward the ends to form the diaphysis.

Step 3: At the same time, periosteum lays down a **collar of bone** (periosteal collar) around the circumference of the shaft.

Step 4: Later, one or more **secondary centres of ossification** develop at each end of the cartilaginous model and form the epiphysis.

Step 5: The **epiphyseal cartilage** separating epiphysis from diaphysis and articular cartilage at each end of bone remain cartilaginous.

Step 6: The epiphyseal plate of cartilage continues to produce new cartilage and thus enables the bone to grow in length. For this reason, epiphyseal plate of cartilage is also called **growth plate.** Once the growth in length is completed, the remaining epiphyseal cartilage ceases to proliferate and becomes ossified leaving only an epiphyseal scar called **epiphyseal line.**

Ossification Centres

These are sites, where bone formation begins. The ossification centres are generally classified into two types: primary and secondary.

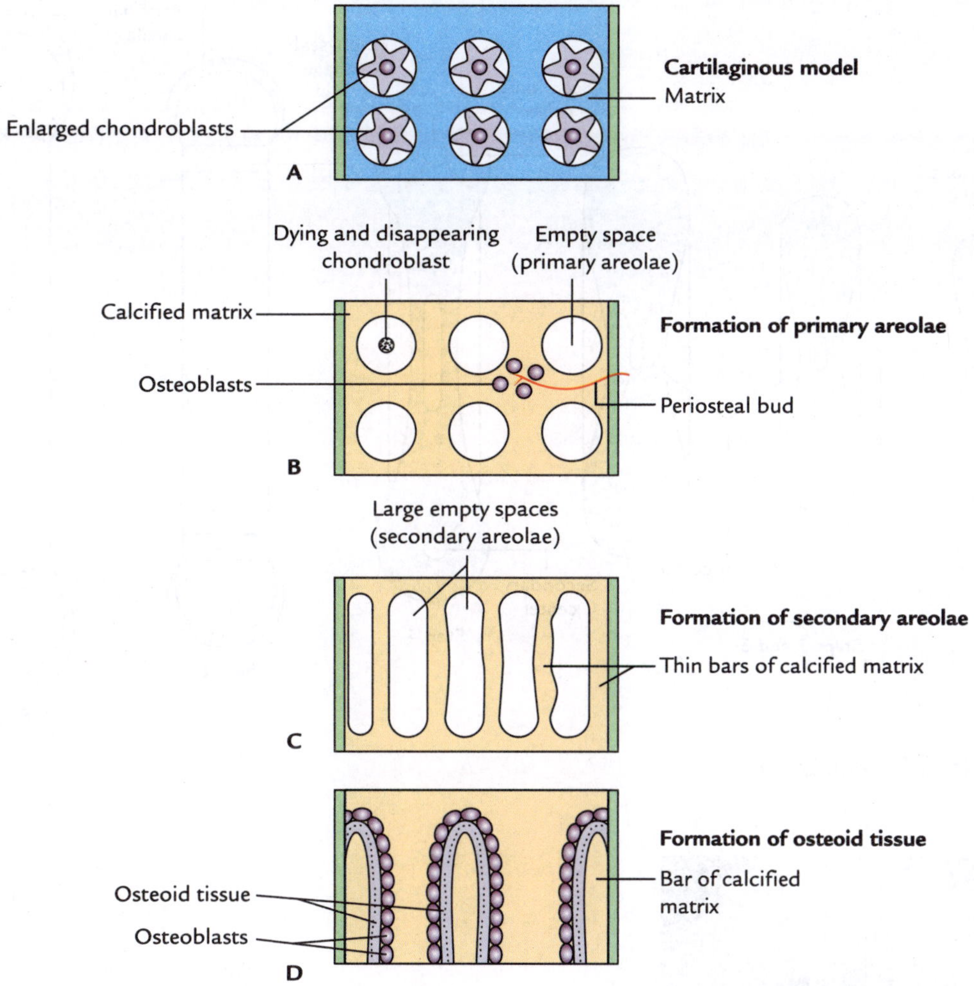

Fig. 6.13 Steps of intracartilaginous ossification (**A** to **D**). (*Source:* Fig. 8.2, Page 86, *Textbook of Clinical Embryology,* Vishram Singh. Copyright Elsevier 2012, All rights reserved.)

1. **Primary centres of ossification,** appear before birth (usually between the 7th to 12th week) with some exceptions (*viz.* primary centers of tarsal and carpal bones appear after birth except those of talus, calcaneum and cuboid).
2. **Secondary centres of ossification,** appear as a rule after birth (usually from the time of birth to 5 years of age).

A primary centre forms centres diaphysis, and the secondary centre form epiphyses. The fusion of epiphysis with the diaphysis starts at puberty and is usually complete by the age of 25 years, therefore after the age of 25 years, no more bone growth can take place.

In general, the appearance of secondary centres and fusion of epiphyses occur about 1 year earlier in females than in males.

N.B.

All the secondary centers appear after birth except the one at the lower end of femur which appears in the 9th month of intrauterine life and sometimes at the upper end of tibia and humerus.

Clinical correlation

- The visibility of centre of ossification in the distal end of femur in radiograph of newborn child found dead is of medicolegal importance because it indicates that the child was full term (Fig. 6.15). In x-ray of newborns, the shaft of long bone presents a white (radiopaque) shadow, whereas ends and joints cast black (radiolucent) shadow. This is because, at birth the shaft of cartilaginous model is ossified, i.e. bony, but ends are still unossified, i.e. cartilaginous.
- On the other hand in x-rays of growing children, the shaft and epiphyses cast white (radiopaque) shadow but the epiphyseal plate between the epiphysis and diaphysis cast a black (radiolucent) shadow.
- **Achondroplasia** (dwarfism): It is a congenital condition with the following clinical features:
  1. Individual is abnormally short (dwarf).
  2. Disproportionately shorter limbs than trunk.
  3. Dorsal kyphosis and lumbar lordosis.

  This condition occurs due to defective endochondral ossification.

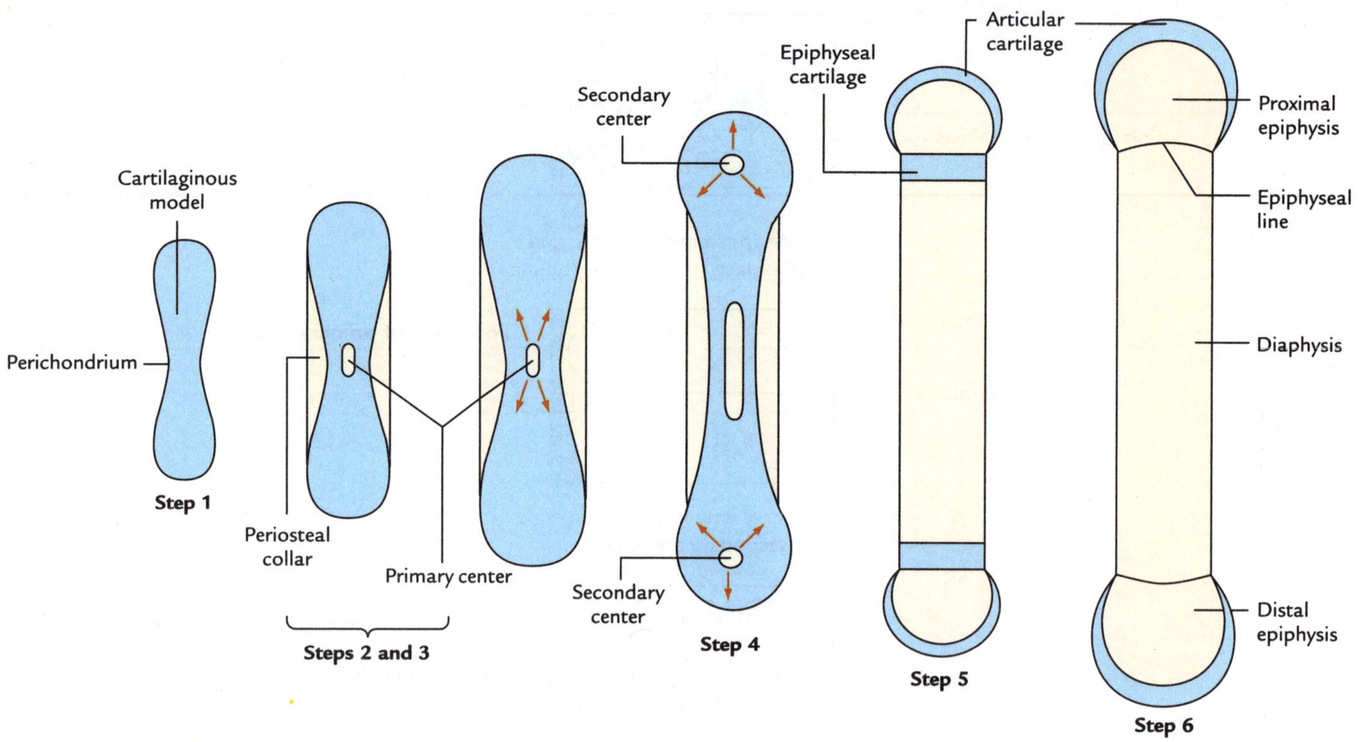

Fig. 6.14 Ossification of a long bone.

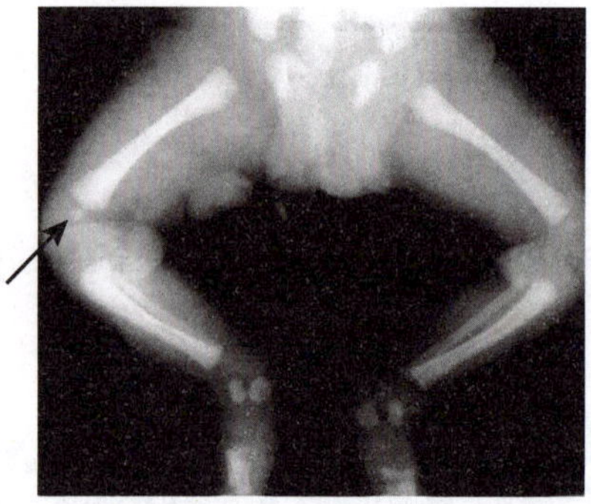

Fig. 6.15 Radiograph of a full term child showing secondary center of ossification at the distal end of the long bone (arrow). (*Source:* Fig. 8.29, Page 99, *Textbook of Clinical Embryology*, Vishram Singh. Copyright Elsevier 2012, All rights reserved.)

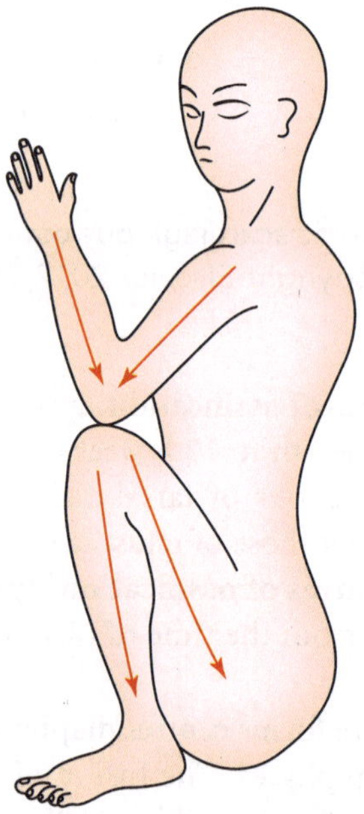

Fig. 6.16 Milking cow position showing direction of nutrient foramina.

Growing End of the Long Bone

In most of the long bones the two epiphyses do not fuse simultaneously. The epiphysis at one end always fuses few years before than that at the other end.

The end at which fusion occurs later is called the **growing end** and this is also the end at which secondary center of ossification appears first.

The growing end is always located opposite to the direction of nutrient foramen.

The direction of nutrient foramen is easily remembered by a '*dictum*' that says, '**To the elbow I go and from knee I flee**'.

In the milking cow position, the direction of nutrient foramina is always downward (Fig. 6.16).

Thus in upper limb, shoulder end of humerus and wrist ends of ulna and radius are growing ends, whereas in the lower limb, the knee ends of femur, tibia and fibula are growing ends.

N.B.

The nutrient foramen in the shaft of all long bones is always directed opposite to the growing end *except* that in the shaft of fibula which is directed toward the growing end.

Law of Union of Epiphyses (Law of Ossification)

According to this law, the epiphyseal centre (secondary centre of ossification) which appears first unites last and the epiphyseal centre which appears later unites first *except* in case of fibula where the epiphyseal centre for lower end appears first and also unites first. On the other hand, the epiphyseal centre for upper end appears late and also unites late (Fig. 6.17). Thus, fibula is the only long bone which violates the law of union of epiphyses.

Growth of a Long Bone

The growth of long bone after birth occurs by two methods:

1. Appositional growth
2. Endochondral growth

N.B.

The bones cannot grow by an interstitial growth like tendons, ligaments and cartilage.

Appositional growth: The appositional growth refers to the addition, i.e. growth, at the periphery of the bones resulting in an increase in the diameter of the long bones.

In appositional growth, the osteoblasts on the surface of bones proliferate. The superficial osteoblasts produced from these divisions remain as such or divide again. The deep osteoblasts resulting from these divisions produce bone matrix, and when they are surrounded by matrix, they become **osteocytes.** Consequently, a new layer of bone is deposited on the surface of the bone.

In cancellous bone, appositional growth adds bone matrix to the outer surface of trabeculae.

Endochondral growth: The endochondral growth is responsible for the increase in the length of long bones.

The endochondral growth occurs due to multiplication of the cells of the epiphyseal plate of cartilage.

The surface of epiphyseal plate facing toward epiphysis gives rise to new cartilage which pushes the epiphysis away from diaphysis.

The amount of new cartilage produced is equal to the amount of cartilage replaced by spongy bone toward the metaphyseal surface of the epiphyseal plate leading to increase in the length of diaphysis. The thickness of epiphyseal plate remains almost the same. The details are as under:

The epiphyseal plate is organized into four zones (Fig. 6.18); from superficial to deep these are:

1. Zone of resting cartilage
2. Zone of proliferation
3. Zone of hypertrophy
4. Zone of calcification

The **zone of resting cartilage** is nearest to the epiphysis and contains randomly arranged chondrocytes which do not divide rapidly.

In the **zone of proliferation**, the chondrocytes proliferate and form longitudinal columns of young cartilage cells resembling stacks of plates or coins.

In the **zone of hypertrophy**, the chondrocytes mature and hypertrophy. They secrete alkaline phosphatase.

Thus, maturation gradient exists in each column of chondrocytes. The cells near the zone of resting cartilage are younger and actively proliferating, whereas cells progressively near the diaphysis are older and are undergoing hypertrophy.

The **zone of calcification** is very thin. It consists of matrix mineralized with calcium carbonate. When the hypertrophied chondrocytes die, the blood vessels from diaphysis grow into this area. The connective tissue surrounding the blood vessels contains osteoblasts from the endosteum. The osteoblasts line up on the surface of the calcified cartilage and deposit bone.

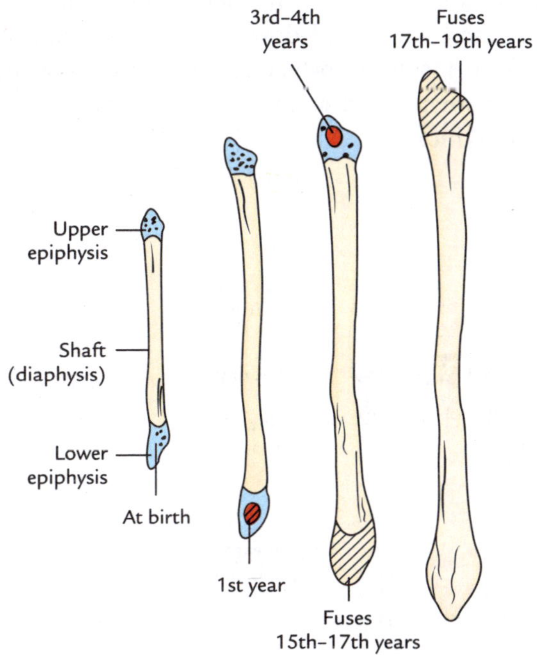

Fig. 6.17 Violation of the law of union of epiphyses by the fibula.

Clinical correlation

Growth in height: The epiphyseal (growth) plates of long bones of upper and lower limbs are responsible for growth in height of an individual. Once the epiphyses unite with diaphyses, the growth in height stops.

The sex hormones stimulate the ossification of epiphyseal plates leading to union of epiphysis with

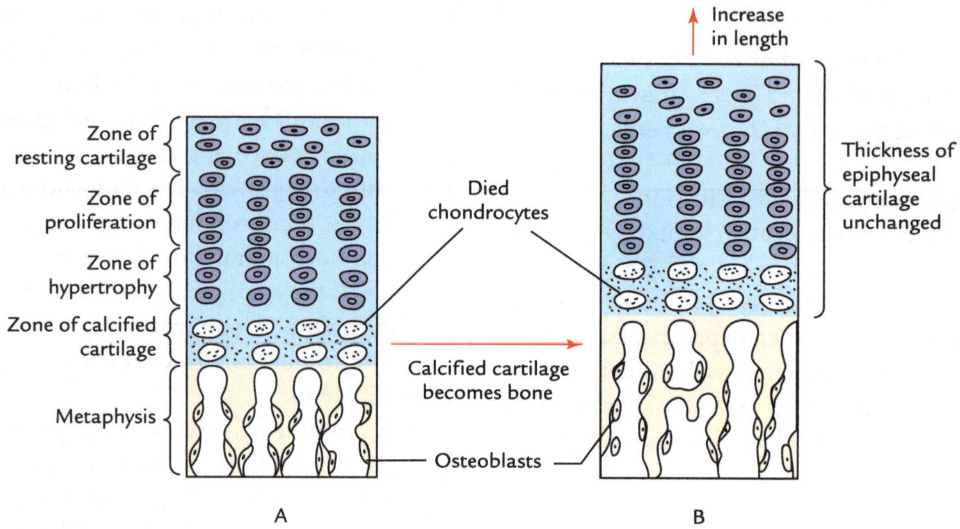

Fig. 6.18 Growth of bone—lengthwise: **A**, four zones of epiphyseal cartilage; **B**, conversion of calcified cartilage into bone.

diaphysis. In females, estrogen causes early closure of epiphyses with diaphysis as compared to that of testosterone. Consequently, females usually do not reach the same height as males.

The damage to the epiphyseal plate at the growing end of long bones of limbs of growing children will lead to shortening of the limb because damage of epiphyseal plate interferes with elongation of that bone.

Remodeling of Bone

The bone does not grow by multiplication of its cells or by increase in its intercellular material (i.e. interstitial growth), hence its shape cannot be maintained.

The bone grows by deposition of new bone by osteoblasts on its ends and on its surface in a random fashion. Therefore to maintain its shape, the unwanted bone is removed by osteoclasts. This process of bone removal is called **remodeling**.

Surface Remodeling

As the bone grows in length, there occurs subperiosteal bone deposition in the shaft while subperiosteal bone resorption occurs in conical region toward the end. Thus diverging regions are straightened to become the part of the shaft (Fig. 6.19).

Internal Remodeling

As the bone grows in diameter by deposition of new layers of bone deep to periosteum, the periosteal bone becomes thicker and thicker which is neither necessary nor desirable. Hence as the bone is laid down outside the shaft, it is removed from inside by osteoclasts. Consequently the shaft grows in diameter, and at the same time its wall does not become too thick.

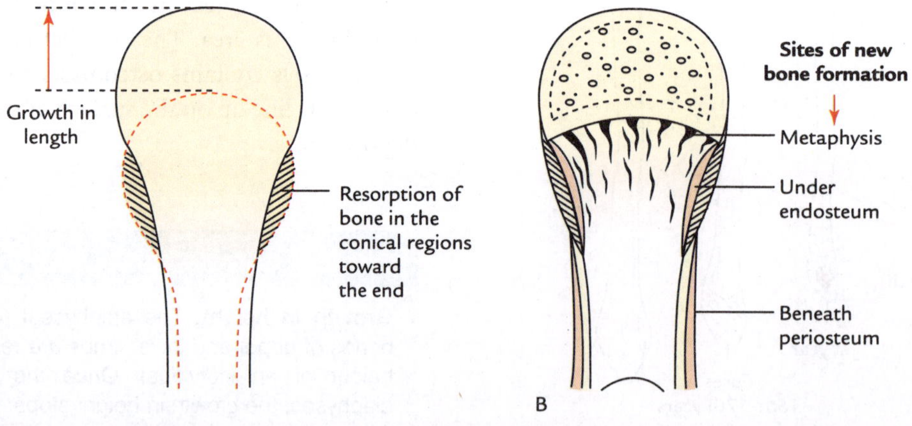

Fig. 6.19 Remodeling of bone: **A**, as the long bone grows, the sites once occupied by expanded ends become part of slender shaft; **B**, sites of new bone deposition (black areas).

The osteoclasts also remove trabeculae in the center of bone that were formed by endochondral ossification. This leads to the formation of **marrow cavity**.

N.B.

Remodeling of developing bone is done by: (a) deposition of bone by osteoblasts and (b) selective absorption of bone by osteoclasts.

Clinical correlation

Paget's disease: Normally the bone is continuously removed and repaired (replaced) by a new bone throughout life. In *Paget's disease* (osteitis deformans) which occurs in later life, there is uncontrolled osteoclast activity causing wide spread bone resorption which is followed by hectic, osteoblastic activity producing woven bone (osteoid) that fills the erosion but the repair stops at the osteoid stage. As a result, the healthy mature bone is gradually replaced by thick, bulky, weak osteoid bone. Consequently in individuals suffering from Paget's disease, the bones are thick and bent, especially the femora, tibiae and spine. The skull is enlarged and thick, the spine is bent forward (kyphosis).

Factors Affecting Growth of Bones

1. Nutritional factors:
   (a) Vitamin A co-ordinates the activity of osteoblasts and osteoclasts. The deficiency of vitamin A slows down the activity of osteoclasts, consequently the size of spinal and cranial foramina is reduced, with eventual compression of nerve roots. On the other hand, the high concentration of Vitamin A causes rarefaction and resorption of bone.
   (b) Vitamin C is essential for the synthesis of organic intercellular matrix (i.e. collagenous fibers and ground substance) by osteoblasts. The deficiency of vitamin A leads to defective development of growing ends of the bone. It also leads to rupture of capillaries producing painful subperiosteal hematoma.
   (c) Vitamin D is essential for the absorption of calcium and phosphate from intestine. Deficiency of vitamin D leads to defective mineralization (calcification) of osteoid tissue. As a result children suffer from **rickets** (characterized by bowing of legs, knobby metaphyseal regions); and adults suffer from **osteomalacia** (i.e. softening of the bones).
2. **Hormonal factors:** The hormones play very important role in bone growth. The hormones which are essential for proper development and growth of bone include pituitary hormones, thyroid hormones, parathyroid hormones and sex hormones. Their defective secretion can cause number of skeletal defects.
3. **Genetic factors:** A clinical condition **'chondrodystrophia foetalis'** occurs due to defective autosomal dominant inheritance. In this condition, endochondral ossification fails to occur properly.
4. **Mechanical factors:** Tensile force helps in bone formation whereas compressive forces favor bone resorption. In practice, orthopedic surgeons provide traction for quick healing of fractures.

CARTILAGE

The cartilage is a specialized connective tissue which provides rigidity along with elasticity. Hence it is found in those areas of the body, where both rigidity and elasticity are required. It consists of chondrocytes embedded in a gel-like matrix.

Phylogenetically, the cartilage tissue is older than bone tissue. Most of the bones in the intrauterine life are preformed in cartilage. The cartilages which are replaced by bones are called **temporary cartilages** and those that persist throughout life are called **permanent cartilages.**

FUNCTION OF CARTILAGE

The following are the functions of the cartilage:

1. Provides rigidity and support to soft tissues.
2. Provides smooth gliding surface for articulation.
3. Enables development and growth of long bones.

N.B.

Both bone and cartilage are specialized connective tissue, but the basic difference between the two is that in bone matrix it is mineralized while in cartilage it is not mineralized.

STRUCTURE

The cartilage has all common features of connective tissue, which include the following:

1. Cells
2. Fibers
3. Ground substance

Cells: Cells of the cartilage are of the following three types:

1. **Chondrogenic cells:** found in the perichondrium, where they undergo mitosis and differentiate into chondroblasts.
2. **Chondroblasts:** young cartilage cells occupying small spaces (lacunae) and may undergo mitosis.
3. **Chondrocytes:** mature cartilage cells which reside in lacunae. They form isogenous cell clusters surrounded by territorial matrix.

Fibers: Cartilage has the following two types of fibers:

1. **Type I collagen fibers** in fibrocartilage.
2. **Type II collagen fibers** in hyaline and elastic cartilages.

Ground substance: It consists of:

1. **Proteoglycans**, specifically chondroitin sulphate and keratan sulphate.
2. **Glycoproteins**, *viz.* chondronectin and chondrocalcin (a calcium-binding protein).
3. **Water (tissue fluid)** contributes to 75% hydration of the ground substance (high degree of hydration).

N.B.

There is no mineral (inorganic) component in the ground substance of cartilage because it is not mineralized.

GROWTH OF CARTILAGE

The cartilage grows by both appositional and interstitial methods.

1. **Appositional growth:** In this, layers of new cartilage are deposited at the surface beneath the perichondrium. The new cartilage is formed by chondroblasts derived from perichondrium. By appositional growth the cartilage increases in width.
2. **Interstitial growth:** It occurs due to increase in size and the number of existing cells and by an increase in the amount of intercellular matrix, due to proliferation of chondrocytes by mitosis in the center of cartilaginous model. By interstitial growth the cartilage increases in length.

N.B.

Adult cartilage grows and repair slowly, after a severe injury.

CHARACTERISTIC FEATURES OF CARTILAGE

The distinguishing features of cartilage are as follows:

1. It is **avascular** and receives its nutrition by diffusion through the ground substance from nearest capillaries. Here thin **cartilage canals** provide nutrition to the deepest core of cartilaginous mass.
2. It has **no lymphatics.**
3. It has **no nerves,** hence it is insensitive.
4. It is **surrounded by perichondrium.**
5. It grows by appositional as well as by interstitial methods of growth.
6. **When cartilage calcifies, chondrocytes die** because they are deprived of nutrition by diffusion.

N.B.

The articular cartilage and fibrocartilage are devoid of perichondrium.

Clinical correlation

- **Cartilage graft:** The cartilage has low antigenicity due to lack of lymphatics and isolation of chondrocytes in separate lacunae within matrix, hence *homogenous transplantation of cartilage* is possible without rejection.
- **Cartilage repair:** Damaged cartilage shows limited *repair* (regeneration) with defects being slowly filled with scar tissue instead of cartilage. Thus, repair of cartilage takes a long time because it is avascular.

TYPES OF CARTILAGE

The cartilages are classified into three types (Fig. 6.20):

1. Hyaline cartilage
2. Elastic cartilage
3. Fibrocartilage

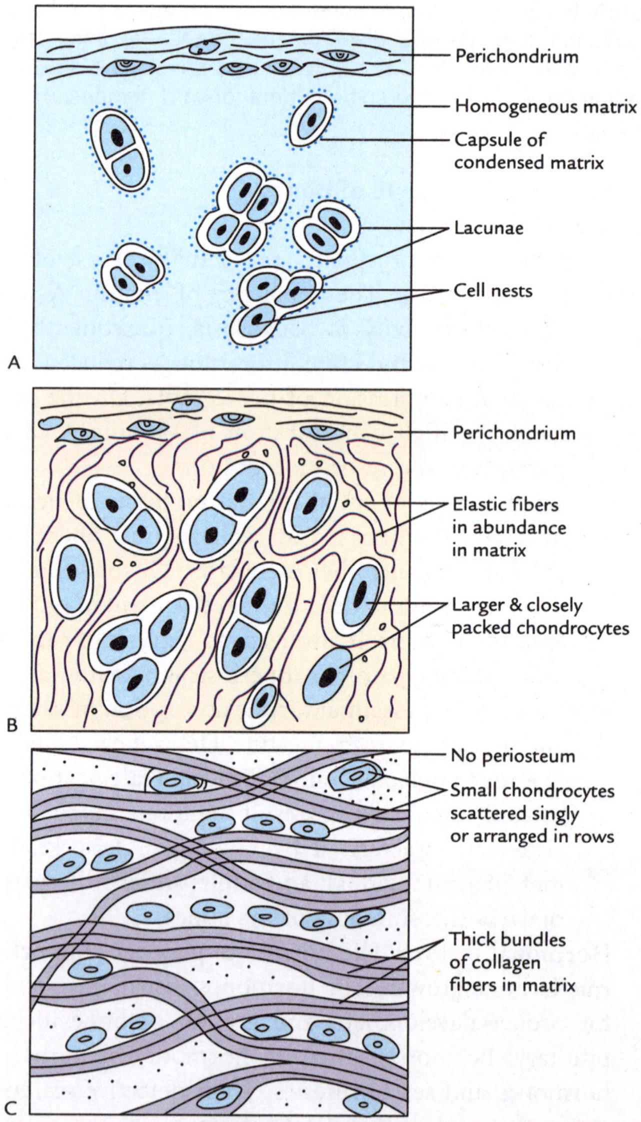

Fig. 6.20 Types of cartilage: **A**, hyaline; **B**, elastic; **C**, fibrocartilage.

Hyaline cartilage (Gk. *hyalos* = **transparent stone**): It appears bluish-white and transparent because it contains very fine collagen fibers having same refractive index as that of ground substance.

It is the most widely distributed cartilage in the body (see Table 6.5). All the long bones in the body are preformed in hyaline cartilage.

N.B.

- All the hyaline cartilages are covered by perichondrium *except* articular cartilages.
- Nonarticular hyaline cartilage has tendency to calcify and to be replaced by bone.

Elastic cartilage: It is made up of numerous chondrocytes embedded in matrix containing rich network of yellow elastic fibers. The sites of distribution of elastic cartilage include pinna of the ear, epiglottis.

Fibrocartilage: It appears white and opaque due to abundance of collagen fibers in it. The collagen fibers are arranged in bundles. The chondrocytes are few, small and scattered singly or arranged in rows. It is formed at sites subjected to great pressure like intervertebral disc.

The key histological features of three types of cartilages (Fig. 6.16) are presented in Table 6.4.

The distribution of the three types of cartilages in the body is enumerated in Table 6.5.

Table 6.4 Salient histological features of the three types of cartilages

Feature	Hyaline cartilage	Elastic cartilage	Fibrocartilage
Color	Glossy bluish, transparent	Yellowish	White, opaque
Perichondrium	Present	Present	Absent
Chondrocytes	Present in large numbers, singly or in groups inside lacunae	Larger, more numerous and packed more closely inside lacunae as compared to hyaline cartilage	Few in number, scattered singly or arranged in rows
Matrix	Homogenous, basophilic, collagen fibers delicate and not visible	Rich in elastic fibers	Thick bundles of collagen fibers run parallel within matrix
Tendency to calcify	Common (in later life)	Less common	Absent

Table 6.5 Sites of hyaline, elastic and fibrocartilages

Hyaline cartilage	Elastic cartilage	Fibrocartilage
Articular cartilages of most of the joints	Pinna of external ear	Intervertebral discs
Thyroid cartilage	Epiglottis	Interpubic disc
Cricoid cartilage	Corniculate cartilage	Menisci of knee joint
Lower part of arytenoids cartilage	Cuneiform cartilage	Articular discs of temporo-mandibular, sterno-clavicular and inferior radio-ulnar joints
Tracheal rings	Apex of arytenoid cartilage	Articular cartilages of temporo-mandibular, sterno-clavicular and acromio-clavicular joints
Costal cartilages	Auditory tubes	Glenoid labrum, acetabular labrum, etc.
Bronchial cartilage	External auditory meatus	
Nasal cartilages		

Golden Facts to Remember

➢ Total number of bones in the body	206
➢ Largest bone in the body	Femur
➢ Smallest bone in the body	Stapes
➢ Longest bone in the body	Femur
➢ Smallest long bone in the body	Malleus
➢ Most slender long bone in the body	Fibula
➢ Largest flat bone in the body	Hip bone
➢ Largest sesamoid bone in the body	Patella
➢ Most actively growing area of long bone	Metaphysis
➢ Most vascular area of a long bone	Metaphysis
➢ Most commonly fractured bone in the body	Clavicle in children and adults, radius in people over 50 years of age
➢ Largest nutrient artery in the body	Nutrient artery of tibia
➢ Commonest site of osteomyelitis in a long bone	Metaphysis
➢ All the long bone of body lie vertically *except*	Clavicle which lies horizontally
➢ All the bones in the body are covered by periosteum *except*	Sesamoid bones and ear ossicles
➢ All the bones in the body are made up of both compact and spongy bone *except*	Inferior nasal concha
➢ All the bones in the body form joint/joints *except*	Hyoid bone
➢ Commonest site of bone marrow aspiration	Manubrium sternum in adults and iliac crest in children
➢ First bone to ossify in the body	Clavicle
➢ Commonest congenital anomaly due to defective endochondral ossification	Achondroplasia (dwarfism)
➢ Commonest congenital anomaly due to defective membranous ossification	Cleidocranial dysostosis
➢ Most common site of accessory bones	Lambdoid suture of skull
➢ All the long bones in the body follow law of ossification *except*	Fibula
➢ Most abundant cartilage in the body	Hyaline cartilage
➢ Most durable cartilage in the body	Fibrocartilage
➢ Largest yellow elastic cartilage in the body	Cartilage of ear auricle
➢ Largest hyaline cartilage in the body	Thyroid cartilage of larynx

Multiple Choice Questions

1. **Part of growing long bones commonly involved in osteomyelitis is:**
   (a) Epiphysis
   (b) Metaphysis
   (c) Diaphysis
   (d) Epiphyseal plate

2. **The scapula is an example of:**
   (a) Long bone
   (b) Flat bone
   (c) Irregular bone
   (d) Short bone

3. **All of the following bones are pneumatic bones *except*:**
   (a) Maxilla
   (b) Mandible
   (c) Frontal
   (d) Sphenoid

4. **Primary center of ossification appears in:**
   (a) Epiphysis
   (b) Metaphysis
   (c) Diaphysis
   (d) Epiphyseal plate

5. **The secondary center of ossification appears in:**
   (a) Epiphysis
   (b) Metaphysis
   (c) Diaphysis
   (d) Epiphyseal plate

6. **In adults, the red bone marrow is found in all of the following sites *except*:**
   (a) Sternum
   (b) Ribs
   (c) Vertebrae
   (d) Medullary cavity of long bones

7. **In advanced age, gelatinous bone marrow may be found in:**
   (a) Hip bones
   (b) Skull bones
   (c) Scapula
   (d) Vertebrae

8. **All of the following bones ossify partly in membrane and partly in cartilage *except*:**
   (a) Temporal
   (b) Parietal
   (c) Mandible
   (d) Clavicle

9. **The coracoid process of scapula is an example of:**
   (a) Traction epiphysis
   (b) Pressure epiphysis
   (c) Atavistic epiphysis
   (d) Aberrant epiphysis

10. **All of the following are examples of traction epiphysis *except*:**
    (a) Greater trochanter of femur
    (b) Greater tubercle of humerus
    (c) Lesser tubercle of humerus
    (d) Coracoid process of scapula

11. **All of the following bones are examples of sesamoid bone *except*:**
    (a) Patella
    (b) Fabella
    (c) Os trigonum
    (d) Pisiform
    (e) Cartilage

12. **All of the following statements are true about hyaline cartilage *except that it*:**
    (a) Covers articular surfaces of bones
    (b) Forms epiphyseal plates
    (c) Forms most of the laryngeal cartilages
    (d) Has abundant elastic fibers in its matrix

13. **All of the following are examples of white fibrocartilage *except*:**
    (a) Intervertebral discs
    (b) Articular cartilages of temporo-mandibular joint
    (c) Cartilage of pinna of the ear
    (d) Acetabular labrum

14. **All of the following statements are true regarding elastic cartilage *except* that it:**
    (a) Has abundant elastic fibers in its matrix
    (b) Is adapted to withstand tension and compression
    (c) Has yellowish appearance
    (d) Is found in external auditory canal

15. **All statements are true regarding hyaline cartilage *except* that it:**
    (a) Has a homogeneous bluish-stained matrix
    (b) Has a clear glassy appearance
    (c) Forms cartilaginous model of most of the long bones
    (d) Forms menisci of knee joint

Answers

1. *b*, **2.** *c*, **3.** *b*, **4.** *c*, **5.** *a*, **6.** *d*, **7.** *b*, **8.** *b*, **9.** *c*, **10.** *d*, **11.** *c*, **12.** *d*, **13.** *c*, **14.** *b*, **15.** *d*

CHAPTER 7

Joints

Learning Objectives

After studying this chapter, the student should be able to:

- classify the joints according to their structure and function
- state the different types of synovial joints and describe the characteristic features of a typical synovial joint
- outline the different types of fibrous joints and describe their characteristic features
- describe the features of primary and secondary cartilaginous joints. Discuss the secondary cartilaginous joints in detail
- compare and contrast the features of rheumatoid arthritis and osteoarthritis
- classify levers and discuss functional significance of each type
- describe the close-packed and loose-packed positions of major joints of the limbs
- discuss the factors maintaining the stability of the joint
- correctly solve the review questions given at the end of the chapter

INTRODUCTION

In general usage, the term **joint** means a place where two things are joined together. In anatomical usage, a joint is a junction between two or more bones. The long bones articulate by their ends, the flat bones by their margins and short or irregular bones by their surfaces. It is important for a medical student to know various synonyms which are commonly used in clinical medicine. The term **articulation or arthrosis** means a joint in Latin. The term **arthrology** (i.e. study of joints) or term **arthritis** (i.e. inflammation of a joint) are derived from the term *arthron* which means a joint in Greek. Basically, a joint is a device to permit movements; however, some joints are immovable. The *dislocation* is defined as loss of contact (partial or complete) between two articulating bones.

CLASSIFICATION OF JOINTS

The joints can be classified according to their structure and function.

For the sake of convenience of presentation, functional classification is described first.

FUNCTIONAL CLASSIFICATION

It is based upon the degree of mobility of the joint. They are of three types:

1. Immovable joints (synarthroses)
2. Slightly movable joints (amphiarthroses)
3. Freely movable joints (diarthroses)

Immovable joints (synarthroses) show no mobility, e.g. cranial sutures in adults, primary cartilaginous joints in growing children.

Slightly movable joints (amphiarthroses) show some degree of mobility, e.g. secondary cartilaginous joints, syndesmoses.

Freely movable joints (diarthroses) show maximum degree of mobility, e.g. synovial joints.

STRUCTURAL CLASSIFICATION

It is based upon the type of connecting tissue and the presence or absence of a joint cavity. The joints are classified into three types (Fig. 7.1):

1. Fibrous
2. Cartilaginous
3. Synovial

In clinical practice, the structural classification is most commonly followed, hence will be discussed in detail.

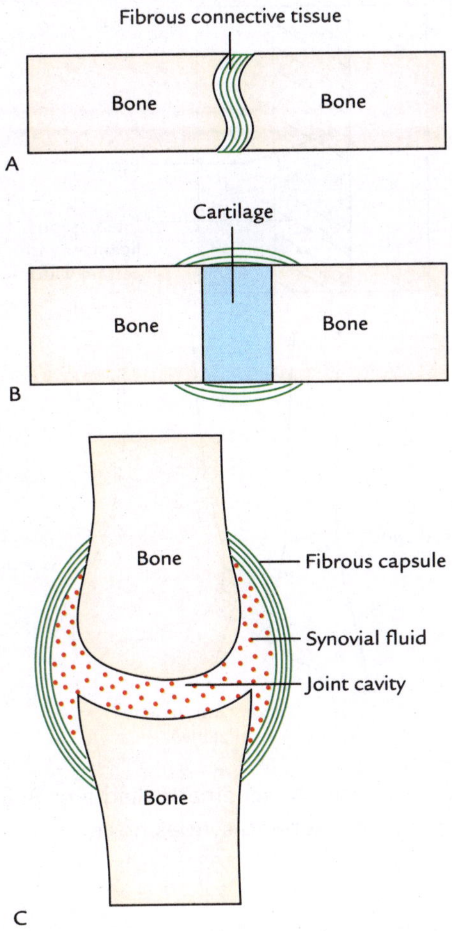

Fig. 7.1 Types of joints: **A**, fibrous; **B**, cartilaginous; **C**, synovial.

Fibrous joints: Here the bones forming the joint are united by fibrous connective tissue. These joints are either immovable or permit only a slight degree of movement. A fibrous joint lacks joint cavity.

The fibrous joints are of three types—sutures, syndesmoses and gomphoses.

1. **Sutures:** The articular surfaces are connected by a thin layer of connective tissue (sutural ligaments). These joints are confined to the skull (i.e. they are peculiar to the skull) and are immovable (Fig. 7.2). In growing children, they may permit a little mobility.

Depending upon the shape of the articular surfaces and margins of the articulating bones, these joints are further divided into the following subtypes (Fig. 7.3):

(a) *Plane suture*: The articular surfaces are plane and fairly smooth, e.g. median palatine suture, where the paired maxillary and palatine bones articulate to form the hard palate.
(b) *Serrate or limbus suture*: The articular surfaces of the sutures are reciprocally serrated and interlock with each other in a jigsaw fashion, e.g. sagittal suture.
(c) *Denticulate suture*: The margins of the sutures interlock with each other like teeth of a saw, e.g. lambdoid suture.
(d) *Squamous suture*: The articulating surfaces of the sutures are relatively flat and overlap each other, e.g. suture between temporal and parietal bones.
(e) *Schindylesis*: It is a specialized suture where a ridge of one bone fits into the groove of the other bone, e.g. joint between the rostrum of sphenoid bone and the cleft between the alae of vomer bone.

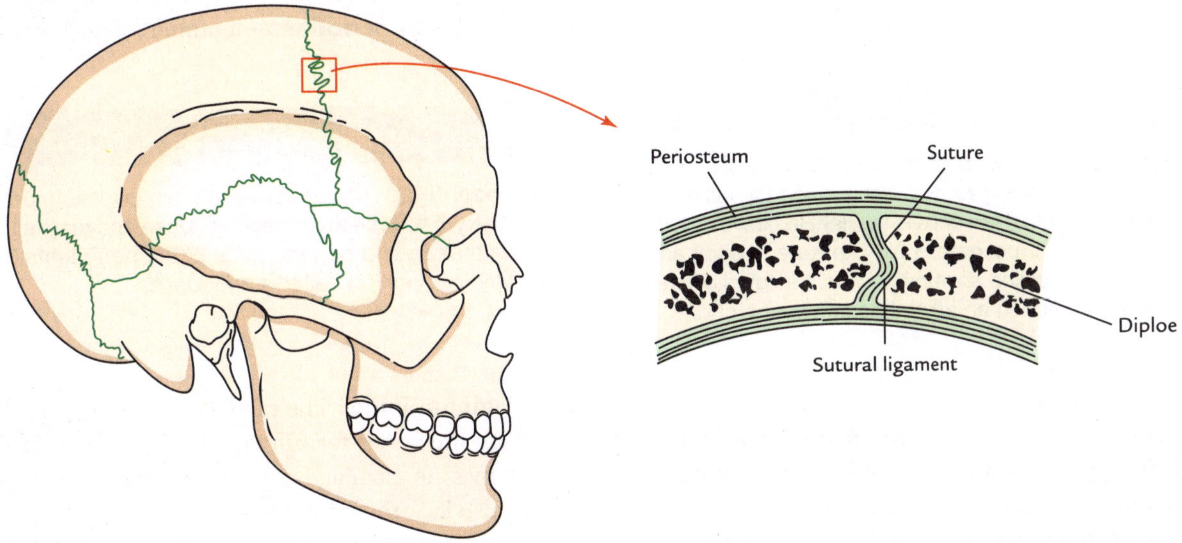

Fig. 7.2 A suture.

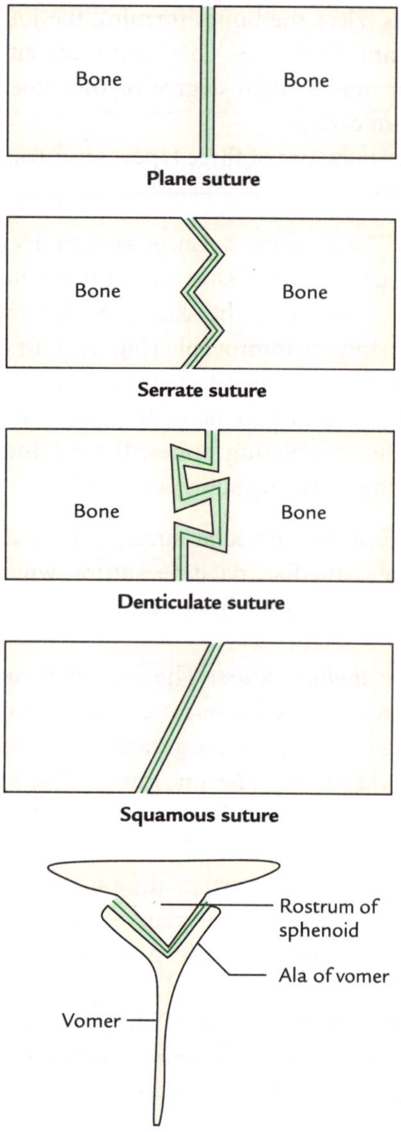

Fig. 7.3 Subtypes of sutures.

Clinical correlation

Synostosis: In the elderly, most of the sutures of the skull undergo ossification leading to rigid bony union (*synostosis*). For this reason the skull of the child is resilient to blows but not so in adults. In adults it becomes rigid like an egg shell and frequently splinters following an impact. Thus, fractures of skull are much more common in an adult than in a young child.

2. **Syndesmoses:** These are joints where two adjacent bones are linked together by a considerably greater amount of connective tissue than in sutures in the form of interosseous ligaments and membranes (Fig. 7.4), e.g. interosseous radio-ulnar joints, interosseous tibiofibular joints, inferior tibiofibular joints, joints between adjacent laminae of vertebrae (being connected by ligamenta flava), tympano-stapedial joints.

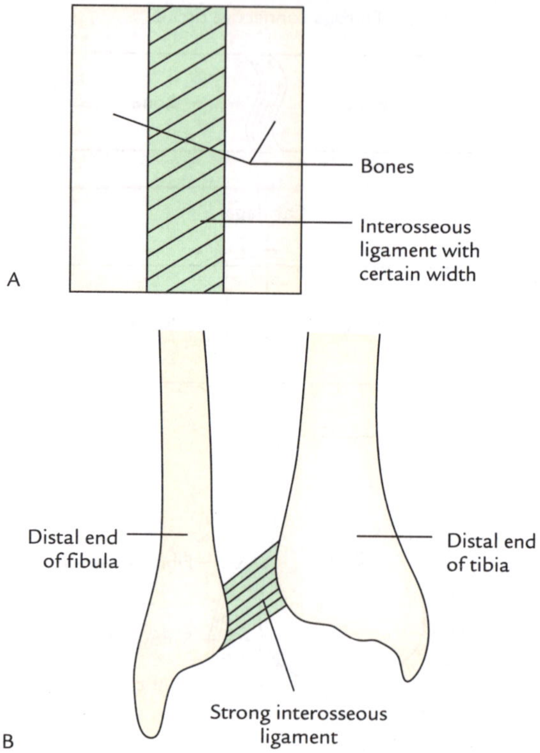

Fig. 7.4 Syndesmosis: **A**, schematic diagram; **B**, inferior tibiofibular joint representing syndesmosis.

Slight movement is permitted at these joints, *viz.* rotation or radius around ulna in movements of supination and pronation.

3. **Gomphoses (peg and socket joint):** These are specialized fibrous joints restricted to the fixation of teeth in alveolar sockets of the mandible and the maxillae. The root of the tooth is attached to the socket within the alveolus by **periodontal ligament** (Fig. 7.5).

Clinical correlation

Periodentitis: The gomphoses have clinical importance in dentistry, because teeth become loose and may fall following inflammation and degeneration of the periodontal ligament, a clinical condition called *periodontitis*

Cartilaginous joints: The cartilaginous joints are those joints in which the bones forming the joint are united by means of either hyaline cartilage or fibrocartilage. The cartilaginous joints also lack the joint cavity.

The cartilaginous joints are of two types—primary cartilaginous joints (**synchondroses**) and secondary cartilaginous joints (**symphyses**):

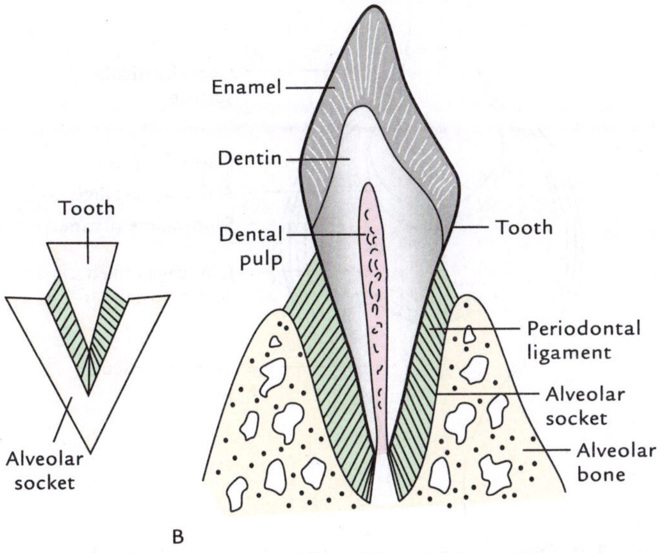

Fig. 7.5 Gomphosis (peg and socket variety): **A**, diagrammatic representation; **B**, tooth in alveolar socket representing gomphosis.

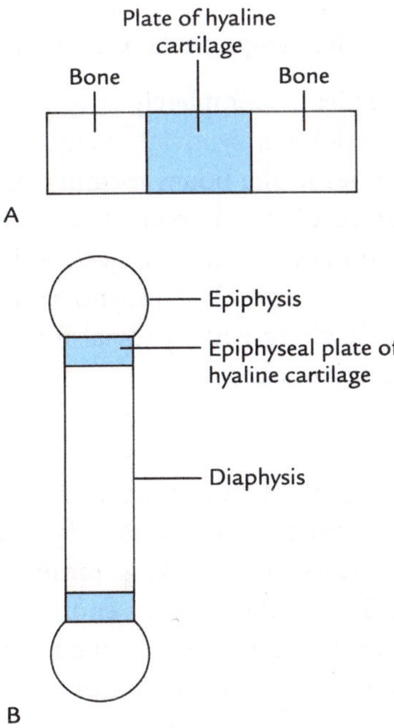

Fig. 7.6 Primary cartilaginous joint (synchondrosis): **A**, schematic diagram; **B**, primary cartilaginous joint between epiphysis and diaphysis representing synchondrosis.

1. **Primary cartilaginous joints (synchondroses)** (Fig. 7.6): The bones or parts of the bones forming the joint are joined by a plate of hyaline cartilage, e.g.:
   (a) Joint between epiphysis and diaphysis of growing long bone.
   (b) Joint between basisphenoid and basiocciput (sphenoccipital joint).
   (c) First costosternal joint.

These joints are immovable and mostly temporary in nature. As the growth ceases they undergo synostosis (i.e. plate of hyaline cartilage is completely replaced by bone).

Clinical correlation

The joints between the epiphysis and diaphysis of a growing long bone are of great clinical significance because:

(a) Piece of hyaline cartilage between the epiphysis and diaphysis allows the growth of long bone in length hence it is also called growth plate and as growth is completed in height, these joints ossify.
(b) Growth plate is clearly seen as a radiolucent shadow between epiphysis and diaphysis in radiographs.
(c) Damage of the epiphyseal plate, particularly at the growing end, following fracture of a long bone in child may lead to shortening of the limb.

2. **Secondary cartilaginous joints (symphyses):** In these joints, the articular surfaces of bones forming the joint are covered by thin plates of hyaline cartilage, which are connected by a disc or a pad of fibrocartilage (Fig. 7.7), e.g.
   (a) *Symphysis pubis*, between two pubic bones.
   (b) *Intervertebral discs*, between bodies of adjacent vertebrae.
   (c) *Manubriosternal joint*, between manubrium and body of sternum.
   (d) *Symphysis menti*, between two halves of fetal mandible (not true symphysis).

The differences between the primary and secondary cartilaginous joints are given in the box below:

Primary cartilaginous joint	Secondary cartilaginous joint
Bones are connected by hyaline cartilage	Bones are covered by hyaline cartilage and connected by fibrocartilage
Immovable	Slightly movable
Disappear with age	Do not disappear with age
Rarely occurs in midline	Always occur in midline

N.B.

- Secondary cartilaginous joints typically occur in the midline.
- All the symphyses belong to the axial skeleton *except* the pubic symphysis which belongs to the appendicular skeleton.
- These joints permit limited movement due to compressible pad of fibrocartilage.
- The term symphysis menti is a misnomer.

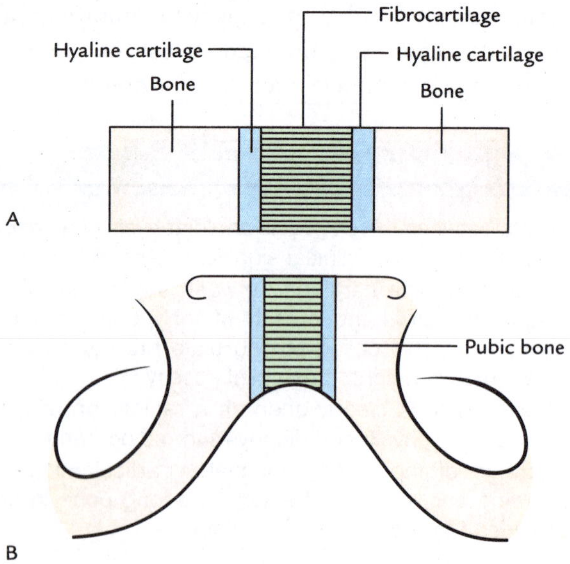

Fig. 7.7 Secondary cartilaginous joint (symphysis): **A**, schematic diagram; **B**, pubic symphysis representing symphysis.

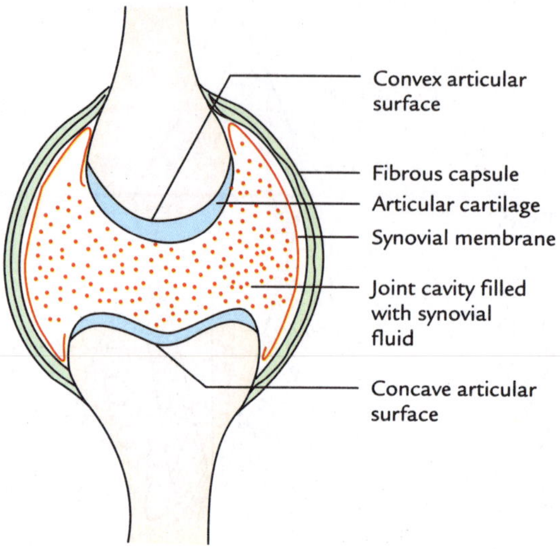

Fig. 7.8 Diagrammatic representation of a typical synovial joint.

Synovial joints: Out of all the types of joints, the synovial joints are most common and by far the most important clinically. Therefore, they have been described here in detail.

SYNOVIAL JOINTS

These joints possess a cavity and the articular ends of bones forming the joint are enclosed in a **fibrous capsule**. As a result they are separated by a narrow cavity, the **articular cavity** (or the joint cavity), which is filled with a fluid called **synovial fluid**. The synovial fluid is like an egg albumin, hence the name synovial joint. *The synovial joints are the most evolved and freely movable joints*. They are often termed as **diarthrodial joints.**

The characteristic features of synovial joints (Fig. 7.8) are as follows:

1. The articular surfaces are covered by a thin plate of hyaline cartilage.
2. The joint cavity is enveloped by an *articular capsule* which consists of an *outer fibrous capsule* and *inner synovial membrane.*
3. The cavity of the joint is lined everywhere by synovial membrane *except* over the articular cartilages.
4. The cavity is filled with synovial fluid secreted by synovial membrane which provides lubrication of the articular surfaces and nutrition to the articular cartilages.
5. Sometimes joint cavity is incompletely or completely divided by articular disc/meniscus.
6. Some additional structures are present within the joint cavity, e.g.: (a) fat pads, (b) tendons, etc.

COMPONENTS OF SYNOVIAL JOINTS AND THEIR FUNCTIONAL SIGNIFICANCE

The following are the components of synovial joints:

1. **Fibrous capsule:** It completely invests the joint like a sleeve and encloses a synovial cavity. It is attached by continuous lines to the bones forming the joint close to the articular cartilages. It consists of longitudinal and interlacing bundles of white connective tissue fibers. It is lined on its inner aspect by the synovial membrane. The fibrous capsule along with synovial membrane together forms the **articular capsule**.

Functions:

(a) The fibrous capsule stabilizes the joint in such a way that it permits movements but resists dislocation.
(b) Numerous sensory nerve endings ramify on the capsule. The stimulation of these nerve endings produce reflex contraction of muscles acting on the joint in such a way that joint is brought in a position of maximum comfort to protect the joint. This is known as **'Watch-dog'** action of the capsule.

2. **Ligaments:** These are thickened bands of collagen fibers. They are of two types: true ligaments and accessory ligaments (Fig. 7.9).
   (a) *True ligaments* are the local thickenings of parallel fiber bundles of capsular ligament, hence not separate from the capsular ligament, therefore they are also called **intrinsic ligaments**, e.g. medial and lateral collateral ligaments of knee joint.
   (b) *Accessory ligaments* are separate from fibrous capsule and may be extracapsular or intracapsular. The stylomandibular and spheno-mandibular are the examples of extracapsular accessory ligaments and

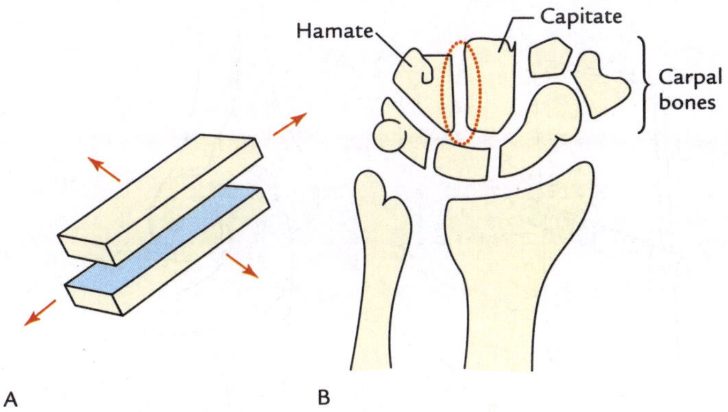

Fig. 7.9 Plane (gliding) joint: **A**, diagrammatic representation of the joint; **B**, joint between capitate bone and hamate bone representing the plane joint.

anterior and posterior cruciate ligaments of knee joint are the examples of intracapsular accessory ligaments.

True ligaments permit the movements in one plane and prevent unwanted movements in other plane. In addition, they also stabilize the joint.

Accessory ligaments provide additional reinforcement to the joint and limit the range of movements.

A tear in the ligament is called *sprain* which leads to swelling and pain in the joint.

3. **Synovial membrane:** It is a thin highly vascular membrane of connective tissue lining the inside of the fibrous capsule. It is reflected from the fibrous capsule onto the bone, which it covers right up to the articular cartilage. Note that articular cartilages are not covered by synovial membrane.

Function: The synovial membrane produces synovial fluid in sufficient quantity to keep the surfaces properly lubricated.

The synovial fluid is slippery like an egg-white. It is a dialysate of blood plasma plus a mucin called hyaluronic acid. *The viscosity and lubricating properties of the synovial fluid are better than those of commercial lubricants.*

4. **Articular cartilage:** With few exceptions the articular cartilage is made up of hyaline cartilage.

The cartilage consists of proteoglycan-hyaluronic acid aggregates. The hyaluronic acid retains water which resists compression. The cartilaginous articular surface has a low coefficient of friction.

Function: The articular cartilage provides smooth friction-free movements and resists compression forces.

N.B.

The articular cartilages of all the synovial joints in the body are thin plates of hyaline cartilage *except* those of temporo-mandibular, sterno-clavicular and acromio-clavicular joints, which are thin plates of fibrocartilage, therefore these joints are called *atypical synovial joints*.

Sometimes a noise (cracking sound) is produced in the joint when the articular surfaces are separated forcefully. The sound is produced due to the development of vacuum within the joint due to forceful separation of articular surfaces.

5. **Articular disc or meniscus:** The articular discs are pads of fibrocartilage interposed between the articular surfaces of some joints, e.g. temporo-mandibular, sterno-clavicular, acromio-clavicular, radio-ulnar and knee joints.

Functions:

(a) Helps in lubrication of a joint by maintaining an interval between the articular surfaces.
(b) Divides the joint completely into two compartments.
(c) Acts as a ligament to modify certain joint movements.
(d) Prevents wear and tear of articular cartilages by providing a cushioning effect.

6. **Bursae:** These are pouch-like sacs of connective tissue filled with synovial fluid, found near certain synovial joints. They are commonly located between tendon and bone, between muscle and bone, between skin and bone and between tendon and skin.

The bursae reduces the friction of one structure moving over the other.

Function: The function of bursae is to cushion certain muscles and to facilitate the movement of tendons or muscles over bony or ligamentous surfaces.

The **synovial tendon sheath** is a modified bursa that surrounds and lubricates the tendons of certain muscles, particularly those that cross the wrist and ankle joints.

7. **Fat pads (Haversian glands):** These are pads of fat placed between synovial membrane and fibrous capsule or between synovial membrane and bone, e.g. acetabular fat of hip joint, infrapatellar fat-pad of knee joint. As fat is very pliant, the pads can accommodate themselves to changing condition of the joint during different movements.

Clinical correlation

The tissues involved in diseases of the synovial joints are hyaline cartilage, bone and synovial membrane.

- **Osteoarthritis:** Under normal conditions, the articular surfaces of bones of synovial joints do not come in contact with each other, because articular surfaces of bones are capped by articular cartilages and synovial fluid within the joints provides lubrication to these cartilages.

If articular cartilages are damaged due to trauma or disease or if the synovial fluid is reduced, the articular bones come in contact with each other and undergo attrition. The bones begin to degenerate. There is abnormal bone repair and articular surfaces become uneven (misshapen) causing *osteoarthritis*. It affects large weight-bearing joints, e.g. hip and knee joints are most commonly involved in osteoarthritis. Sometimes there is formation of *osteophytes*.

- ***Formation of osteophytes:*** The zone of articular bone at the junction of articular cartilage, synovial membrane and periosteum is highly vascular. It is endowed with immense proliferative power and hence the site for formation of osteophytes (pseudo bone formation) which leads to lipping of articular margins.
- ***Rheumatoid arthritis:*** It is a chronic progressive inflammatory autoimmune disease involving synovial membrane.

This leads to hypertrophy and hyperplasia of synovial cells and fibrinous inflammatory effusion into the joint. If disease progresses, it will cause erosion of articular cartilage and growth of granulation tissue that separates the bones and distorts the shape of the joint. Rheumatoid arthritis commonly affects small joints of hands and feet.

Table 7.1 highlights differences between osteoarthritis and rheumatoid arthritis.

Arthroplasty: It is a surgical repair or replacement of joints. Recent advancement in soft tissue repair involves the use of artificial ligaments made up of carbon fibers coated with plastic (polylactic acid).

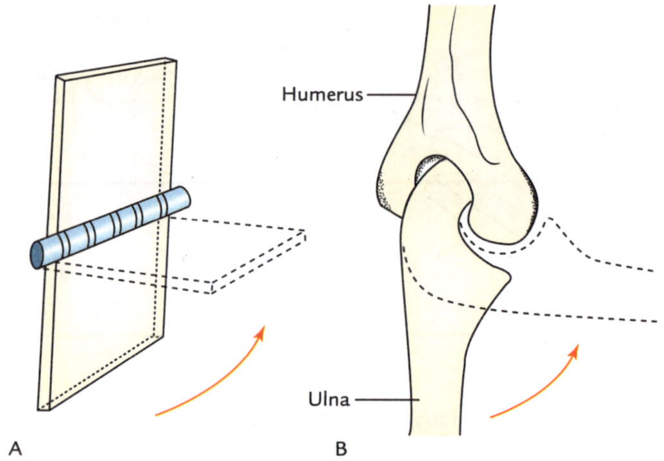

Fig. 7.10 A hinge joint: **A**, diagrammatic representation of the joint showing bending movement; **B**, humero-ulnar joint representing a hinge joint.

CLASSIFICATION OF SYNOVIAL JOINTS

A. According to the shape of articular surfaces

1. **Plane joints** (Fig. 7.9)**:** The articular surfaces are nearly flat (plane). They permit gliding movements in various directions, i.e. side to side, back and forth movements with slight rotation. These are the simplest type of joint movements. The examples are:
   (a) *Intercarpal joints*
   (b) *Intertarsal joints*
   (c) *Intermetatarsal*
   (d) *Intermetacarpal*
   (e) *Joints between the articular processes of adjacent vertebrae* (zygapophyseal joints)
2. **Hinge or Ginglymus joints** (Fig. 7.10)**:** The articular surfaces are pulley shaped. Movements are permitted only in one plane around a transverse axis much like the hinge of the door. These joints have strong collateral ligaments to prevent the other movements. The hinge joints are the most common type of synovial joints. The examples are:
   (a) *Elbow joint* (strictly speaking humero-ulnar joint)
   (b) *Interphalangeal joints*
   (c) *Knee joint*
   (d) *Ankle joint*
3. **Pivot or trochoid joints** (Fig. 7.11)**:** The articular surface of one bone is rounded and fits into the concavity of another bone. Further, the rounded part is surrounded by a ligamentous ring, i.e. the rod surrounded by a ring. The movement in a pivot joint has limited rotation around a central axis, i.e. either the rod rotates in a osteo-ligamentous ring, e.g. superior radio-ulnar joint or osseo-ligamentous ring rotates around the rod such as median atlanto-axial joint. The superior radio-ulnar joint permits rotation of forearm and median atlanto-axial joint allows the rotational movements of the head.
4. **Condylar joints** (Fig. 7.12)**:** The round articular surface of one bone fits into socket-type articular surface of another bone. The end of bone bearing round articular surface is called condyle. These joints permit movements in two directions (biaxial), i.e. up and down and side-to-side. The examples are:
   (a) *Right and left temporo-mandibular joints*
   (b) *Knee joints*
5. **Ellipsoidal joints** (Fig. 7.13)**:** The elliptical convex surface of one bone articulates with the elliptical concave surface of another bone. The movements are permitted in two directions (biaxial), i.e. flexion and extension around a transverse axis and abduction and adduction around the

Table 7.1 Features of osteoarthritis and rheumatoid arthritis

	Osteoarthritis	Rheumatoid arthritis
Nature of disease	Degenerative and inflammatory	Inflammatory and autoimmune
Tissue affected	Articular cartilage	Synovial membrane
Joints affected	Weight bearing, e.g. hip, knee, joints of cervical and lumbar spine	Small joints of hands and feet

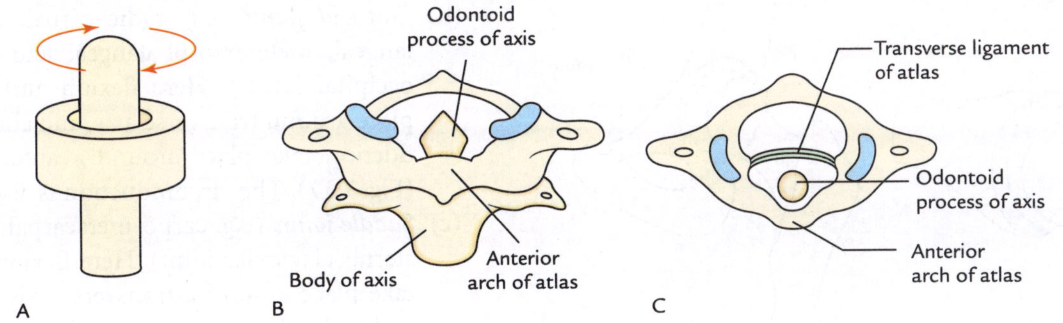

Fig. 7.11 Pivot joint: **A**, diagrammatic representation of the joint; **B** and **C**, median atlanto-axial joint representing pivot joint.

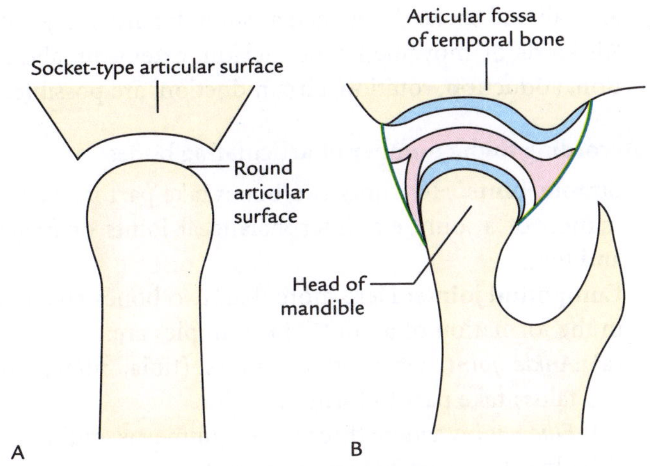

Fig. 7.12 Condylar joint: **A**, diagrammatic representation of the joint; **B**, temporo-mandibular joint representing a condylar joint.

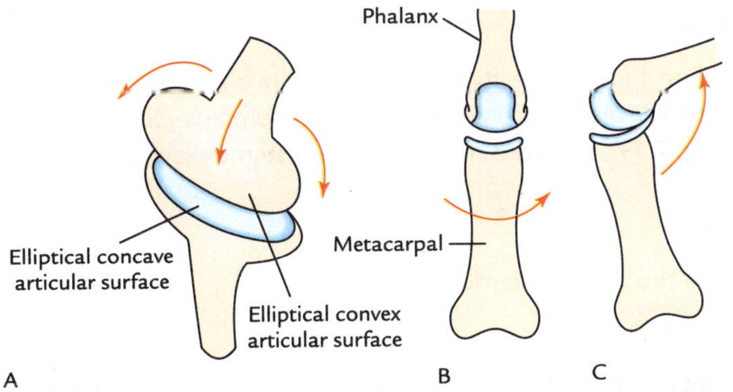

Fig. 7.13 Ellipsoid joint: **A**, diagrammatic representation of the joint; **B** and **C**, metacarpo-phalangeal joint representing ellipsoid joint.

anteroposterior axis. The combination of these movements produces **circumduction**. The examples are:
(a) *Radio-carpal joint* (wrist joint)
(b) *Atlanto-occipital joints*
(c) *Metacarpo-phalangeal joints*
(d) *Metatarso-phalangeal joints*

6. **Saddle or sellar joints** (Fig. 7.14)**:** The articular surfaces are reciprocally saddle shaped, i.e. concavo-convex. This unique articulation is modified condyloid joint that allows a wide range of movement. The examples are:
   (a) *First carpo-metacarpal joint*
   (b) *Sterno-clavicular joint*
   (c) *Calcaneo-cuboid joint*
   (d) *Incudo-malleolar joint* (smallest saddle joint)
7. **Ball and socket or spheroidal joints** (Fig. 7.15)**:** Rounded convex surface of one bone fits into the cup-like socket of another bone. The movements occur around an indefinite number of axes which have one common center. This type of articulation provides the greatest range of movement of all the synovial joints. The movements include flexion, extension, adduction, abduction, medial rotation, lateral rotation, and circumduction. The examples are:
   (a) *Hip joint* (largest ball and socket joint)
   (b) *Shoulder joint*
   (c) *Incudo-stapedial joint* (smallest ball and socket joint)

The examples of various types of synovial joints (according to the shape of their articular surfaces) are summarized in Table 7.2.

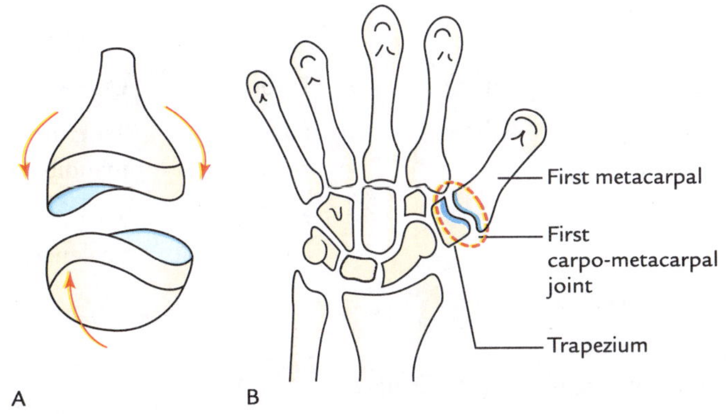

Fig. 7.14 Saddle joint: **A**, diagrammatic representation; **B**, first carpo-metacarpal joint representing saddle joint.

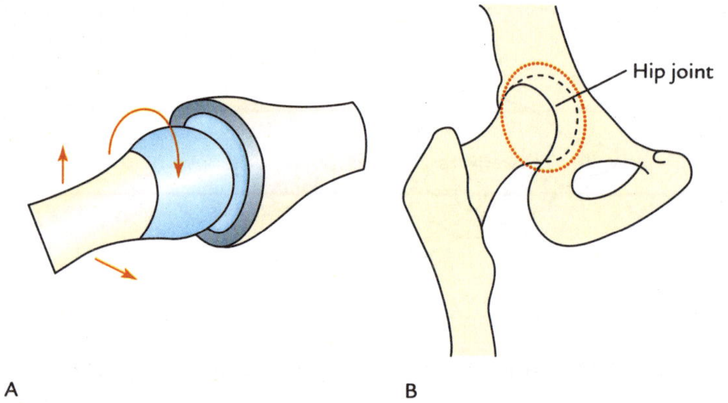

Fig. 7.15 Ball and socket joint: **A**, diagrammatic representation of the joint showing directions of possible movements; **B**, hip joint representing ball and socket joint.

B. According to the plane/planes of movements

1. **Uniaxial joints:** In these joints the movements occur in only one plane or axis. The examples are:
   (a) *Hinge joints* (e.g. elbow, ankle and interphalangeal joints). Here movements take place around a transverse axis. Hence only flexion and extension is possible.
   (b) *Pivot joints* (e.g. superior radio-ulnar (Fig. 7.16) and median atlanto-axial joints). Here movements take place around a vertical axis, hence only rotation is possible.
2. **Biaxial joints:** In these joints the movements occur in two planes or axes. The examples are:
   (a) *Condylar joints* (e.g. knee and temporo-mandibular joints). These are modified hinge joints, where not only flexion and extension take place around a transverse axis but slight rotation also takes place around a vertical axis.
   (b) *Ellipsoid joints* (e.g. radio-carpal, metacarpo-phalangeal, metatarso-phalangeal and lateral atlanto-occipital joints). Here flexion and extension take place around transverse axis, and abduction and adduction take place around a anteroposterior axes (Fig. 7.17). The circumduction is also possible.
   (c) *Saddle joints* (e.g. carpo-metacarpal joint of thumb, sterno-clavicular joint). Here flexion and extension take place around a transverse axis, and abduction and adduction take place around an anteroposterior axis. Some rotation is also associated with aforesaid movements. This is known as **conjunction rotation.**
3. **Multiaxial (polyaxial) joints:** In these joints movements occur in three planes or axes (Fig. 7.18). The examples are ball and socket joint such as shoulder and hip joints. All kinds of movements, i.e. flexion, extension, abduction, adduction, rotation, circumduction, are possible.

C. According to the number of articulating bones

1. **Simple joints:** Here only two bones take part in the formation of a joint, e.g. interphalangeal joints of fingers and toes.
2. **Compound joints:** Here more than two bones take part in the formation of a joint. The examples are:
   (a) *Ankle joint*, where three bones (tibia, fibula and talus) take part to form this joint.
   (b) *Elbow joint*, where three bones (humerus, radius and ulna) take part to form this joint.
   (c) *Radio-carpal (wrist) joint*, where four bones (radius, scaphoid, lunate and triquetral) take part in the formation of this joint.

N.B.

When the joint cavity is divided into two compartments by a articular disc or meniscus it is called *complex joint*, e.g. knee (Fig. 7.19), temporo-mandibular and sterno-clavicular joints.

Table 7.2 Examples of various types of synovial joints according to the articular surfaces

SYNOVIAL JOINTS						
Plane	**Hinge**	**Pivot**	**Condylar**	**Ellipsoidal**	**Saddle**	**Ball and socket**
Intercarpal	Elbow	Superior radio-ulnar	Temporo-mandibular	Radio-carpal (wrist)	First carpo-metacarpal	Hip joint (largest)
Intertarsal	Knee	Median atlanto-axial	Metacarpo-phalangeal	Atlanto-occipital	Sterno-clavicular	Shoulder joint
Intermetatarsal	Ankle			Metacarpo-phalangeal	Calcaneo-cuboid	Incudo-stapedial (smallest)
Intermetacarpal	Interphalangeal			Metatarso-phalangeal	Incudo-malleolar (smallest)	
Zygapophyseal						

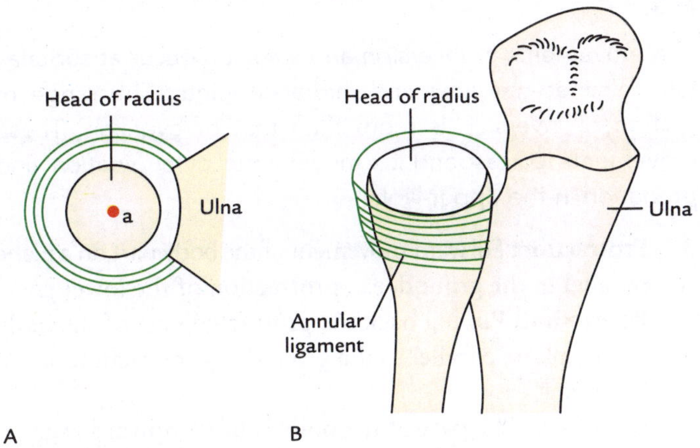

Fig. 7.16 Superior radio-ulnar joint: **A,** diagrammatic representation of the joint showing vertical axis; **B,** actual superior radio-ulnar joint.

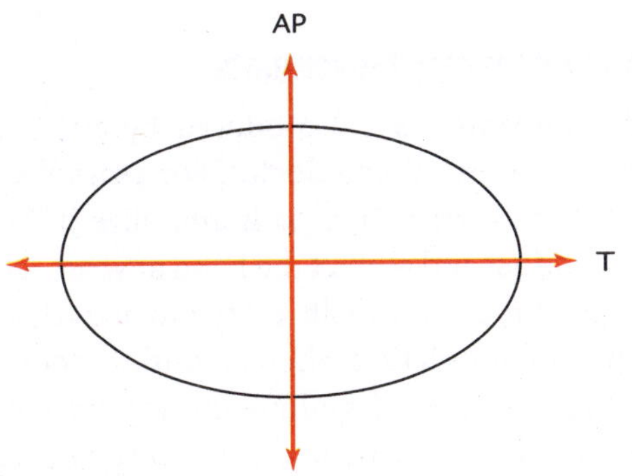

Fig. 7.17 Two axes of a multiaxial joint. (AP = anteroposterior axis producing abduction and adduction; T = transverse axis producing flexion and extension.)

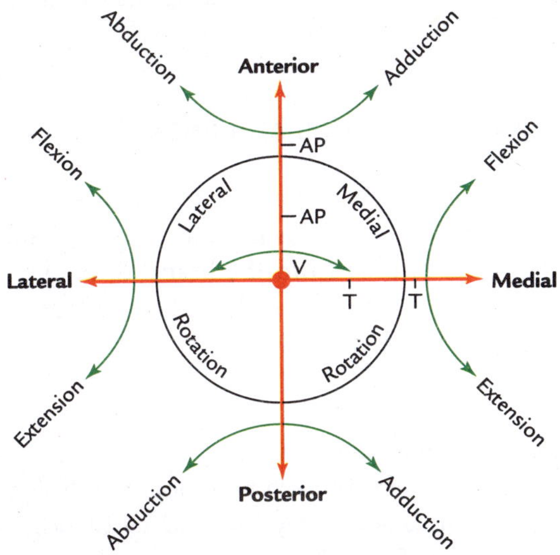

Fig. 7.18 Axes and movements of a polyaxial joint. (AP = anteroposterior axis; T = transverse axis; V = vertical axis.)

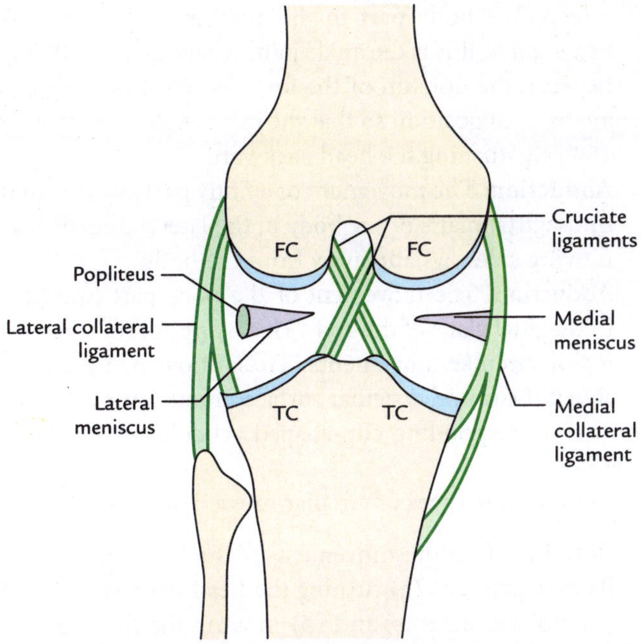

Fig. 7.19 Knee joint—an example of a complex joint. (FC = femoral condyle; TC = tibial condyle.)

MOVEMENTS OF SYNOVIAL JOINTS

Active Movements

Three types of **active movements** occur at the synovial joints:

1. Gliding or slipping movements
2. Angular movements
3. Rotary or circular movements

Gliding or slipping movements: These movements occur in plane joints, where one bone slips over the other in a particular direction. Such movements are limited. The series of gliding movements in small joints of hand, foot and vertebral column provide an efficient buffer against a force.

Angular movements: These movements increase or decrease the joint angle produced by the articulated bones. The four types of angular movements are as follows:

1. **Flexion:** It is the movement that decreases the joint angle in an anteroposterior plane, e.g. bending of elbow and knee. The flexion of elbow joint is a forward movement, whereas flexion of knee is a backward movement.

N.B.

In ankle joint, the flexion occurs when the dorsum of foot is elevated. This movement is termed as *dorsiflexion*. The rising on toes is *plantar flexion*. In flexion of shoulder joint the arm is brought forward.

2. **Extension:** This movement is reverse of flexion and in it the joint angle is increased. In an extended joint, the angle between the articulating bones is 180°. The extension

returns the body part to the anatomical position. The *exception* to this is the ankle joint where there is 90° angle between the dorsum of the foot and the lower leg in an anatomical position so that the joint angle is greater than 180°, e.g. turning the head backward.

3. **Abduction:** The movement of a body part away from the midsagittal plane of the body in the lateral direction, e.g. moving sideways and away from the body.
4. **Adduction:** The movement of the body part toward the midsagittal plane of the body. This is opposite of abduction.

Rotary or circular movements: These movements are only possible if the round articular surface of one bone articulates with the corresponding cup-shaped articular surface of the other bone.

The two basic types of circular movements are as under:

1. **Rotation:** It is the movement of the body part around its own axis, e.g. (a) turning the head from side-to-side, i.e. 'no' movements, and (b) moving the forearm from palm up position to palm down position and vice-versa.
   (a) *Supination*: Rotation of forearm from midprone position in such a way that the palm of the hand is turned forward (anteriorly).
   (b) *Pronation*: Rotation of forearm from midprone position in such a way that the palm of the hand is directed backward.

N.B.

The rotation around a longitudinal axis is called *rotation proper* which may be adjunct or conjunct. The *adjunct rotation* takes place actively by some muscles whereas *conjunct rotation* occurs passively due to configuration of articular surfaces or tension of some ligaments. For example, the rotation of hip is an adjunct rotation whereas rotation of knee during locking and unlocking is a conjunct rotation.

2. **Circumduction:** It is a combination of four angular movements: flexion, extension, abduction and adduction in successive order, describing a cone. In other words, it is a circular, cone-like movement of the body part (segment). The distal-free segment forms the circular movement and the proximal attached segment forms the pivot. Such movements are possible at shoulder, wrist, hip and ankle joints.

Special Active Movements

These are as follows:

1. **Inversion:** Movement in which the sole of the foot faces inward and medially. It occurs when the medial border of the foot is raised.
2. **Eversion:** Movement in which the sole of the foot faces outward and laterally. It occurs when the lateral border of the foot is raised.

N.B.

The movements of *inversion and eversion* occur at subtalar, talo-calcaneo-navicular and midtarsal joints. The range of motion of inversion is more than that of eversion. These movements correspond to movements of *supination* and *pronation* in the upper limb.

3. **Protraction:** Forward movement of the body part on a plane parallel to the ground, e.g. protraction of the lower jaw.
4. **Retraction:** Pulling back the protracted part of the body on the plane parallel to the ground, e.g. retraction of the lower jaw.
5. **Elevation:** The part of the body is lifted upward, e.g.
   (a) Elevation of the mandible to close the mouth.
   (b) Lifting of the scapula to shrug the shoulder.
6. **Depression:** The part of body is moved downward e.g. depression of mandible to open the mouth.

The active movements possible at synovial joints are summarized in Table 7.3.

Passive and Accessory Movements

The **passive movements** are produced by an external force such as gravity or examining doctor. For example, the doctor holds the patient's wrist so as to immobilize it. He can then flex, extend, adduct and abduct the hand at wrist. These movements, the patient can normally carry out actively by himself.

By careful manipulation, the examining doctor can also produce a slight degree of gliding and rotation at the wrist. These movements the patient cannot carry out actively by himself, hence they are called **accessory movements**.

Clinical correlation

The assessment of passive and accessory movements is of great value in testing and diagnosing muscle and joint disorders in clinical practice.

BLOOD SUPPLY TO SYNOVIAL JOINTS

It is derived from the periarticular network of arteries (**circulus articularis vasculosus**) that surround the joint. This network is formed from the branches of the arteries lying in the vicinity of the joint. It supplies the capsule, synovial membrane and epiphysis.

N.B.

- Articular cartilages are avascular.
- Fibrous capsule and ligament have poor blood supply.
- Synovial membrane is richly supplied by blood. The rich vascular plexus of synovial membrane also helps to supply nutrition to the periphery of the articular cartilages.

Table 7.3 Movements possible at synovial joints

Movement	Definition
Angular movements	
Flexion	Bending (decreasing joint angle) the joint occasionally backward, e.g. knee joint
Extension	Straightening the joint (increasing the joint angle)
Abduction	Movement away from the midline of the body
Adduction	Movement toward the midline of the body
Circumduction	Combination of flexion, extension, abduction and adduction
Special movements	
Rotation	Movement round the long axis of the bone
Supination	Turning the palm of the hand forward or upward
Pronation	Turning the palm of the hand backward or downward
Inversion	Turning the sole of the foot inward
Eversion	Turning the sole of the foot outward
Protraction	Forward movement parallel to ground
Retraction	Pulling back the protracted part
Elevation	Lifting upward
Depression	Moving downward

NERVE SUPPLY TO SYNOVIAL JOINTS

The synovial joints have rich nerve supply. The nerve fibers supplying the joint are of three types:

1. Sensory nerve fibers conveying pain.
2. Sensory nerve fibers conveying proprioceptive sensations.
3. Autonomic fibers which have vasomotor effects.

The innervation of various structures of a joint is as under:

(a) Capsule is innervated by encapsulated nerve endings (**Ruffini's corpuscles**) and free nerve endings:
  (i) **Encapsulated nerve endings** are sensitive to proprioceptive sensations, *viz.* postural reflexes and position of the joint sense.
  (ii) **Free nerve endings** are sensitive to pain.
(b) Ligaments are supplied by pain sensitive-free nerve endings.
(c) Synovial membrane is innervated by vasomotor sympathetic fibers and pain sensitive-free nerve endings.
(d) Articular cartilage has no nerves.
(e) Articular discs are insensitive *except* at the attached margins.

***Hilton's Law*:** The Hilton's law states that the nerves supplying the joint also supply the muscles regulating the movements of the joint and skin over the joint (Fig. 7.20).

Clinical correlation

If the joint is excessively stretched or suffers from a disease or injury, the irritation of nerves supplying the joint causes muscles acting on the joint to contract in such a way that the joint is brought in a position of maximum comfort to protect the joint. The pain of the joint is referred to skin overlying the joint.

***Gardner's observation*:** The part of the joint capsule which is rendered taut by the contraction of a group of muscles is supplied by a nerve which innervates their antagonist muscles. This is essential to ensure the stability of the joint.

Last's formulation of segmental innervation of muscles regulating joint movements of the limb (Fig. 7.21): According to Last's formulation:

(a) Four consecutive spinal segments regulate the movements of each joint in the limb. The upper two segments regulate one movement and the lower two segments regulate the opposite movement.

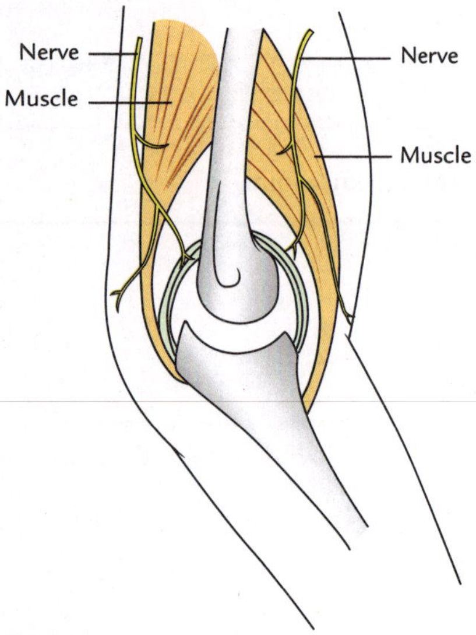

Fig. 7.20 Innervation of synovial joint to depict Hilton's law.

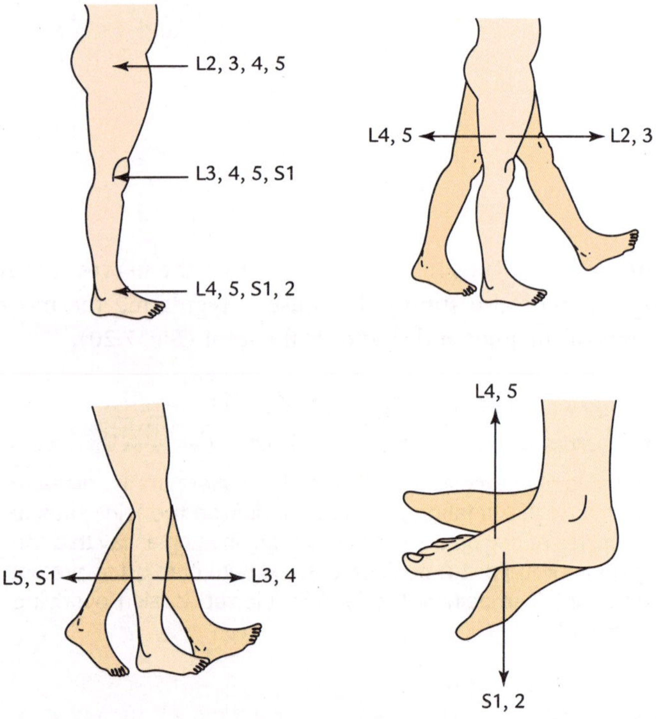

Fig. 7.21 Segmental innervation of muscles regulating the movements of the lower limb.

(b) The joint, one segment distal in the limb is supplied by the centers one segment (en block) lower in the spinal cord.

To cite an example, the innervation and movements of the major joints of lower limbs are as follows:

(a) *Segmental innervation of the joints*

Joint	Segmental innervation
Hip	L2, 3, 4 and 5
Knee	L3, 4, 5 and S1

(b) *Segments regulating the joint movements*

Joint	Segmental regulation
Hip	Flexion L2, 3 Extension L4, 5
Knee	Extension L3, 4 Flexion L5, S1
Ankle	Dorsiflexion L4, 5 Plantar flexion S1, 2

FACTORS MAINTAINING THE STABILITY OF SYNOVIAL JOINTS

The stability of synovial joints is maintained by the following structures:

1. **Bones:** The bones play an important role in providing the stability to certain joints, e.g.
   (a) In hip joint the head of femur is perfectly fitted into the socket of the hip bone, hence acquired dislocation of the hip joint is rare.
   (b) In ankle joint the talus is caught in tibiofibular mortice formed by medial malleolus, inferior surface of the lower end of tibia and lateral malleolus.
2. **Ligaments:** The intracapsular and extracapsular ligaments not only provide stability to the joint to prevent its dislocation but also guide and prevent the unwanted movement, e.g.
   (a) Cruciate ligaments within the knee joint provide anteroposterior stability.
   (b) The collateral ligaments of knee joint provide side-to-side stability.

N.B.

Most of the ligaments are made up of bundles of collagen fibers, hence they do not help against a continuous strain because once stretched they tend to remain elongated.

3. **Muscles:** The tone and strength of different group of muscles acting on the joint provide *most important and indispensible factor to maintain the stability of the joint.* Once these muscles become weak, flabby or paralyzed, the joint becomes unstable and likely to dislocate.

Clinical correlation

Dislocation of a joint: The lack of support by ligaments, poor shape of articular surfaces, or lack of adequate support by muscles leads to dislocation of a joint. Once the joint is dislocated, the bones forming the joint no longer remain in their normal anatomical relationship with each other.The commonly dislocated joints of the body are: shoulder joint, acromio-clavicular joint and temporo-mandibular joint.

BIOMECHANICS OF BODY MOVEMENTS

LEVERAGE

A lever is a rigid bar that can rotate about a fixed point (**fulcrum**) where force is applied to overcome the resistance. The levers are generally associated with machines but can equally apply to other mechanical structures such as human body.

In human body the synovial joint represents the fulcra (F); the bones form the rigid lever arms that move the resisting object like weight of the part being moved, gravity or an external weight (R); the muscles provides the force or effort (E) that causes the lever to move.

Classes of Levers

According to the arrangement of the fulcrum (F) in relation to the effort/force (E), and resistance (R), three kinds of levers are classified:

1. First class
2. Second class
3. Third class

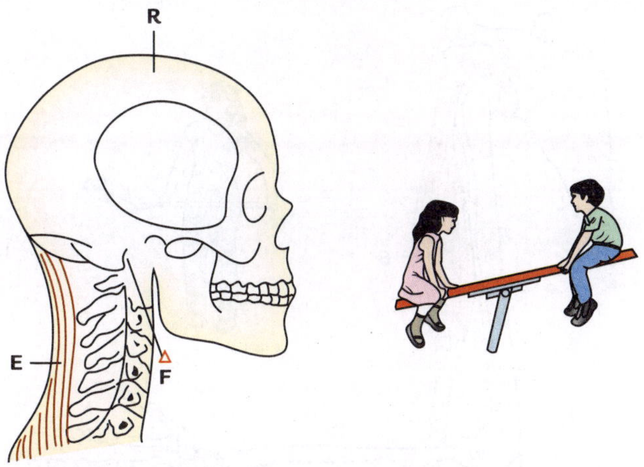

Fig. 7.22 First class lever. (E = effort; F = fulcrum; R = resistance.)

First class lever (Fig. 7.22): The fulcrum (F) is located between the effort (E) and the resistance (R). Playground see-saw is a good example of the first lever, where the fulcrum (crossbar) is located between a child sitting on one end of the board and pushing it down against the ground (effort) and weight of other child sitting at the other end of the board (resistance).

The first lever is best designed for balance. An example of first class lever in the human body will be the head sitting on the first (atlas) vertebra and moving forward and backward. Here, atlanto-occipital joint acts as the fulcrum (F), the weight of the cranium and the facial portion of the head acts as resistance (R), and posterior neck muscles that contract to maintain the balance of head on the joint are the effort (E).

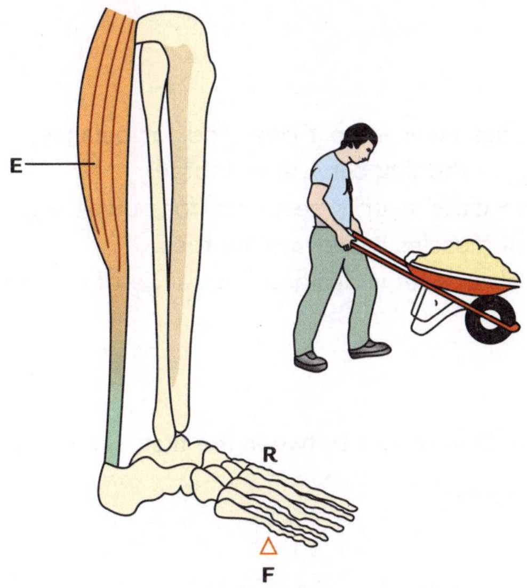

Fig. 7.23 Second class lever. (E = effort; F = fulcrum; R = resistance.)

Second class lever (Fig. 7.23): In second class lever, resistance is positioned between the fulcrum and the effort, an example of second class lever is a wheel barrow. The wheel at the front end acts as the fulcrum (F), the contents of the wheel barrow act as the resistance (R) and person pushing the wheel barrow acts as the effort (E). The best example of a second class lever in the human body is contraction of the calf muscle (E) to elevate the body (R) on toes with balls of the foot (metatarsal phalangeal—MP joints) acting as the fulcrum (F).

Third class lever (Fig. 7.24): In third class lever, the effort (E) lies between the fulcrum (F) and the resistance (R). An example of second class lever is a person using a shovel. The hand placed on the part of the handle closest to the blade acts as the force/effort (E) to lift the weight, *viz.* shovel full of dirt acts as resistance (R) and the hand placed near the end of the handle acts as the fulcrum (F). An example of third class lever in the human body is the flexion of the elbow joint: during flexion of elbow, the contraction of biceps brachii muscle (E) pulling the radius (R) to flex the elbow (F).

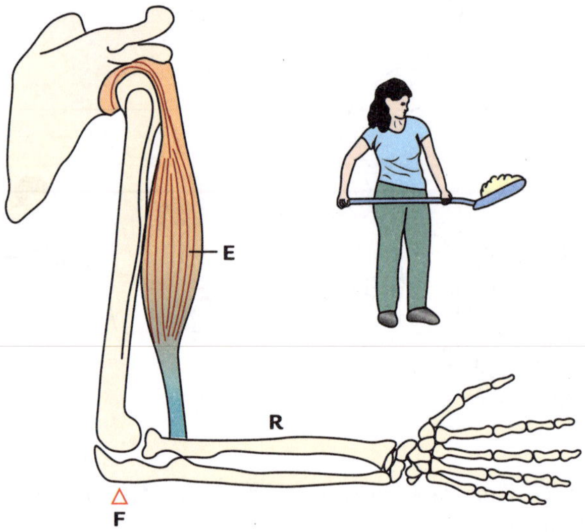

Fig. 7.24 Third class lever. (E = effort; F = fulcrum; R = resistance.)

N.B.

- First class lever is best designed for balance, e.g. head sitting on the first cervical vertebrae.
- Second class lever is best used for power, e.g. action of the calf muscles to elevate the toes.
- Third class lever is designed for range of motion.

The differences between the three types of levers are listed in Table 7.4.

POSITION OF THE JOINTS

CLOSE PACKED POSITION

It is the position of the joint, in which the articular surfaces are fully congruent and have maximum area of contact.

All the ligaments are taut and so arranged that they force the articular surfaces to come together in the closed packed position in such a way that they cannot be pulled apart. Thus, two bones forming the joint functionally become one.

In close packed position, the joint is most firm and rigid. Hence, usually there is no dislocation in this position but if it does take place, the damage to intraarticular structure is most likely to occur. The close packed position of some of the joints are shown in Table 7.5.

LOOSE PACKED POSITION

The position in which articular surfaces are incongruent is called loose packed position. The joint space is freely mobile in this position and hence prone to dislocation.

The loose packed position of some of the joints are enumerated in Table 7.6.

Table 7.4 Differences between the first, second and third class levers

First class lever	Second class lever	Third class lever
	Features	
Fulcrum (F) located between effort (E) and resistance (R)	Resistance located between effort and fulcrum	Effort located between fulcrum and resistance
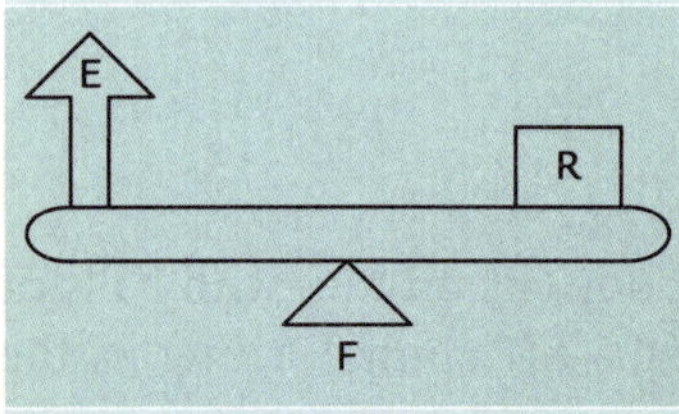	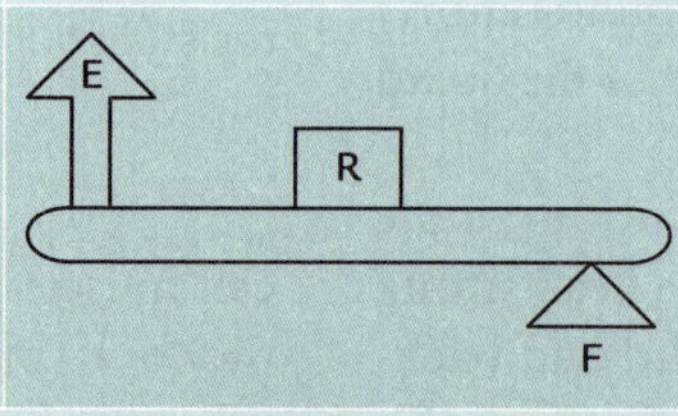	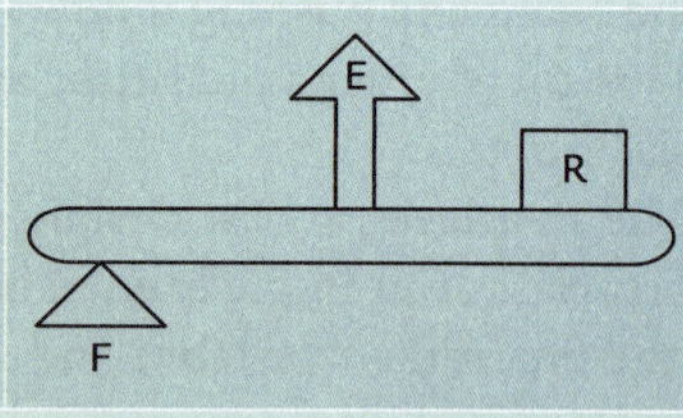
	Uses	
Best suited for balance	Best suited for power	Best suited for range of motion
Requires small amount of effort to lift the weight	Can lift reasonable amount of weight but to a lesser extent	Can lift great weight to a greater extent
	Example in human body	
Forward and backward movements of head on atlanto-occipital joint	Elevation of foot and entire weight of body when person stands on his toes (MP) joints	Flexion of forearm on elbow joint

Table 7.5 Close packed position of major joints of the body

Joint	Close packed position
Hip	Extended and medially rotated
Knee	Fully extended
Ankle	Fully extended (dorsiflexed)
Shoulder	Abducted and laterally rotated
Elbow	Fully extended

Table 7.6 Loose packed position of major joints of the body

Joint	Loose packed position
Hip	Semiflexed
Knee	Semiflexed
Ankle	Plantar flexed
Shoulder	Semiabducted

Golden Facts to Remember

➢ Largest joint in the body/most complex joint in the body	Knee joint
➢ Largest ball and socket joint in the body	Hip joint
➢ Smallest ball and socket joint in the body	Incudostapedial joint
➢ Most common variety of joints in the body	Hinge joints
➢ Largest symphyses joint in the body	Joint between the bodies of L5 and S1 vertebrae
➢ All the symphyses in the body belong to axial skeleton *except*	Pubic symphysis which belongs to appendicular skeleton
➢ Smallest saddle joint in the body	Incudomalleolar
➢ Articular cartilages of all the synovial joints are made up of hyaline cartilage *except*	Those of temporo-mandibular, sterno-clavicular and acromio-clavicular joints which are made up of fibrocartilage
➢ Thickest articular cartilage in the body	Articular cartilage of patella
➢ Most mobile joint in the body	Shoulder joint
➢ Joint exhibiting maximum types of movements	First carpometacarpal joint
➢ Most commonly dislocated joint in the body	Shoulder joint (in adults), pulled elbow (in children)
➢ Most commonly sprained joint in the body	Ankle joint
➢ Most commonly sprained ligament	Anterior talofibular ligament
➢ Most common joint to undergo recurrent dislocation	Shoulder joint
➢ Joint most commonly involved in osteoarthritis	Knee joint
➢ Joint which disappear after a growth of an individual ceases	Primary cartilaginous joint
➢ Joint most commonly involved in congenital dislocation	Hip Joint
➢ Most common joint disease	Osteoarthritis
➢ Most stable position of a joint	Close packed position
➢ Most unstable position of a joint	Loose packed position
➢ Most unstable joint in the body	Shoulder joint
➢ Most important factor to maintain the stability of a joint	Muscles around the joint
➢ Strongest ligament in the body	Iliofemoral ligament (also called Bigelow's ligament)
➢ Most common type of lever in the body	Third class lever

Multiple Choice Questions

1. **All of the following are the examples of the fibrous joint *except*:**
   (a) Suture
   (b) Syndesmosis
   (c) Symphysis
   (d) Gomphosis

2. **All of the following secondary cartilaginous joints belong to axial skeleton *except*:**
   (a) Manubriosternal joint
   (b) Intervertebral discs
   (c) Symphysis pubis
   (d) Symphysis menti

3. **All of the following are characteristic features of a synovial (diarthrodial) joint *except*:**
   (a) Articular surfaces are covered by an articular cartilage
   (b) Have a joint cavity filled with synovial fluid for lubrication
   (c) Mostly are freely movable joints
   (d) Articular cartilage are covered by synovial membrane

4. **Most important factor for the stability of joint is:**
   (a) Fibrous capsule
   (b) Ligaments
   (c) Atmospheric pressure
   (d) Surrounding muscles

5. **All of the following are the examples of synovial joint *except*:**
   (a) Pivot
   (b) Saddle
   (c) Syndesmosis
   (d) Ellipsoid

6. **All of the following are seen in diarthrosis *except*:**
   (a) Fibrous capsule
   (b) Synovial fluid
   (c) Little or no movement
   (d) Articular cartilage capping the articular surfaces of the bones

7. **All of the following are the examples of saddle joint *except*:**
   (a) Sterno-clavicular joint
   (b) Wrist joint
   (c) Calcaneo-cuboid joint
   (d) Incudo-malleolar joint

8. **All of the following are the examples of closed packed position of different joints *except*:**
   (a) Extended and medially rotated hip joint
   (b) Abducted and laterally rotated shoulder joint
   (c) Dorsiflexed ankle joint
   (d) Plantar flexed ankle joint

9. **Articular cartilages of all of the following joints are made up of thin plates of fibrocartilage *except*:**
   (a) Temporo-mandibular joint
   (b) First carpo-metacarpal joint
   (c) Sterno-clavicular joint
   (d) Acromio-clavicular joint

10. **Manubriosternal joint is an example of:**
    (a) Symphysis
    (b) Synchondrosis
    (c) Syndesmosis
    (d) Synovial joint

11. **Xiphisternal joint is an example of:**
    (a) Syndesmosis
    (b) Synchondrosis
    (c) Symphysis
    (d) Synovial joint

12. **Which of the following joint is not a fibrous joint:**
    (a) Syndesmosis
    (b) Gomphosis
    (c) Symphysis
    (d) Schindylesis

Answers

1. *c*, **2.** *c*, **3.** *d*, **4.** *d*, **5.** *c*, **6.** *c*, **7.** *b*, **8.** *d*, **9.** *b*, **10.** *a*, **11.** *b*, **12.** *b*

CHAPTER

8

Vertebral Column

Learning Objectives

After studying this chapter, the student should be able to:

- describe the structure of the vertebral column
- write down the characteristics of a typical vertebra
- outline the cardinal features of typical cervical, thoracic and lumbar vertebrae
- describe the structure of intervertebral discs and discuss their prolapse
- identify the differences in the zygapophyseal joints in cervical, thoracic and lumbar regions
- explain the movements of vertebral column
- state the functions of vertebral column
- describe the curvatures of the vertebral column and discuss their abnormalities
- present an overview of actions of postvertebral muscles on the vertebral column
- correctly solve the review questions given at the end of the chapter

INTRODUCTION

The vertebral column consists of vertebrae and intervening intervertebral discs (Fig. 8.1). The vertebrae contribute three-fourth to the total length of the column, whereas intervertebral discs contribute one-fourth to the total length. The length of vertebral column amounts to about two-fifth of the total height of the body.

The vertebral column serves the dual purpose of affording protection to the spinal cord and of supporting the trunk, and transmitting the body weight to the pelvis and lower limbs.

The flexibility and mobility are served by its unique architecture, for it is composed of a series of individual and movable segments, placed one over the other and separated by soft tissue pads—the **intervertebral discs**.

In the recent times, there is alarming increase in the injuries of vertebral column due to road-traffic accidents and in its degenerative changes due to sedentary habits. Therefore, detailed knowledge of vertebral column is utmost essential to all the medical professionals.

Functions of the Vertebral Column

The functions of vertebral column are

1. Forms the axis of the trunk.
2. Supports the trunk and transmits the body weight to the pelvis and lower limbs.
3. Its intervertebral discs act as a shock-absorber during running and jumping.
4. Supports the skull.
5. Provides protection to the delicate spinal cord and passage to the spinal nerves.
6. Serves as surface for the attachment of the muscles.
7. Provides attachment to the ribs, shoulder and pelvic girdles.

VERTEBRAE

The vertebral column consists of 33 vertebrae: 7 cervical, 12 thoracic, 5 lumbar, 5 sacral and 4 coccygeal (Fig. 8.2). The 24 movable presacral vertebrae comprise 7 cervical, 12 thoracic and 5 lumbar.

The 5 sacral vertebrae immediately below the lumbar are fused in the adult to form the **sacrum**. The lowermost 4 coccygeal vertebrae are fused in later life to form the **coccyx**, respectively. Thus the number of separate movable vertebrae in vertebral column is only 24.

True and False Vertebrae

In the cervical, thoracic and lumbar regions, the vertebrae are separate and movable, and are known as **true vertebrae**. In the sacral and coccygeal regions, they are fused and are known as **false vertebrae**.

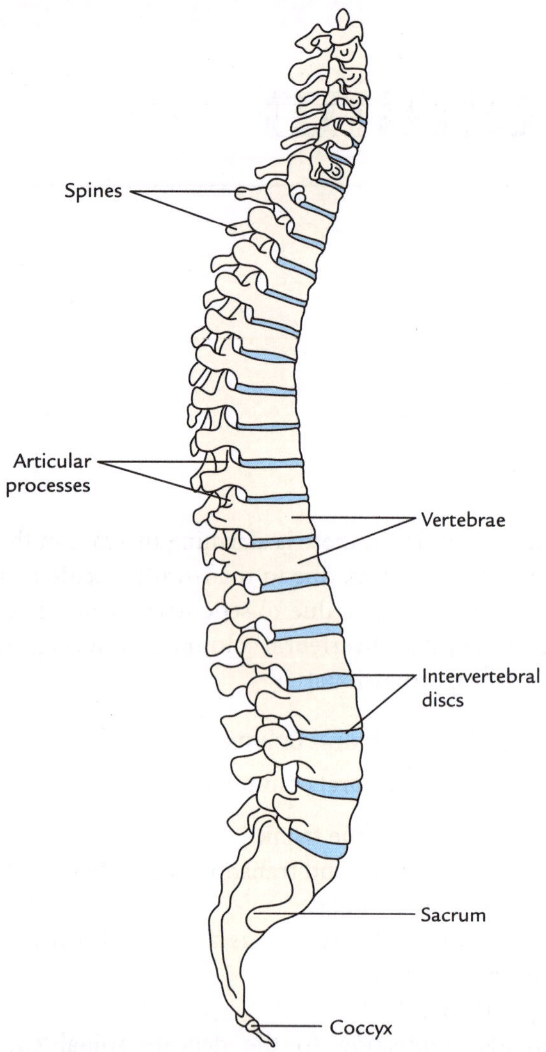

Fig. 8.1 Architecture of vertebral column (right lateral view).

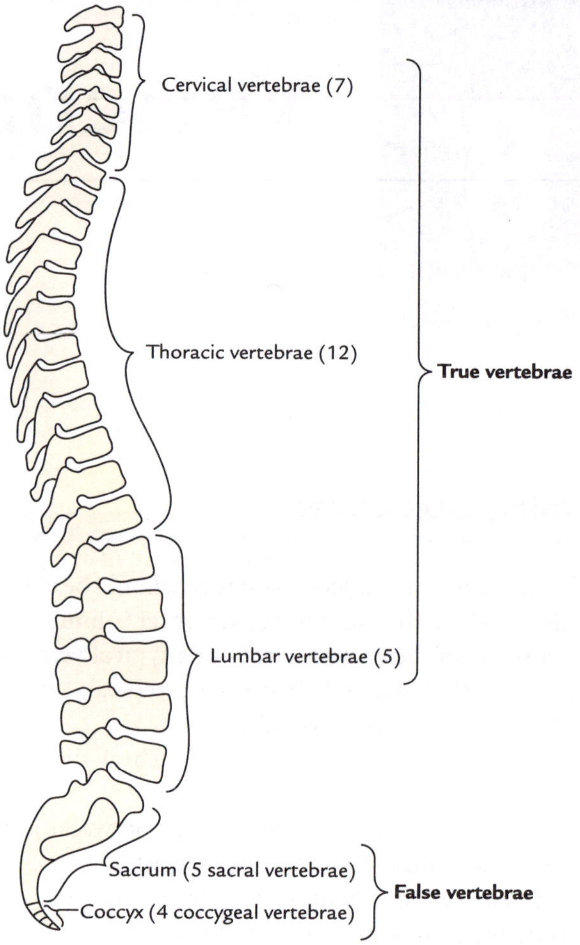

Fig. 8.2 Bony components of vertebral column (lateral view).

The vertebrae in each region not only have features characteristic to that region but also every vertebra in each region has one or more distinguishing features of its own. However, each vertebra is built on the same general plan and therefore has many characteristics in common. The 'typical characters' of a vertebra are seen best in the mid-thoracic region.

CHARACTERISTICS OF A TYPICAL VERTEBRA

The following description deals with the typical thoracic vertebra of mid-thoracic region.

Each vertebra is composed of the following parts (Fig. 8.3):

1. **Body**, the weight bearing part.
2. **Vertebral arch** that protects the spinal cord.
3. **Spinous process** that acts as a lever.
4. Right and left **transverse processes** that act as levers.
5. **Articular processes** (two superior and two inferior) that help to restrict the movements.

Body

The body of vertebra is situated anteriorly. It gives strength and supports the weight. It consists mostly of spongy bone covered by an outer shell of compact bone. The spongy bone contains red bone marrow. The body is separated from the bodies of the vertebrae above and below by an intervertebral disc. The size of vertebral bodies varies with the site. It is smallest in the cervical region and becomes larger and longer towards the lumbar region.

In the cervical region, the superior surfaces of the vertebral bodies are saddle-shaped with flange-like lips arising from most of their lateral circumference. These flange-like lips are called **uncinate or neurocentral processes.** Between C3 and C7 vertebrae, the neurocentral processes of inferior vertebral body articulate with the beveled lateral border of the superior body forming **neurocentral joints of Luschka.**

These joints are synovial in nature and commonly involved in **cervical spondylosis** (osteoarthritis of cervical spine).

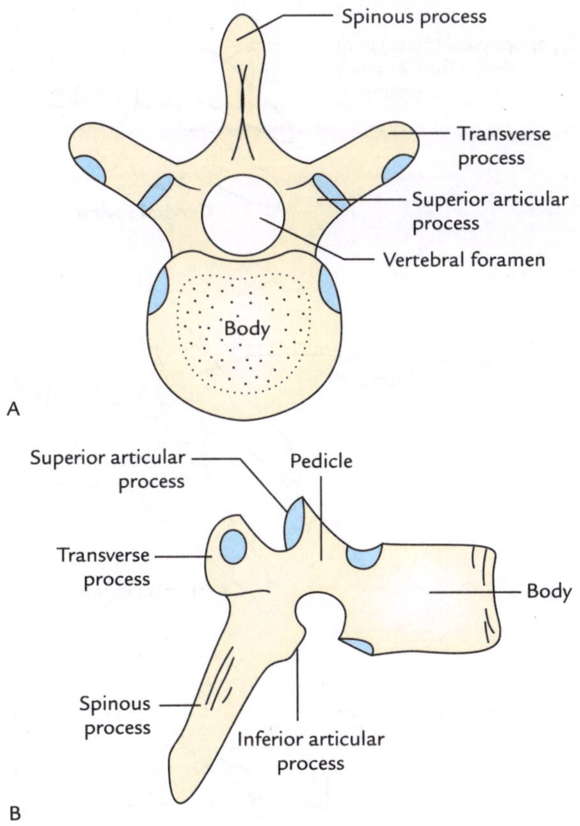

Fig. 8.3 A typical thoracic vertebra showing parts of a vertebra: A, superior view; B, lateral view.

> **Clinical correlation**
>
> **Cervical spondylosis:** It is the most common condition affecting the neck. The degenerative changes appear during third decade of life. The earliest changes are confined to the intervertebral disc but soon the facet and uncovertebral joints are also involved. The disc space between C5 and C6 is most frequently involved. The spondylosis causes restriction of movements and nerve root pain.

Vertebral (Neural) Arch

It is posterior to the body. Each vertebral arch with posterior surface of the body encloses a large vertebral foramen. The series of arches along with vertebral bodies form the **vertebral canal.** In the adult, the upper two-third of the vertebral canal is occupied by the spinal cord. Each half of vertebral arch is divided into two parts, a **pedicle** and a **lamina.**

The two laminae meet in the midline posteriorly to form the **spinous process.** Each lamina is attached to the posterolateral aspect of the body by a rounded bar of bone called **pedicle.** The **ligamenta flava** connect the laminae of adjacent vertebrae.

The pedicle is notched superiorly and inferiorly forming **superior and inferior vertebral notches,** respectively. The inferior vertebral notch is deeper than the superior vertebral notch.

Spinous Process

It projects posteriorly from the site of union of right and left laminae of vertebrae. The spinous processes are interconnected by **ligamentum nuchae, supraspinous** and **interspinous ligaments.**

Transverse Processes

The transverse processes project laterally on each side from the junction of a pedicle and a lamina.

N.B.

The movement of one vertebral body over the other is affected in part by the actions of muscles on the lever-like transverse and spinous processes.

In the cervical region, the transverse processes possess a foramen called *foramen transversarium.* The upper 6 foramina transversaria transmit all the important vertebral artery.

In the thoracic region, the transverse processes act as struts for the ribs. Consequently, they are strong and stout. Their tips bear articular facets for the ribs except for the transverse processes of the 11th and 12th vertebrae because they do not articulate with the 11th and 12th ribs (called floating ribs).

In the lumbar region, the transverse processes are thin and flat, and in conformity to the rounded shape of the abdominal cavity, they are directed slightly posteriorly.

Morphology of the Transverse Processes

As mentioned earlier, the transverse processes project laterally from the vertebral arch at the pediculo-laminar junctions.

The costal elements (*pleurapophyses*) develop as basic parts of the vertebral arches in mammalian embryos, but become independent only in thoracic vertebrae as ribs. Elsewhere they remain less developed and fuse with the transverse processes of descriptive anatomy.

Thus, except in thoracic region, a transverse process consists of two elements, a **costal element** and a **true element** (morphological transverse process; Fig. 8.4).

Articular Processes

The neural arch has four articular processes: two superior and two inferior. The superior processes project rather more from pedicles and articulate with the inferior articular processes of the vertebra above. The inferior articular processes spring from laminae and articulate with superior articular processes of the vertebra below.

The superior and inferior articular processes are above and below the junction of pedicle and lamina, and the

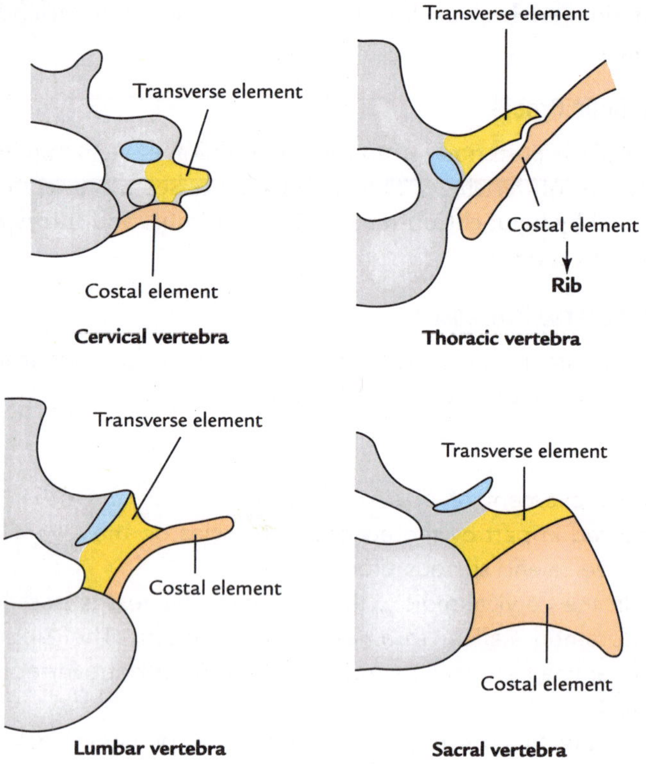

Fig. 8.4 Transverse and costal elements of transverse processes of cervical, thoracic, lumbar and sacral vertebrae.

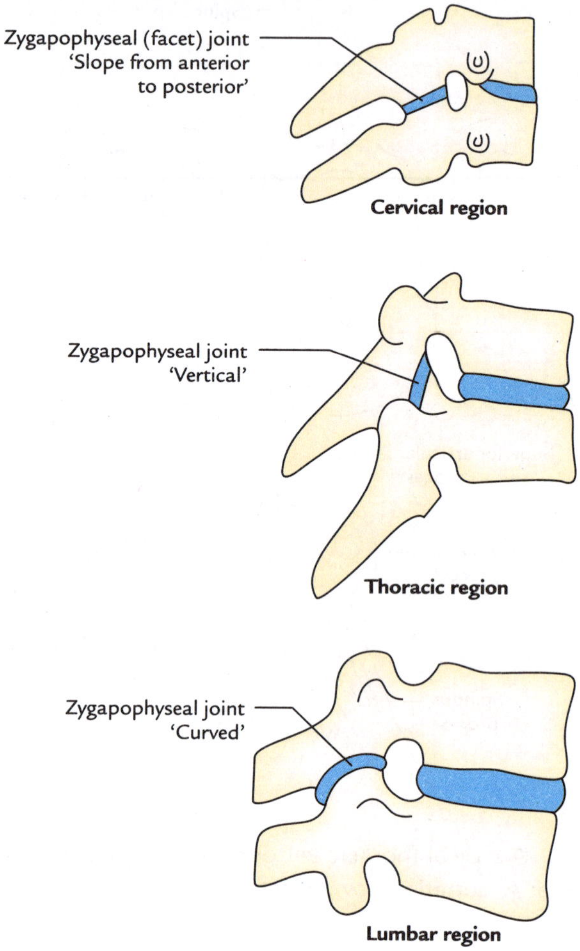

Fig. 8.5 Direction of zygapophyseal joints in cervical, thoracic and lumbar regions of the vertebral column is shown in lateral view.

part of arch which separates these processes, is called **pars interarticularis.**

Direction of Articular Surfaces of the Articular Processes

The direction of articular surfaces differs in cervical, thoracic and lumbar region.

The articular surfaces of superior articular processes face:

(a) backwards and upwards in the **cervical region,**
(b) backwards and laterally in the **thoracic region,** and
(c) backwards and medially in the **lumbar region.**

The articular surfaces of inferior articular processes are directed opposite to those of superior articular processes.

Zygapophyseal Joints

The joints between the superior and inferior articular processes of adjacent vertebrae are called **zygapophyseal joints.** They are synovial joints. A thin articular capsule attached to the margins of the articular facets encloses the joint cavity.

In cervical region, the zygapophyseal joints slope inferiorly from anterior to posterior. This allows one to look sideways and upwards. The direction of these joints differs in cervical, thoracic and lumbar regions (Fig. 8.5).

In the thoracic region, the zygapophyseal joints are oriented vertically. This limits flexion and extension but facilitates rotation.

In the lumbar region, the joint surfaces of zygapophyseal joints are curved and adjacent articular processes interlock. This limits the range of movements in this region, though flexion and extension still remains the major movements in the lumbar region.

N.B.

In all three regions (cervical, thoracic and lumbar), the zygapophyseal joints prevent the vertebrae from slipping forward, but allow the flexion and extension of the vertebral column.

INTERVERTEBRAL FORAMINA

The two adjacent vertebral notches together form an intervertebral foramen which can be seen when two adjacent vertebrae are viewed from the side (Fig. 8.6). Encircling the vertebral foramen are two pedicles, an intervertebral disc, two articular processes forming facet joint and a capsule uniting them.

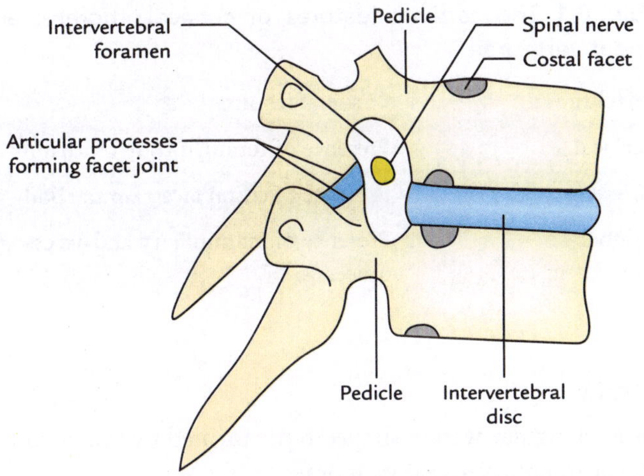

Fig. 8.6 Location and boundaries of intervertebral foramen.

Throughout the length of the vertebral column, intervertebral foramina provides passage to the spinal nerves. Each spinal nerve is attached to the spinal cord by a posterior and an anterior root (Fig. 8.7). The close relationship of spinal nerve to intervertebral disc is very important for it is compressed in disc prolapse producing neurological signs and symptoms.

SPACES BETWEEN VERTEBRAL ARCHES

The laminae and spinous process of adjacent vertebrae overlap in most parts of the spine, however, in lumbar region where they leave big gap between them. These spaces are widened further by flexion of spine to allow easy access to vertebral canal to perform clinical procedures, *viz.* lumbar puncture.

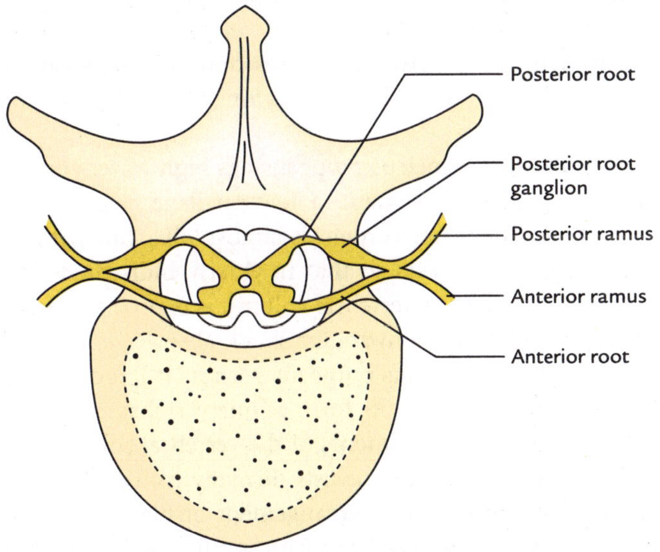

Fig. 8.7 Location of spinal cord and roots of spinal nerves in vertebral canal and intervertebral foramen, respectively.

N.B.

- Nucleus pulposus of intervertebral disc usually herniates posterolaterally, compressing a nerve root.

Clinical correlation

- Radiographs of vertebral column: They are usually taken in anteroposterior and lateral views.
  (a) In *anteroposterior views,* the spinous processes appear as ovoid or somewhat elongated shadows and pedicles appear as ovoid shadows.
  (b) In *lateral view,* the bodies and intervertebral discs are clearly seen.

SPECIAL FEATURES OF VERTEBRAE IN DIFFERENT REGIONS

Cervical Vertebrae

The transverse processes of cervical vertebrae possess a foramen called foramen transversarium for the passage of a vertebral artery (except for C.V.7) to supply the brain (Fig. 8.8). The foramen transversarium is the cardinal feature of the cervical vertebrae.

The first cervical vertebra consists simply of a ring of bone with two short transverse processes. Remember, first cervical vertebra has neither body nor spine. The anterior part of large vertebral foramen is occupied by the dens (also called odontoid process), a tooth-like projection from the body of axis. The odontoid process of axis is held in position by the transverse ligament of the atlas. The posterior part of vertebral foramen is occupied by the spinal cord.

The two superior articular facets on the superior aspect of atlas form the joints with the condyles of the occipital bones called atlanto-occipital joints. The nodding movements ('yes' movements) of the head take place at these joints.

N.B.

The first cervical vertebra is called *atlas* and supports the head. It is named after *Atlas*, a famous Greek Titan, who according to a Greek myth was reputed to support the heavens on his shoulders.

The second cervical vertebra has a small body with an upward projecting tooth-like process—the dens or odontoid process that articulates with the first cervical vertebra—the atlas to form the median atlanto-occipital joint. Presence of *odontoid process* is the *cardinal feature* of the second cervical vertebra. This joint allows the side-to-side movements ('no' movements) of the head.

The second cervical vertebra is called *axis* because it forms the pivot around which atlas (carrying head) rotates like a wheel. The term 'axis' is derived from Sanskrit word *aksha* meaning pivot.

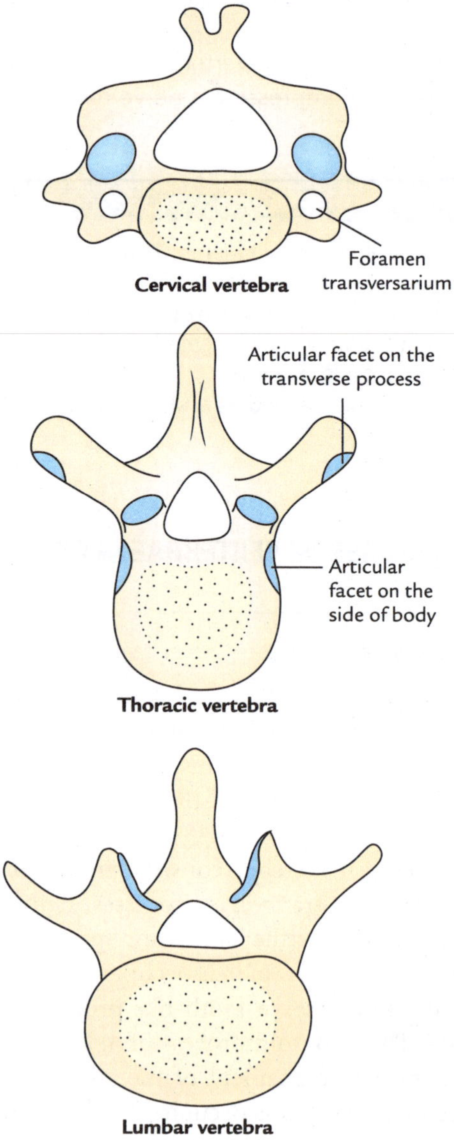

Fig. 8.8 Special features of vertebrae in cervical, thoracic and lumbar regions.

Thoracic Vertebrae

The bodies and transverse processes of thoracic vertebrae possess the articular facets for articulation with the ribs. The **articular facets** on the sides of the body form the cardinal feature of thoracic vertebrae (Fig. 8.8).

Lumbar Vertebrae

The lumbar vertebrae have large kidney-shaped bodies. The spinous processes are broad and hatchet-shaped. The special feature of lumbar vertebrae is the presence of mammillary and accessory processes; they are, however, visualized only on careful examination (Fig. 8.8).

The **cardinal features** of cervical, thoracic and lumbar vertebrae are given in Table 8.1.

Table 8.1 The cardinal features of cervical, thoracic and lumbar vertebrae

Vertebrae	Cardinal feature
Cervical	Presence of foramen transversarium
Thoracic	Presence of costal facets on the body
Lumbar	Presence of mammillary and accessory processes

Sacrum

It is a triangular wedge-shaped bone formed by the fusion of five rudimentary sacral vertebrae.

The upper aspect of the body of the first sacral vertebra articulates with the body of the fifth lumbar vertebra. On each side, the upper part of sacrum articulates with the ilium to form the strong sacroiliac joint. The inferior tip of the sacrum articulates with the base of the coccyx. The cavity within the sacrum (**sacral canal**) contains the roots of sacral and coccygeal nerves.

Coccyx

It is a small triangular bone formed by the fusion of four terminal rudimentary vertebrae. The broad base of coccyx articulates with the tip of the sacrum. The coccyx represents the tail in the human beings.

INTERVERTEBRAL DISCS

The bodies of adjacent vertebrae are united by intervertebral discs (Fig. 8.9). The disc consists of two parts: (a) an outer rim of fibrocartilage called annulus fibrosus and (b) a central core of soft gelatinous (jelly-like) material called **nucleus pulposus** (remnant of embryonic notochord) which acts as cushion or shock-absorber.

Although the nucleus pulposus is central in cervical and thoracic regions, in the lumbar region it lies slightly more posteriorly.

In children, the nucleus pulposus has high water content, a small collagenous element, a few cartilage cells. In new born infants, the water content is almost 90%, but with advancing age it decreases so that in elderly individuals, it is under 70%. When the vertebral column is exposed to an increased load, it acts as a hydraulic shock-absorber. The semifluid character of nucleus pulposus permits it to adapt itself readily to the changes in its form as one vertebra rocks over another during the movements of the vertebral column.

The **annulus fibrosus** consists of many concentric layers of collagenous fibers. This arrangement of fibers limits the rotation between the vertebrae. The annulus is slightly thinner posteriorly than what it is anteriorly and can rupture, particularly in the lumbar region.

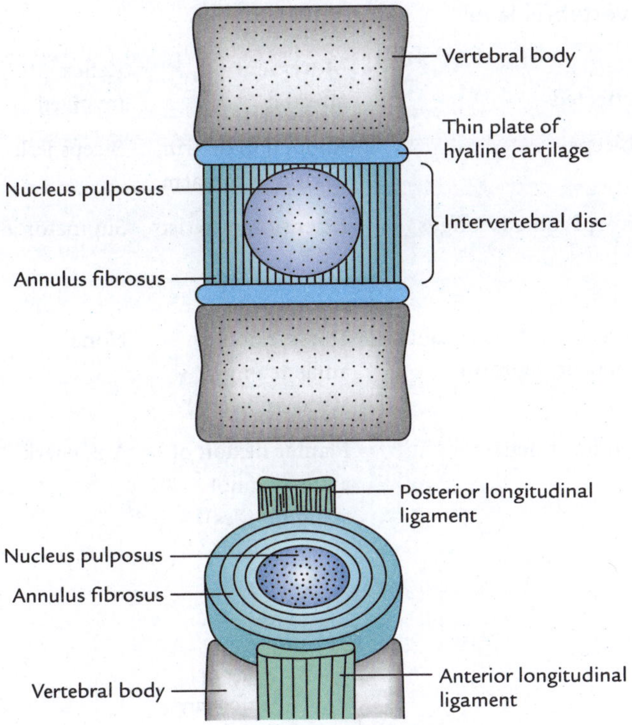

Fig. 8.9 Structure of an intervertebral disc: **A**, anterior view; **B**, superior view of transverse section.

In the lumbar region, the discs become somewhat thicker anteriorly especially between L4 and L5, and between L5 and S1.

The degenerative changes in annulus fibrosus can lead to herniation of nucleus pulposus, inappropriately called **slipped disc.**

Along with the plate of hyaline cartilage covering the vertebral bodies, the intervertebral disc forms a secondary cartilaginous joint (symphysis). The intervertebral discs are kept in position by the anterior and posterior longitudinal ligaments of the vertebral column.

The **anterior longitudinal ligament** extends the whole length of the column and lies in front of the vertebral bodies.

The **posterior longitudinal ligament** also extends the whole length of the vertebral column and lies inside the vertebral canal in close contact with the vertebral bodies.

The anterior longitudinal ligament is a broad strong band whereas posterior longitudinal ligament is weak and narrow.

Clinical correlation

Slipped disc: The protrusion of nucleus pulposus through a tear in the annulus fibrosis is termed as slipped disc (Fig. 8.10). The prolapse generally occurs posterolaterally, but sometimes it occurs posteriorly.

Posterior prolapse directly presses the spinal cord, whereas posterolateral protrusion presses on the roots of the spinal nerves and their sensitive covering leading to pain in the area of distribution of nerve root (root pain).

The disc prolapse is generally seen in cervical and lumbar regions:

1. **Cervical disc prolapse**. The prolapse of disc in cervical region is less common than in lumbar region. The disc between C5/C6 or C6/C7 is most susceptible.
2. **Lumbar disc prolapse**. The prolapse of disc is common in lumbar region. The discs between L4/L5 and L5/S1 are more susceptible. The commonest presenting symptom is **low backache** (*lumbago*).

The important features of a prolapsed disc at various vertebral levels are presented in Table 8.2.

The disc between L5 and S1 is most commonly herniated. It compresses the S1 nerve root.

The herniated disc can be well located by an MRI (Fig. 8.11). Sometimes the plate of hyaline cartilage covering the body of

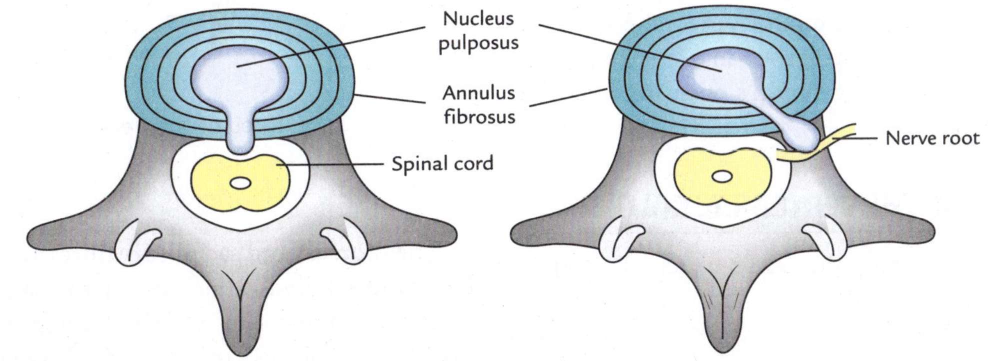

Fig. 8.10 Prolapse (herniation) of nucleus pulposus **A**, posterior; **B**, posterolateral.

Table 8.2 Neurological deficits due to prolapsed disc at various vertebral levels

Herniated disc	Compressed nerve root	Area of sensory loss/pain	Muscles affected	Movement affected	Reflex involved
Between C4/C5	C5	Shoulder and lateral aspect of arm	Deltoid, biceps	Abduction of arm, flexion of forearm	Biceps jerk
Between C5/C6	C6	Lateral aspect of forearm and hand	Extensor carpi radialis longus, brachioradialis	Extension of wrist	Supinator jerk
Between L4/L5	L5	Lateral aspect of thigh, leg and dorsum of foot	Tibialis anterior, extensor hallucis longus, extensor digitorum longus	Dorsiflexion of ankle (cannot stand on heels)	None
Between L5/S1	S1	Posterolateral aspect of calf, lateral border of foot	Gastrocnemius, soleus	Plantar flexion of ankle (cannot stand on toes)	Ankle jerk

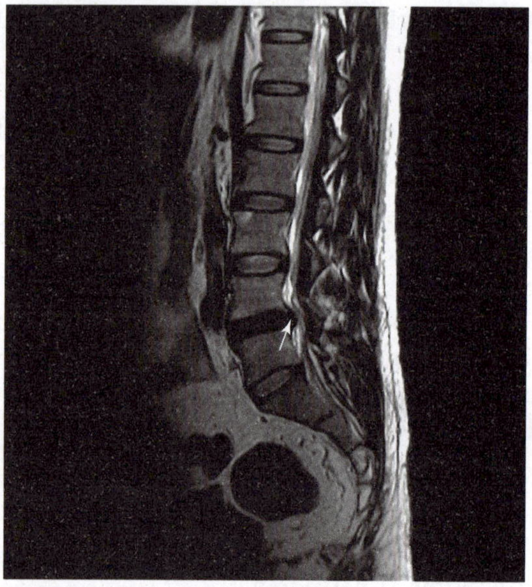

Fig. 8.11 MRI of lumbar region showing herniation of intervertebral disc between L4/L5 (arrow).

vertebra cracks following the fracture of vertebral body. This leads to herniation of nucleus pulposus into a spongy part of the body forming a nodule (Schmorl's node) that may be detected in a radiograph.

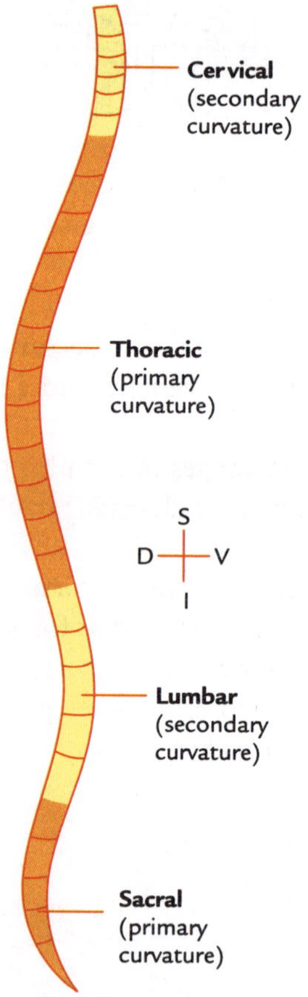

Fig. 8.12 Curvatures of the vertebral column.

CURVATURES OF THE VERTEBRAL COLUMN

When viewed from the side, the adult vertebral column presents four curvatures (Fig. 8.12):

1. Cervical
2. Thoracic
3. Lumbar
4. Sacral

The thoracic and sacral curvatures are termed as **primary curvatures** because they are in the same direction as the curvature of the fetal vertebral column. The cervical and lumbar curvatures are termed as **secondary curvatures** as they develop after birth. The secondary curvatures are concave posteriorly and therefore compensate for and counteract the primary curvatures.

DEVELOPMENT OF CURVATURES

In prenatal (before birth) life, the vertebral column is uniformly curved with concavity facing ventrally with the result that the head and neck are more or less touching each other (Fig. 8.13). This position shows primary curvature/fetal curvature. The secondary curvatures appear after birth as follows:

1. **Cervical curvature** with convexity facing forwards develops when an infant learns to hold his/her head erect and directs his/her visual axes forward at about the age of 3 months.
2. **Lumbar curvature** with convexity facing forwards develops when the child acquires the art of standing and walking erect at about the age of 18 months.

In the thoracic and sacral regions, the ventral concavities persist as in prenatal life; hence called **primary curvatures.**

ABNORMALITIES OF THE VERTEBRAL CURVATURES

These are as follows:

1. **Kyphosis (hunchback):** This is an exaggeration of posterior convexity of thoracic curvature. It can occur in old age due to osteoporosis or disc degeneration.
2. **Lordosis (swayback):** This is an exaggeration of anterior convexity of the lumbar curve. It can occur as a result of pregnancy or a pot-belly.
3. **Scoliosis (crookedness):** This is an abnormal lateral curvature of the vertebral column either to the right or to the left. It is commonest in the thoracic region. It can be caused by poliomyelitis, a short leg or a hip disease.

Clinical correlation

Decrease in height of an individual

- The height of an individual, particularly the one who carries heavy load on his head, may be shorter in the evening than in the morning because with fatigue:
  (a) Curvatures of the spine are increased.
  (b) Turgor of the nucleus pulposus of the intervertebral discs is decreased.
  (c) Height of the arches of the feet is decreased.

  After recuperative rest at night, the person regains normal height in the morning.
- The height of an individual in old age becomes less due to flattening of the intervertebral discs following desiccation and dehydration of the nucleus pulposus.

LINE OF GRAVITY

The line of gravity passes through the body of the axis vertebra, anterior to the sacrum, posterior to the center of the hip joints, anterior to the center of knee joints and anterior to the center of ankle joints. Since the greater part of the body weight lies anterior to the vertebral column, the deep muscles of the back are important in maintaining the normal curvatures of the vertebral column in the standing position (Fig. 8.14).

Clinical correlation

Backache and legache in females: In females who wear high-heeled shoes, the posture becomes unnatural. There is forward tilt of their bodies, their knees are excessively bent, and their spine is thrust forward at the lumbar curvature to maintain balance. Consequently there is a shift in the line of center of gravity of their body putting an undue strain on muscles and ligaments of the back and leg to maintain erect posture. This leads to backache and legache. Thus females who wear high-heeled shoes have perpetual backache and legache.

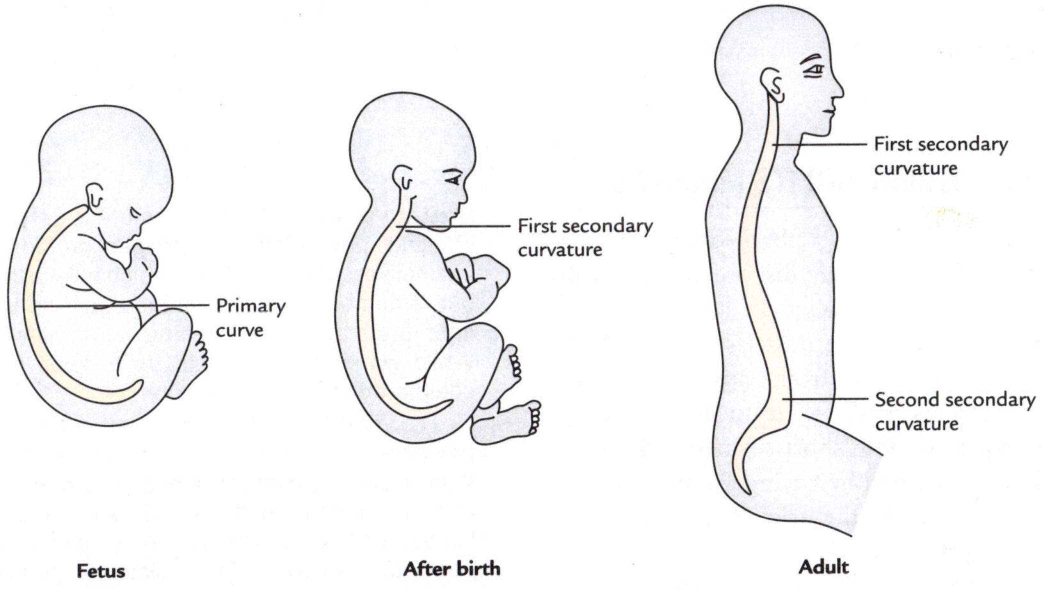

Fig. 8.13 Development of curvatures of the vertebral column.

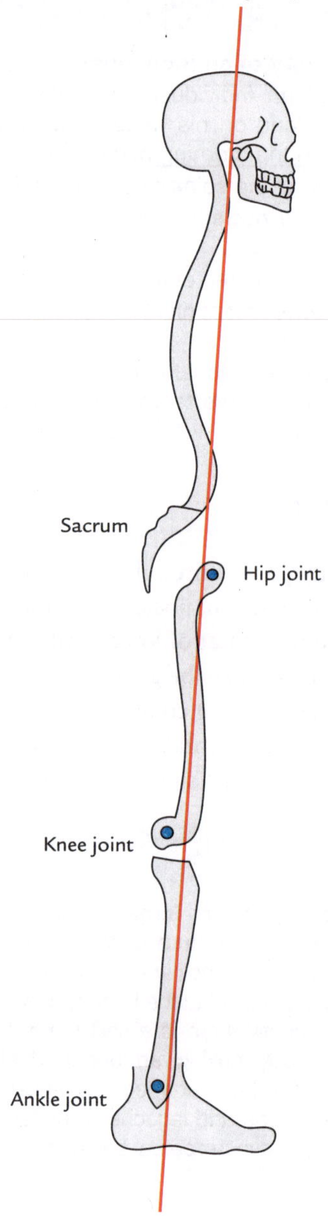

Fig. 8.14 Line of gravity.

VERTEBRAL COLUMN AND ITS MUSCLES

The posture and flexibility of the vertebral column are controlled by groups of muscles that are disposed (a) vertically parallel to the column and (b) obliquely surrounding the trunk on the back. These groups of muscles form a discontinuous layer or sheet that extends from base of skull to the sacrum, i.e. this muscle sheet is broken up into short segments. Although broken up into short segments, the functional unity of whole is secured by having the insertions of one short group overlapped by the origins of another in a relay-race fashion.

The muscle groups have specific actions when they act against the resistance such as gravity. Due to influence of gravity upon the muscle action, when the trunk is bent forward, the extensor muscles of the back get tense and control bending. Similarly when the column bends slightly to one side, the contralateral muscles become tense to control this movement. Thus there is an ever-shifting balance of power between different muscle groups to steady the column and oppose the influence of gravity.

Due to increasing incidence of backache, students should have some working knowledge of the muscles of the back. The muscles of the back are divided into two columns called **erector spinae** (true muscles of back). Each column consists of superficial long muscles and deeper short muscles.

The long muscles passing across many vertebrae and deeper shorter muscles join adjacent vertebrae. The longer muscles maintain normal posture, i.e. maintain normal spinal curvature while the smaller deeper muscles constantly adjust the position of one vertebra to another.

The erector spine has aponeurotic attachment to the back of sacrum, adjacent iliac crest and lumbar spinous processes. As it ascends, it splits into three columns—lateral, intermediate and medial, known as iliocostalis, longissimus and spinalis, respectively.

Each of these columns is divided into three relays (Fig. 8.15), according to their level, as follows:

Column	Relays
1. Iliocostalis	(a) Iliocostalis lumborum (b) Iliocostalis thoracis (c) Iliocostalis cervicis
2. Longissimus	(a) Longissimus thoracis (b) Longissimus cervicis (c) Longissimus capitis
3. Spinalis	(a) Spinalis thoracis (b) Spinalis cervicis (c) Spinalis capitis

Clinical correlation

Posture at work: Normal posture is very important while working particularly for longer period. Some people instinctively adopt postures which relieve the tired muscles but remember it throws undue strain on the ligaments of intervertebral joints, leading to continuous backache. While working one should try to keep his/her vertebral column erect (i.e. in extension).

The flexion of the vertebral column increases the pressure on the anterior portion of the intervertebral disc, thus pushing the nucleus pulposus posteriorly where the annulus fibrosus is thinner. This is especially so in the lumbar portion of the vertebral column. Any weakness posteriorly allows the nucleus pulposus to herniate posterolaterally causing disc prolapse.

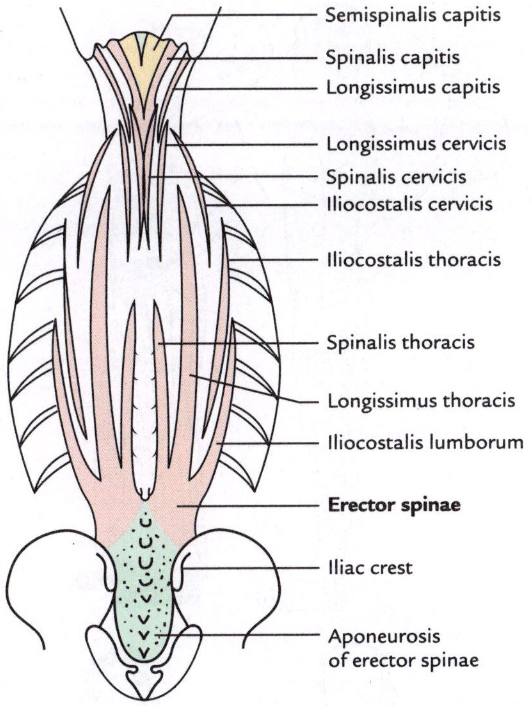

Fig. 8.15 Erector spinae muscles (true muscles of back).

MOVEMENTS OF THE VERTEBRAL COLUMN

The amount of movement between any two adjacent vertebrae is very small, but when these movements are put together, the movements of the column as a whole becomes quite extensive.

The movements of the vertebral column include the following:

1. Flexion (bending forward)
2. Extension (bending backward)
3. Lateral flexion (bending to the side)
4. Rotation (twisting on either side)

The movement between the two vertebrae is most free where the disc is thickest (vertical height), namely in the cervical and lumbar regions. Conversely, the movement is least where the disc is thinnest such as in the mid-thoracic region.

The movements of vertebral column, flexion, extension, lateral flexion and rotation are self-explanatory but the degree of movement in cervical, thoracic and lumbar regions requires further consideration (Fig. 8.16). While considering the degree of movement, the three principal features that should be taken into account are:

(a) zygapophyseal joints,
(b) rib-cage and
(c) elasticity of the intervertebral discs.

In the **cervical region,** all the movements are possible and they are enhanced by the movements occurring between the atlas and the axis and between the atlas and the base of the skull.

The head and neck have a considerable range of movements which are controlled to a fine degree. This is in keeping with the need to accurately position the organs of sight, hearing and smell.

Clinical correlation

Whiplash injury: The movements of flexion and extension of cervical spine diminishes from the superior to the inferior half of the cervical region. Accordingly, the inferior half is likened to the handle of the whip and superior half to the lash. Therefore, sudden changes of momentum produce the so called *whiplash injury*, roughly at the mid-cervical region. The whiplash injury occurs classically as a result of rear impact when a slightly moving vehicle strikes another vehicle in front. The whiplash injuries are now a common cause of persistent cervical pain.

In the ***thoracic region***, the movements of vertebral column are handicapped by the rib-cage. However, the zygapophyseal joints are designed to allow maximum rotation, as if to compensate for the limitation imposed by the rib-cage. The maximum rotation occurs in the mid-thoracic region.

In the ***lumbar region***, little rotation occurs due to nature of configuration of the zygapophyseal joints in this region.

The flexion, extension and lateral flexion are the principal movements of the lumbar spine.

Clinical correlation

Forward bending of lumbar spine includes the movement at the hip joints. An orthopedic surgeon/physiotherapist while analyzing the flexion of lumbar spine must take into account the flexion at hip joints.

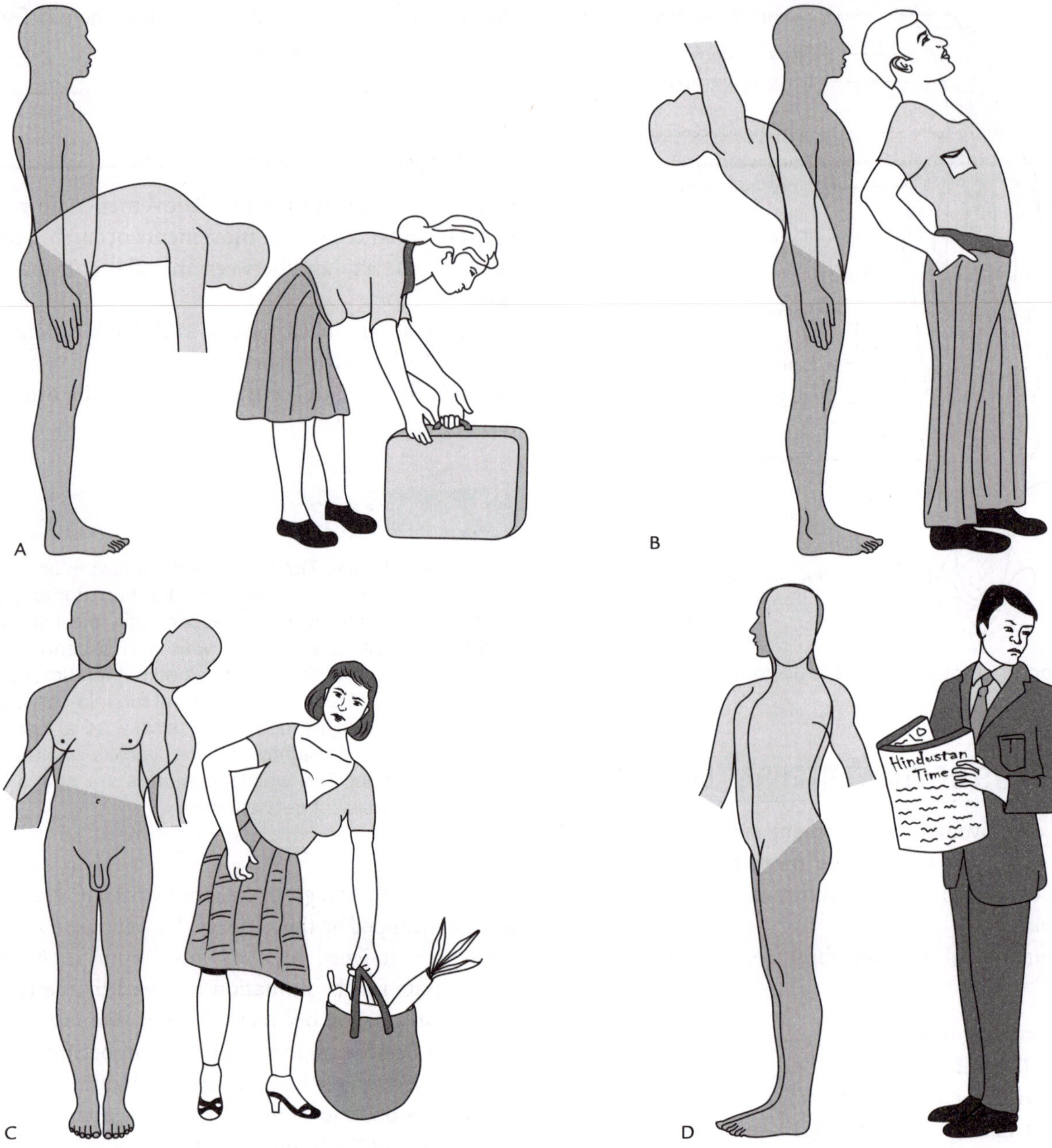

Fig. 8.16 Movements of vertebral column: **A**, flexion; **B**, extension; **C**, lateral flexion; **D**, rotation.

Golden Facts to Remember

➢ Total number of vertebrae in the vertebral column	33
➢ Total number of true vertebrae in the vertebral column	24
➢ Largest vertebra	Fifth lumbar (L5)
➢ All the true vertebrae have body except	First cervical vertebra
➢ Thickest intervertebral disc	Disc between L5 and S1 vertebrae
➢ Commonest site of disc prolapse	Intervertebral disc between L5 and S1
➢ Most susceptible disc for herniation in the cervical region	Disc between C5 and C6
➢ Most important investigation to confirm disc prolapse	MRI (magnetic resonance imaging)
➢ Commonest site of spondylosis	Cervical region
➢ Commonest site of 'whiplash injury'	Mid-cervical region
➢ Most commonly fractured thoracic vertebra	Twelfth (T12) thoracic vertebra
➢ Commonest site of scoliosis	Thoracic region
➢ Commonest site of spondylolisthesis	Between L5 and S1 vertebrae (slipping of one vertebra over the other)
➢ Commonest congenital anomaly of vertebral column	Spina bifida
➢ Commonest site of fracture dislocation in the vertebral column	Dorsolumbar region between T12 and L1 vertebrae
➢ Most common site of compression fracture of vertebra	Lumbar region
➢ Most common tumors of vertebral column	Secondaries (metastatic tumors)
➢ Commonest site of tuberculosis of vertebral column	Cervical region
➢ Schmorl's node	Extrusion (i.e. herniation) of nucleus pulposus into the body of vertebra

Multiple Choice Questions

1. **Select the incorrect statement about the vertebral column:**
   (a) It consists of 33 vertebrae
   (b) It has 24 separate movable vertebrae
   (c) It possess 2 curvatures
   (d) It forms the axis of the trunk

2. **All of the following statements are true about vertebral column *except*:**
   (a) Vertebrae contribute three-fourth of its total length.
   (b) Intervertebral discs contribute one-quarter of its total length
   (c) Provides firm support to the body
   (d) Vertebral bodies act as shock-absorber during running and jumping

3. **Select the incorrect statement about the zygapophyseal joints:**
   (a) They are joints between laminae of two adjacent vertebrae
   (b) They slope inferiorly from anterior to posterior in the cervical region
   (c) They are oriented vertically in the thoracic region
   (d) Their articular surface curve and interlock with each other in the lumbar region

4. **Select the incorrect statement about the direction of articular surfaces of superior articular processes:**
   (a) Directed backwards and upwards in the cervical region
   (b) Directed backwards and downwards in the thoracic region
   (c) Directed backwards and laterally in the thoracic region
   (d) Directed backwards and medially in the lumbar region

5. **All of the following statements are true about the intervertebral discs *except* that:**
   (a) Their outer rim is formed by the fibrocartilage
   (b) Their center is filled with the nucleus pulposus
   (c) They take past in the formation symphyses between the adjacent vertebral bodies
   (d) They are thickest in the thoracic region

6. **The functions of intervertebral discs include all *except* that they:**
   (a) Act as a shock-absorber
   (b) Contribute to the height of vertebral column
   (c) Contribute to the flexibility of the vertebral column
   (d) Enhance the rotation between the vertebrae

7. **Select the incorrect statement regarding the movements of the vertebral column:**
   (a) Little rotation occurs in the lumbar region
   (b) Movements are facilitated by rib-cage in the thoracic region
   (c) Movements are enhanced in the cervical region by movements occurring at atlanto-axial and atlanto-occipital joints
   (d) None of the above

8. **Select the incorrect statement about the disc prolapse:**
   (a) It occurs due to rupture of annulus fibrosus
   (b) It mostly occurs anterolaterally
   (c) The disc between L5 and S1 is most commonly herniated
   (d) It mostly occurs posterolaterally

Answers

1. *c*, **2.** *d*, **3.** *a*, **4.** *b*, **5.** *d*, **6.** *d*, **7.** *b*, **8.** *b*

CHAPTER 9

Muscular System

Learning Objectives

After studying this chapter, the student should be able to:

- define muscles and describe their four basic properties, differentiate skeletal, cardiac and smooth muscles
- describe the gross features of a typical skeletal muscle and discuss the lubricating device which facilitates movements of muscle tendons
- compare and contrast the red and white fibers in the skeletal muscle
- describe the various types of muscle fiber architecture and biomechanical advantage of each type
- discuss the microscopic features of a skeletal muscle
- define 'motor unit' and explain why motor units are considered as basic functional units of muscle contraction
- use examples to describe the various ways in which the muscles are named
- discuss group action of muscles and explain what is meant by synergistic and antagonistic muscle groups
- correctly solve the review questions given at the end of the chapter

INTRODUCTION

The muscle is a contractile tissue of the body, derived from the mesodermal layer of embryonic germ cells.It forms the red flesh of the body and accounts for about 40% of the body weight.

The muscles tissue is composed of differentiated cells containing contractile proteins. The structural biology of these proteins generates the forces necessary for cellular contraction. Thus muscles are responsible for bringing about movements within the certain organs and the body as a whole. Hence they are regarded as the '**motors of the body**' (Fig. 9.1).

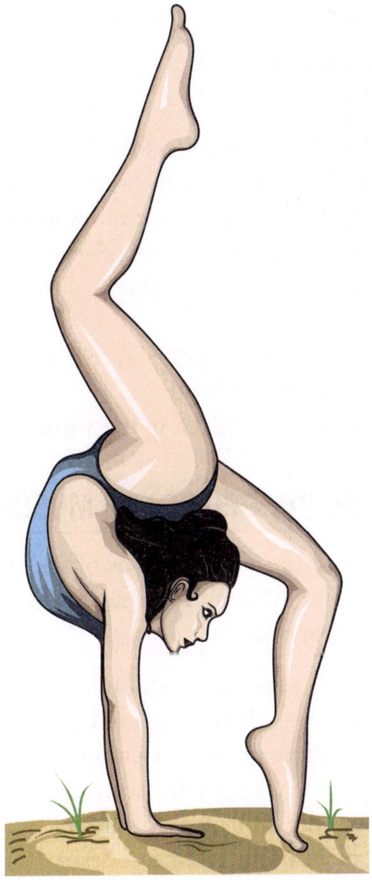

Fig. 9.1 Muscles, the motors of the body moving its various parts.

Thus muscle can be defined as follows: It is a contractile tissue which brings about the movements of organs and body as whole.

N.B.

All the muscles of the body develop from mesenchyme except arrectores pilorum, muscles of iris, and myoepithelial cells of glands which develop from ectoderm.

TYPES OF MUSCLES

On the basis of morphological and functional characteristics, the muscles are classified into three types:

1. Skeletal muscles (voluntary)
2. Smooth muscles (involuntary)
3. Cardiac muscles (involuntary)

The **skeletal muscles** are attached to the skeleton, the **smooth muscles** form the walls of the viscera and the **cardiac muscles** form the wall of the heart (myocardium).

These three types of muscles differ considerably from each other (Fig. 9.2). The differences between these three are enumerated in Table 9.1.

Apart from skeletal, cardiac and smooth muscles, there are contractile cells which function as single cell units, *viz.*:-

1. Myoepithelial cells
2. Myofibroblasts

Myoepithelial cells are spindle-shaped epithelial cells containing contractile protein in the form of **actin filaments**. They are present at the bases of secretory acini of glands (e.g. salivary, lacrimal, mammary and sweat glands) between basement membrane and peripheral surface of epithelial cells of acini.

The contraction of myoepithelial cells helps in the expulsion of secretion from the acini.

Myofibroblasts are involved in the wound healing.

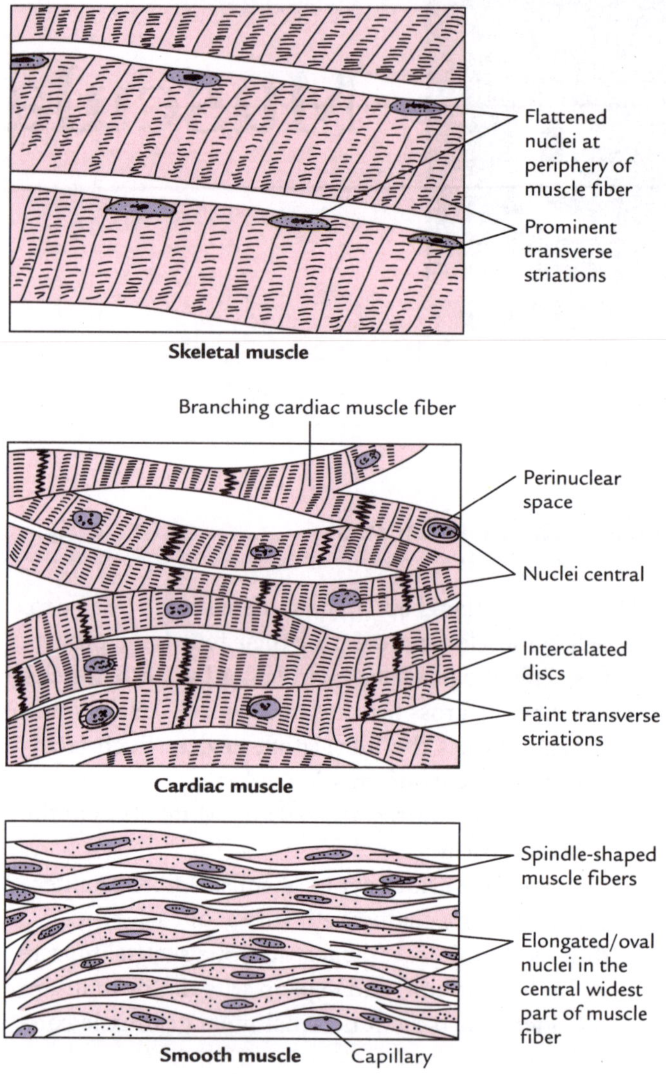

Fig. 9.2 Types of muscles.

BASIC PROPERTIES OF MUSCLES

Although the structure and functions of skeletal, cardiac and smooth muscles are different from each other, they share the following basic properties:

1. **Irritability**, i.e. sensitive to stimuli.
2. **Contractility**, i.e. when stimulated, the muscle contracts lengthwise leading to its shortening.
3. **Extensibility**, i.e. once the stimulus is removed, the muscle fibers return to their original length.
4. **Elasticity**, i.e. muscle assumes a desired shape regardless of how it might be stretched.

The structure and functions of smooth muscles are better understood when studying the involuntary organs of the body and those of the cardiac muscle when studying the heart.

The following knowledge is restricted only to the skeletal muscle as they are clinically more relevant.

SKELETAL MUSCLES

The skeletal muscles are most abundant. They are located superficially and mostly found attached to the skeleton. They are displayed by students during dissection of cadavers. The skeletal muscles perform the function of levers to move the body and its appendages to perform day-to-day activities. An overview of layout of major superficial skeletal muscles in the body is shown in Figure 9.3.

Clinical correlation

The skeletal muscles are:

- Commonly *paralyzed* and hence tested routinely by the clinicians in clinical practice.
- Often injured particularly in athletes.
- Commonly used for **intramuscular injections**, *viz.* deltoid muscle in shoulder region, gluteus medius muscle in gluteal region, and vastus lateralis muscle in thigh region.

The sites of intramuscular infection are given in Table 9.2 and in Figure 9.4. For above region they are described in detail in the following text.

Table 9.1 Difference between the three types of muscles: skeletal, cardiac and smooth

Characteristic features	Skeletal muscle	Cardiac muscle	Smooth muscle
Synonyms	Somatic or voluntary or striated	Myocardium	Involuntary or nonstriated or smooth
Location	Usually attached to the skeleton	Present in the wall of the heart	Present in the wall of hollow viscera, *viz.* gastrointestinal tract, respiratory tract, urogenital tract
Control	Voluntary	Involuntary	Involuntary
Muscle fibers	(a) Unbranched cylindrical (b) Multinucleated, nuclei located peripherally (c) Cross-striations present	(a) Branched cylindrical with characteristic intercalated discs (junctions between the muscle fibers) (b) Single nucleus, nuclei located centrally (c) Cross-striations faint	(a) Unbranched—spindle shaped (b) Single nucleus, nuclei located centrally (c) No cross-striations
Rhythmicity	Absent	Present	Present
Function	Movement of body parts	Pumping of blood from heart	Movement of viscera
Nerve supply	Somatic	Autonomic	Autonomic
Stretch receptors	Present	Absent	Absent
Neuromuscular junction	Present	Absent	Absent

FUNCTIONS

The skeletal muscles perform the following general functions:

1. Motion
2. Heat production
3. Posture and body support

Motion: It is the most obvious function when the skeletal muscles contract. The muscles move the body and/or its appendages, i.e. walking, running, etc.

Heat production: Metabolism within the muscle cells releases heat as an end product. The rate of heat production increases immensely when a person performs strenuous exercises.

Posture and body support: The skeletal muscles maintain posture by providing support around the flexible joints. Postural muscles are at work even when you think that you are relaxed, e.g. when one is sitting, the head is balanced at the atlanto-occipital joint by muscles at the back of the neck. When one gets sleepy, the head suddenly nods forward as postural muscles relax and the weight (resistance) overcomes the effort.

MICROSCOPIC STRUCTURE

The skeletal muscle is made up of muscle fibers and supporting connective tissue (Fig. 9.5).

Supporting Tissue

Each fiber is surrounded by a delicate connective tissue called **endomysium**. Each bundle of muscle fibers (i.e. *fasciculus*) is surrounded by a coarser connective tissue called **perimysium**. The dense connective tissue surrounding the entire muscle is called **epimysium**.

N.B.

At the junction of a muscle belly with a tendon, the fibers of **endomysium, perimysium** and **epimysium** become continuous with the fibers of the tendon.

Muscle Fibers

The skeletal muscle fibers are longer than those of smooth muscle. The length ranges from 1 to 40 mm and diameter from 10 to 100 m.

Each muscle fiber (myocyte) is multinucleated, cross-striated and cylindrical. The nuclei are oval and located at the periphery of the fiber, under the plasma membrane or sarcolemma. The cytoplasm of muscle fiber is called **sarcoplasm**. The sarcoplasm contains longitudinally oriented bundles of **myofibrils**, which are made up of contractile proteinaceous filaments called **myofilaments**. The myofilaments are of two types: thin and thick. The regular arrangement of myofilaments within the muscle fiber gives it a characteristic cross-striated appearance.

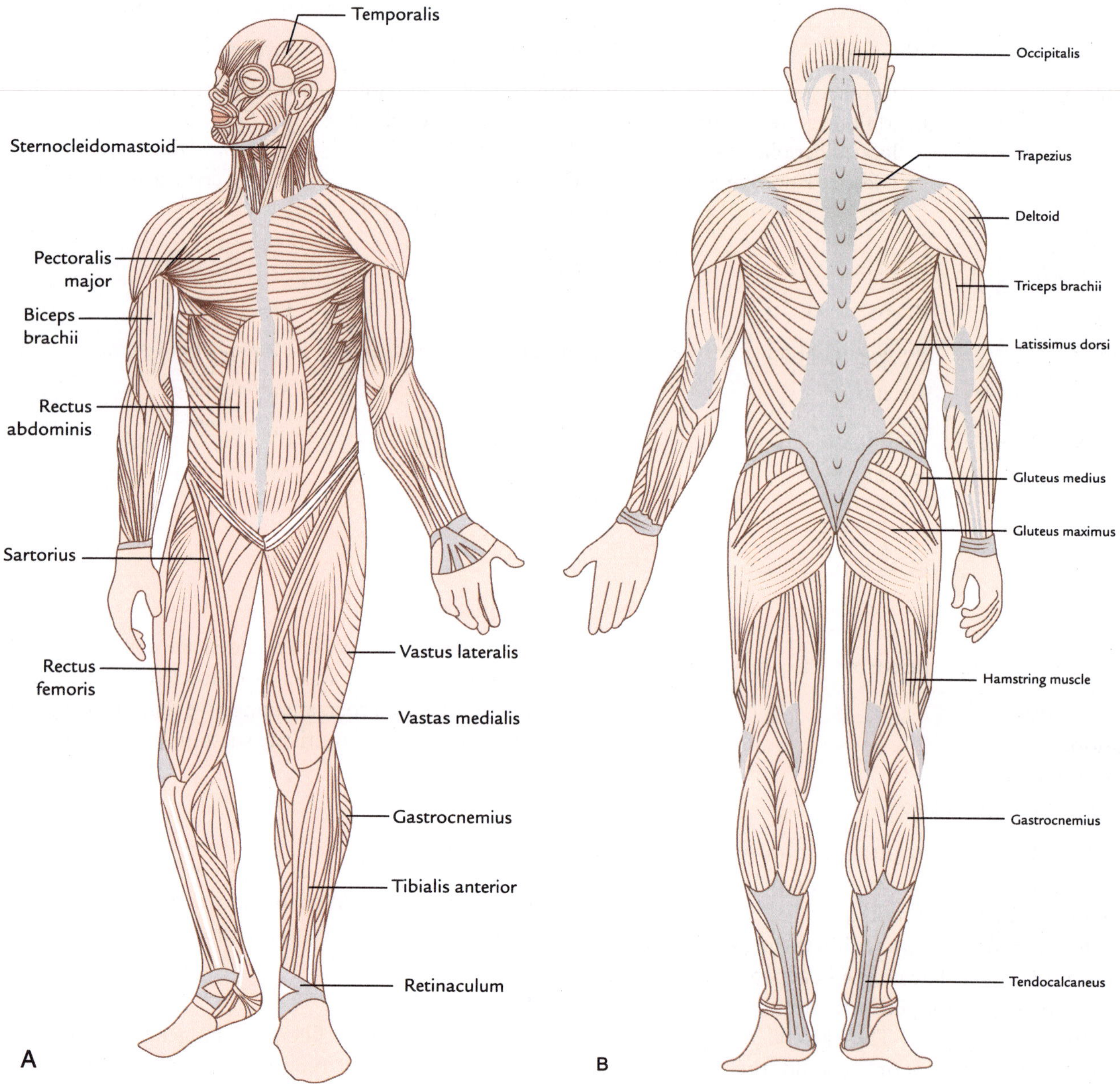

Fig. 9.3. Major superficial muscles of the body: **A,** anterior view; **B,** posterior view.

Table 9.2 Common sites of the intramuscular infections

Muscle	Site
1. Deltoid	Upper and outer quadrant of shoulder region
2. Gluteus medius	Upper and outer quadrant of gluteal region
3. Vastus lateralis	Anterolateral aspect of mid-thigh

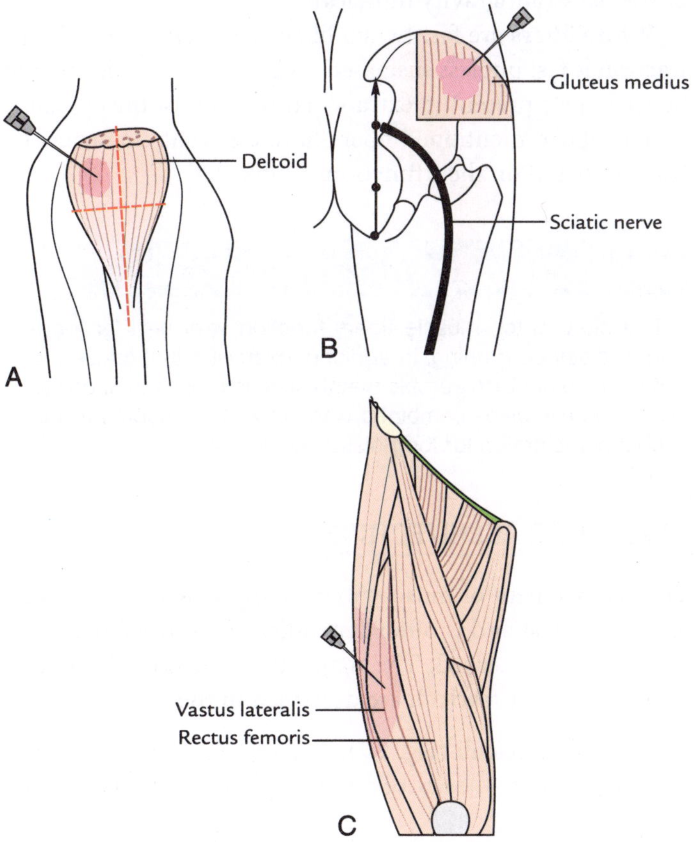

Fig. 9.4. Common sites of intramuscular infections. **A,** shoulder region; **B,** gluteal region; **C,** thigh.

The cross-striated appearance is due to the cytoplasm of the fibers, which shows alternating dark and light bands. With polarized light, the bands that appear darker with light microscope are anisotropic while those that appear light with light microscope are isotropic. Accordingly, the darker bands are called **A bands** and the lighter bands the **I bands**. The middle of A band is dissected by a less dense line called **H line** [Fig. 9.5 (D) and 9.6 (1)]. The I bands are dissected by a thin dark line called **Z line**.

- In the region of dark A band, the thin and thick myofilaments partially overlap each other.
- The I band contains only thin myofilaments.
- The H band present in the center of the A band contains only thick myofilaments.
- The M line is a dark line seen in the center of the H band, where the thick filaments are held together.

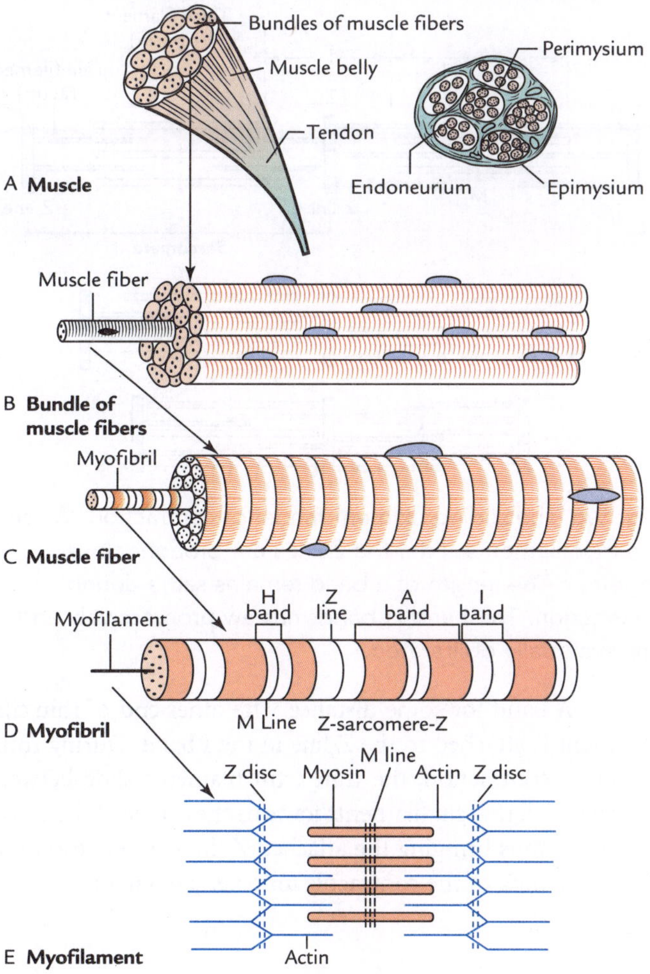

Fig. 9.5 Structure of muscle at gross **(A),** microscopic **(B–D)** and submicroscopic **(E)** levels.

- The region of thick and thin myofilaments between the two Z lines is called sarcomere. It is the contractile unit of the myofibril.

Myofibrillar Proteins

They are of two types:

1. The thick myofilaments consist of protein called **myosin.** The myosin constitutes 60% of the myofibrillar protein and is the most abundant contractile protein.
2. The thin myofilaments consist of proteins called **actin** and **tropomyosin.**

Mechanism of Contraction (Fig. 9.6)

Sarcomere is the basic unit of the contraction. It consists of two types of myofilaments arranged parallel to the long axis of myofibril:

1. **Thick filaments** are composed of protein **myosin** and occupy the A band.
2. **Thin filaments** are composed mainly of protein **actin** and also of **tropomyosin** and **troponin.** One end of each of this filament runs between and parallel to the thick filaments in

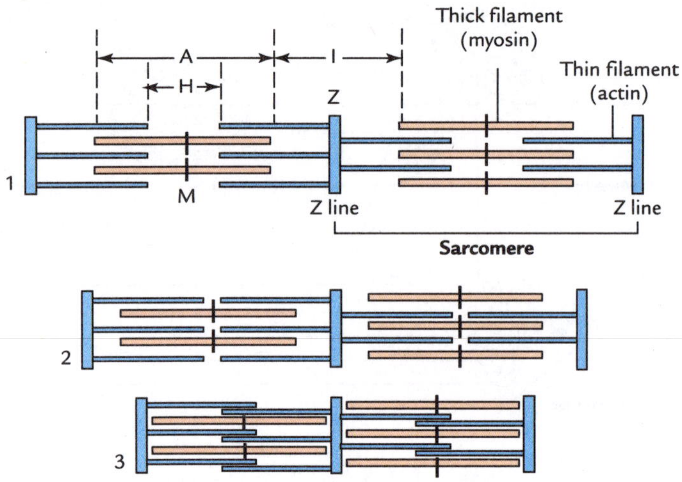

Fig. 9.6 The sliding filament model of contraction. When the myofilaments slide, the Z lines are brought closer together. The length of a band remains same during contraction. The I and H bands narrow progressively and are eventually obliterated.

the A band for some distance. The other end of thin filament is attached to the Z line in the I band. During muscular contraction, the thin actin filaments slide between the thick myosin filaments towards the center of the sarcomere, thus bringing the attached Z lines closer, leading to shortening of the contractile unit, i.e. sarcomere.

N.B.

During contraction, there is no shortening of individual thick and thin filaments.

The sliding of filaments occurs under the influence of energy released from ATP and calcium ions released from sarcoplasmic reticulum.

Clinical correlation

- **Rigor mortis:** It is stiffening of voluntary and involuntary muscles of the body after death. It starts 2 to 4 hours after death and completes after 6 to 12 hours. It gradually disappears within 2 to 4 days. It helps in medicolegal cases to determine the time of death.

The *rigor mortis* occurs due to depletion of adenosine triphosphate (ATP) from the muscle. The mechanism is as under:

(a) ↓ ATP level → stops transport of Ca^{2+} ions into sarcoplasmic recticulum.
(b) Leakage of Ca^{2+} ions from sarcoplasmic reticulum to sarcoplasm due to breakdown of reticulum after cell death.
(c) ↑ Ca level in sarcoplasm → formation of cross bridges between actin and myosin.
(d) Mysosin fails to separate from actin due to lack of ATP and consequently, muscle fails to relax and remain stiff unless tissue degeneration occurs.

TYPES OF SKELETAL MUSCLE FIBERS

The skeletal muscle fibers are classified mainly into two types:

1. Red (type I) fibers
2. White (type II) fibers

Red fibers are slow twitch fibers, i.e. their speed of contraction is slow but more sustained. They are fatigue resistant and hence largely present in postural muscles, long muscles of the back (antigravity muscles).

White fibers are fast twitch fibers, i.e. their speed of contraction is fast but less sustained. They are easily fatigued and hence largely present in extraocular muscles of the eyeball.

The above-mentioned fibers have different characteristic features based on their functions (Table 9.3).

Clinical correlation

The slow twitch muscle fibers function very well for long-long-distance running. In addition, exercises that cause the muscle to perform aerobic metabolism improves their ability. Aerobic exercises combined with slow twitch fibers are the best combination for long-distance running.

FASCICULAR ARCHITECTURE

The arrangement of muscle fibers in individual muscles varies a great deal and is often dependent upon the function of the muscle concerned. The major types of arrangement of muscle fibers or fasciculi are described in the following text:

1. **Parallel fasciculi** (Fig. 9.7): The muscle fibers or fasciculi are parallel to the line of muscle pull. Such muscles contract

Table 9.3 Characteristic features of red and white skeletal muscle fibers

Characteristic features	Red fiber	White fiber
Speed of contraction	Slow	Fast
Fatigability	Fatigue resistant	Fatigue susceptible
Blood supply	Rich	Poor
Myoglobin content	High	Low
Generation of ATP	By aerobic glycolysis	By anaerobic glycolysis
Number of mitochondria	Many	Few
Glycogen content	High	Low
Diameter	Smaller	Larger
Examples	Postural muscles	Extraocular muscles

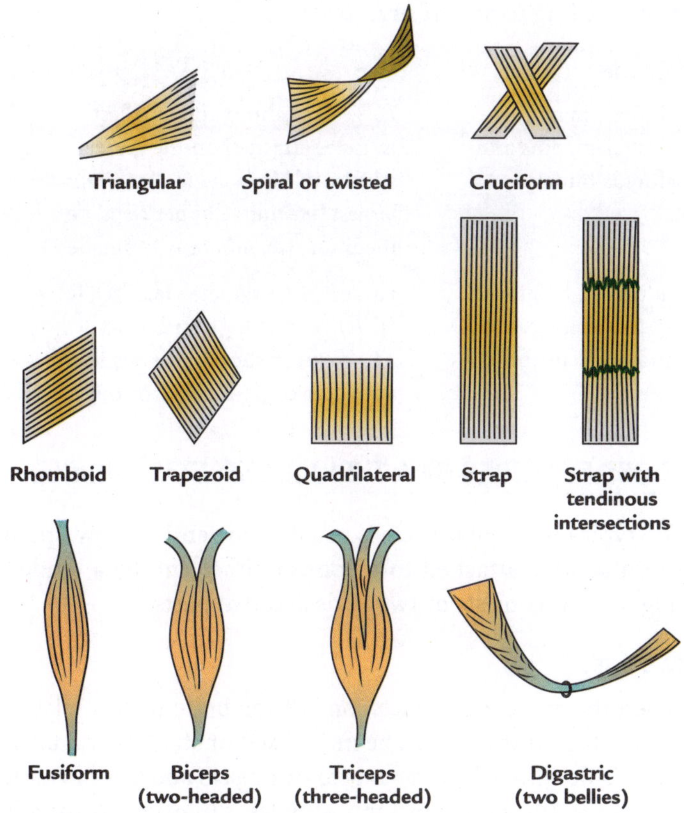

Fig. 9.7 Morphological types of muscles based on their general form and fascicular architecture.

over a great distance (i.e. they have maximum range of movement) and have good endurance. They may be:
(a) *Quadrilateral*, e.g. thyrohyoid, pronator quadratus.
(b) *Strake-like*, e.g. infrahyoid muscles, sartorius.
(c) *Strap-like with tendinous intersections*, e.g. rectus abdominis.
(d) *Fusiform*, e.g. biceps, diagastric.

2. **Convergent fasciculi:** The muscle fibers or fasciculi converge at the insertion point to maximize contraction. This arrangement makes the muscle very powerful, although the range of movement is reduced; such muscles may be:
(a) *Triangular*, e.g. adductor longus.
(b) *Fan-shaped*, e.g. temporalis.
3. **Spiral or twisted fasciculi:** In some muscles, the fibers are twisted or spiraled, e.g. trapezius, latissimus dorsi, pectoralis major, supinator.
4. **Cruciate muscles:** In some muscles, the fibers or fasciculi are arranged in superficial and deep planes and crossed 'X', e.g. sterno-cleidomastoid, masseter, adductor magnus.
5. **Sphincteric fasciculi:** In some muscles, the fibers or fasciculi surround an opening or orifice, thus when they contract, the opening is closed or constricted, e.g. orbicularis oculi around the eye and orbicularis oris surrounding the oral orifice.
6. **Pennate fasciculi** (Fig. 9.8)**:** The pennate-fiber muscles resemble the feather, hence the name pennate. The fleshy fibers correspond to the bars of the feather and the tendon to the shaft, as they are all inserted by tendon. The pennate muscles have many fibers per unit area, and hence they are strong muscles. They may be:
(a) *Unipennate*: when fibers have a linear origin and have the appearance of one-half of a feather, e.g. extensor digitorum longus, flexor pollicis longus, peroneus tertius.
(b) *Bipennate*: when the arrangement of the fibers is that of a whole feather, e.g. flexor hallucis longus, dorsal interossei.
(c) *Multipennate*: when septa (partitions) extend into the origin and the insertion. The arrangement of fibers is such that it provides the appearance of many feathers, e.g. deltoid.
(d) *Circumpennate*: when fibers converge from the walls of a cylindrical space to a buried central tendon, e.g. tibialis anterior.

NAMES OF MUSCLES

The name of muscle can often tell you a lot about that muscle. The muscles are named according to their: (a) location, (b) shape, (c) action, (d) number of heads, (e) attachments (origin and insertion), (f) direction of fibers and (g) size of muscles.

Thus muscle's name tends to fall into one or more of the aforementioned categories.

(a) According to location

Muscle	Location
Tibialis anterior	Anterior aspect of tibia
Temporalis	Temporal fossa
Supraspinatus	Supraspinatus fossa
Infraspinatus	Infraspinatus fossa
Pectoralis	In front of chest (chest = pectus)
Intercostals	Between the ribs

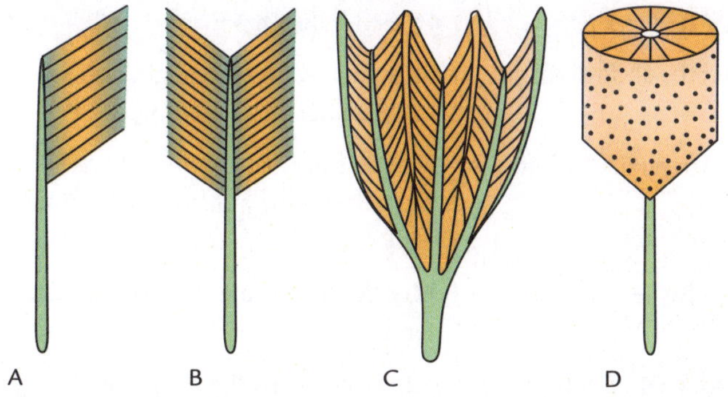

Fig. 9.8 Pennate muscles: **A,** unipennate; **B,** bipennate; **C,** multipennate; **D,** circumpennate.

(b) According to shape

Muscle	Shape
Trapezius	Trapezoid
Serratus anterior	Serrated/jagged-shaped anterior attachment
Quadratus	Quadrangular in shape
Rhomboideus	Rhomboidal in shape

(c) According to action

Muscle	Action
Extensor carpi ulnaris	Extension of wrist (corpus)
Flexor carpi radialis	Flexion of wrist on radial side

(d) According to number of heads

Muscle	Number of heads
Biceps brachii	Two-headed muscle on the front of brachium
Triceps brachii	Three-headed muscle on the back of brachium
Quadriceps femoris	Four-headed muscle on front of femur

(e) According to attachments

Muscle	Attachments
Sterno-cleidomastoid	On sternum, clavicle and mastoid process of skull
Stylohyoid	On styloid process and hyoid bone
Cricothyroid	On cricoid and thyroid cartilage

(e) According to direction of fibers

Muscle	Direction of fibers
Rectus abdominis	Straight (rectus = straight) muscle on the anterior abdominal wall
Transversus abdominis	Muscle running transversely on the front of the anterior abdominal wall
Rectus femoris	Muscle lying straight on the front of femur
External oblique	Superficial (external) muscle having oblique fibers

(f) According to size of muscles

Muscle	Size
Gluteus maximus, gluteus medius and gluteus minimus	Largest, medium and smallest muscles attached on the gluteal surface of hip bone (L. *maximus* = largest, *medius* = in between, i.e. medium size, *minimus* = smallest)
Adductor magnus, adductor longus, and adductor brevis	Largest (L. *magnus* = largest), long (L. *longus* = long), and short (L. *brevis* = short) muscles in the adductor compartment of thigh

GROSS FEATURES OF A TYPICAL SKELETAL MUSCLE

The typical skeletal muscle is usually long and narrow, spans a joint, and is attached to a bone at either end by a tendon (Fig. 9.9). It consists of two ends and two parts.

Two Ends

When the muscle contracts, one of the bone moves relative to the other at the joint. The more fixed or stationary attachment is designated as the **origin** of muscle and the movable end as the **insertion**. In limb muscles, the origin is usually proximal to the insertion.

The inspection of the Figure 9.9 suggests that the upper attachment is the **origin** and the lower attachment is the **insertion**. So that one would expect that the contraction of the muscle would move the distal (lower) bone.

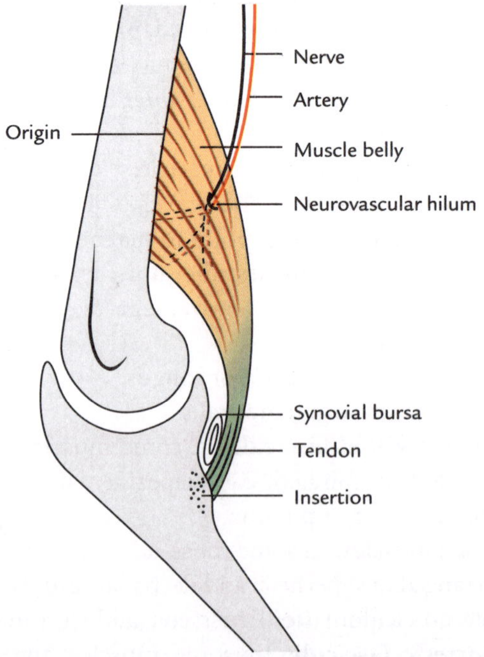

Fig. 9.9 Schematic diagram of a typical skeletal muscle showing origin, insertion (by means of a tendon), nerve supply, blood supply and a lubricating device (synovial bursa).

However, this arrangement can be reversed if the more movable end becomes less movable. For example, what would happen if the hands were holding on to a chinning bar when the biceps contracted? The biceps would still flex the elbow but now the humerus would move towards the insertion. This is because the proximal bone, which is usually more stable, has become more movable. This is termed as the **reversal of muscle action.**

Clinical correlation

Almost every muscle can work with its apparent origin and insertion reversed. For example, the latissimus dorsi is inserted into the floor of the intertubular groove at the upper end of the humerus and is usually described as an adductor and medial rotator of the arm. But if the arm is fixed, the insertion of the muscle will act as the origin and the muscle becomes most important to the patients shifting their position in bed by placing their hands on the bed and lifting the pelvis to the new position.

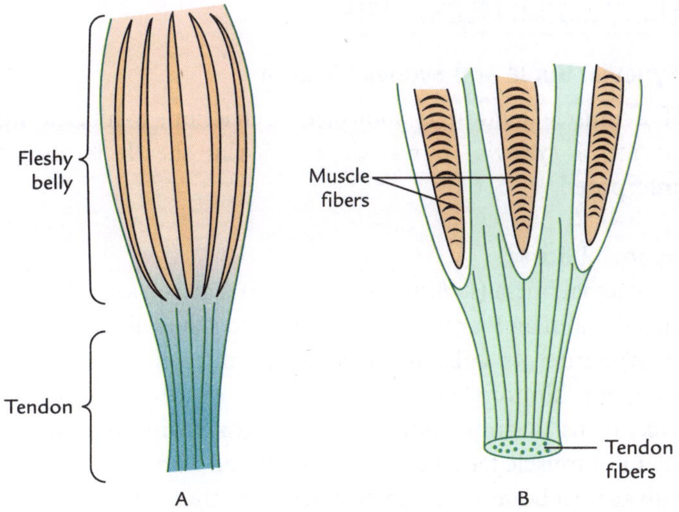

Fig. 9.10 Myotendinous junction: **A,** contiguity of muscle fibers with tendon fibers; **B,** dove-tail type of junction between belly and tendon.

Two Parts

It refers to: (a) a thickened fleshy part called **belly** and (b) a cord- or a rope-like fibrous part called **tendon.**

The word 'muscle' is derived from the Latin word *musculus,* which means little mouse (mus). This is probably due to the fact that some muscles bear fancied resemblance to mice with fleshy part representing the body and tendon representing the tail.

The **belly** is the contractile part and is generally attached to the bone that is proximal to the bone that is to be moved. It is highly vascular with higher metabolic rate. It cannot withstand pressure or friction.

The **tendon** spans the joint and is attached to the bone that is to be moved. When tendon is flattened, it is called *aponeurosis.*

At the myotendinous junction (Fig. 9.10),

(a) the connective tissue framework of muscle belly becomes continuous with connective tissue framework of the tendon and
(b) the muscles fibers of muscle belly are contiguous but not continuous with tendon fibers.

This arrangement at the myotendinous junction resembles the '**dove-tail-arrangement**'.

Tendons

Salient features of tendons are as follows:

1. The tendon is a cord-like structure, formed by dense regular connective tissue that connects the muscle belly to the periosteum of the bone.
2. It functions to transfer the force of contraction from muscle across the joint and on to the bone that is to be moved.
3. The flattened sheets of tendons are called **aponeurosis.**
4. The blood supply of tendon is derived from two sources: (i) from the vessels of its own muscle and (ii) from the periosteal vessels of the bone to which it is attached.
5. In many situations where the tendons are subjected to friction, a lubricating device, a **synovial bursa** or a **synovial sheath** is interposed to enable them to move freely. The synovial sheath consists of two layers: a visceral layer that covers the tendon itself and a parietal layer. The two layers are separated by a thin film of synovial fluid.
6. The tendons serve to withstand pressure. The tendons are immensely strong, e.g. a tendon whose cross-sectional area is 6 cm is capable of supporting a weight of 4000 to 8000 kg.
7. The tendons are supplied by sensory nerve endings; the Golgi tendon organs are those which play a role in tendon reflex.

Clinical correlation

- **Rupture of tendons:** If the tendon of a muscle is severed or ruptured, the muscle becomes ineffective. To assess the integrity of a tendon, one must know the site of its insertion and the movement that contraction of its muscle would normally produce.
- The tendons are ruptured by direct trauma especially when they are weakened by rubbing over a fractured callus or the osteophytes, a new bone produced by arthritis. The tendon of biceps brachii, the Achilles tendon and various tendons in the hands are the ones most often ruptured.
- The tendons have poor blood supply, so if ruptured does not heal itself. Hence, surgical reconstruction is generally needed for the treatment of severed tendon.

LUBRICATING MECHANISMS

Synovial Bursa and Synovial Sheath

If a muscle tendon is subjected to friction, a lubricating device, a synovial bursa; or a synovial sheath is always interposed.

Synovial Bursa

A synovial bursa (L. *bursa* = a purse) is a closed sac differentiated out of areloar tissue. It is similar to synovial membrane in structure. Its walls are separated from each other merely by a thin film of slippery fluid. The bursa, a lubricating device, helps in diminishing friction and allowing free movement of muscle tendons. They are formed whenever tendons rub against bone, cartilage, ligament, or other tendons; hence they are commonest in the limbs. They are also found close to the joints where skin rubs against underlying bony structures, e.g. the *prepatellar bursa* occasionally bursa communicates with the joint cavity, *viz. suprapatellar bursa.*

Types of Bursae

The bursae are of the following three types (Fig. 9.11):

1. Subtendinous
2. Articular
3. Subcutaneous

Subtendinous bursa intervenes between tendon and bone, tendon and ligament, or between two adjacent tendons. Most of synovial bursae of the limbs belong to this type.

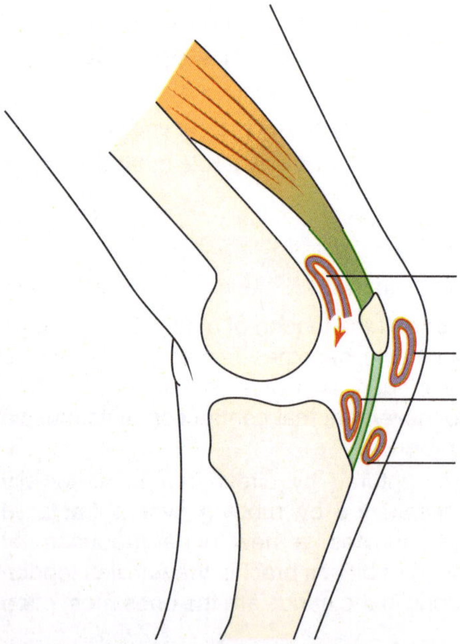

Fig. 9.11 Bursae related to the knee joint. Note that the suprapatellar communicates with the cavity of knee joint.

Articular bursa subserves the function of a joint, e.g. the bursa between the dens of axis (second cervical vertebra) and transverse ligament of atlas (first cervical vertebra).

Subcutaneous bursa intervenes between the skin and bony prominence near the joints, e.g. prepatellar (housemaid's bursa) and superficial infrapatellar bursa (Clergyman's bursa)

N.B.

Subdeltoid/subacromial bursa is the largest synovial bursa in the body.

Clinical correlation

- **Bursitis:** The synovial bursa is commonly inflamed leading to swelling and pain. This clinical condition is called *bursitis*.
- **Adventitious bursa:** Sometimes *adventitious bursa* are formed from tissue spaces of loose areolar tissue subjected to continuous pressure and friction producing clinical conditions. For examples:
  (a) *Porter's shoulder*: The formation of bursa between clavicle and skin in porters.
  (b) *Tailor's ankle*: The formation of bursa between lateral malleolus and skin in tailors

Synovial Sheaths (Fig. 9.12 A, B and C)

When tendons pass through the fibrous bands/osseofibrous tunnels, they are surrounded by **synovial sheaths**. The synovial sheath extends 1 cm on either side of the site of friction. The tendon invaginates the bursa from one side so that the tendon becomes suspended within the bursa by a **mesotendon**. The mesotendon enables blood vessels to enter the tendon. Thus, structurally, the synovial sheath is made up of two concentric layers (parietal and visceral) of synovial membrane. The two layers are separated by a capillary film of synovial fluid, where the range of movement is excessive, the mesotendon either disappears completely, or may be reduced to narrow cords, *viz.* **vinicula** of digital synovial sheaths around the long flexor tendons of the fingers and toes.

BLOOD SUPPLY

The muscle cells have high rate of metabolic activity, hence require extensive vascularity to receive nutrients and oxygen and to eliminate waste products:

1. Small muscles are generally supplied by a single artery and perhaps two veins to return the blood.
2. Large muscles are usually supplied by several arteries and veins.

N.B.

The microscopic capillary exchange between arteries and veins occurs throughout the endomysium that surrounds the individual muscle fibers.

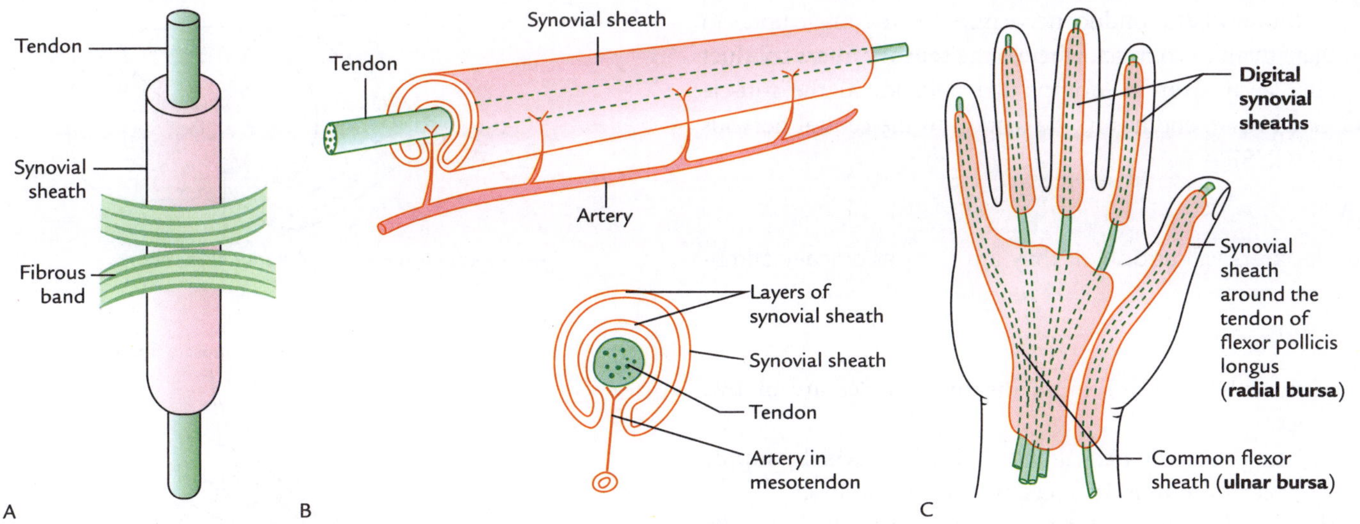

Fig. 9.12 Synovial sheath: **A**, synovial sheath around a tendon passing underneath a fibrous band; **B**, invagination of synovial sheath by a tendon and blood vessels reaching the tendon through mesotendons; **C**, synovial sheath around the long flexor tendons of the fingers.

> **Clinical correlation**
>
> **Stiffness of muscles:** The feeling of stiffness, the day after the strenuous exercise is due to the strain on muscle fibers and the accumulation of lactic acid within the muscle. The *lactic acid* is the waste product of metabolism and is removed by the venous flow from the muscle. If the individual is in a good physical condition, the lactic acid is readily removed and he/she does not suffer from *stiffness.*

Classification of Muscles According to Vascular Pedicles

Muscles are classified into five types according to number of vascular pedicles which enter the muscle and their relative dominance.

- Type I
- Type II
- Type III
- Type IV
- Type V

Type I: These muscles possess a single vascular pedicle, e.g. tensor fascia latae (supplied by ascending branch of the lateral circumflex femoral artery, and gastrocnemius supplied by the sural artery).

Type II: These muscles possess a single dominant vascular pedicle and several minor vascular pedicles, e.g. gracilis (supplied by medical circumflex artery in the dominant pedicle).

Type III: These muscles possess two separate dominant pedicles from different source arteries, e.g. rectus abdominis (supplied by superior and inferior gastric arteries) and gluteus maximus (supplied by superior and inferior gluteal arteries).

Type IV: These muscles possess multiple small vascular pedicles which in isolation are not capable of supplying the entire muscle, e.g. sartorius and tibialis anterior.

Type V: These muscles possess one dominant vascular pedicle and multiple secondary segmental pedicles, e.g. latissimus dorsi (supplied by thoraco-dorsal artery as the dominant pedicle while thoraco-lumbar artery, perforators from lower six posterior intercostal arteries, and lumbar arteries as the secondary segmental supply). The pectoralis major (supplied by pectoral branch of thoraco-acromial trunk as the dominant pedicle and anterior perforators from internal thoracic artery as segmental supply).

> **Clinical correlation**
>
> **Muscle graft:** The classification of muscles according to their blood supply has important surgical relevance in determining which muscles will survive when used as grafting in plastic and reconstructive surgery.

NERVE SUPPLY

Nerves enter the muscles at one or more **neurovascular hila** (Fig. 9.9) which are fairly constant in location. The knowledge of location of these hila is important to physiotherapists since they are the points at which cardiac stimulation of the nerve is most effective.

Generally, the nerve supplying the muscle is called **motor nerve** but strictly speaking it is mixed nerve, i.e. it contains both motor and sensory fibers.

The **motor fibers** conduct nerve impulses to muscle fibers to stimulate them to contract, whereas the **sensory fibers** conduct impulses away from neuromuscular spindles in the muscle and Golgi nerve endings in the tendon to the central nervous system (CNS).

N.B.

Muscle fibers will atrophy if they are not periodically stimulated to contract.

Further details:

1. Motor fibers (60%) supplying the muscles are of two types:
   (a) *Large myelinated alpha (α) fibers* which supply extrafusal muscle fibers of muscle spindles.
   (b) *Small myelinated gamma (γ) fibers* which supply intrafusal fibers of muscle spindles.
2. Sensory fibers (40%) supplying the muscles are of two types:
   (a) *Myelinated fibers* carrying proprioceptive sensations from muscle spindles and tendons.
   (b) *Nonmyelinated fibers* carrying exteroceptive (pain, touch and temperature) sensations.

The relative size of the nerve supplying a muscle depends upon the size of the motor units in that muscle.

Motor Point

It is the point of entry of nerve trunk into the muscle. The nerves mostly enter the muscles from their deep surfaces with few exceptions such as long thoracic nerve supplies serratus anterior muscle from its superficial surface. The motor points corresponds to **neurovascular hila**.

Motor Unit (Fig. 9.13)

A motor unit consists of a single motor neuron (as anterior horn cell), its axon and all the muscle fibers that it supplies.

The muscles that have precise and accurately controlled action, *viz.* extraocular muscles, have smaller motor units with an innervation ratio of 1:10. But muscles that have generalized functions (gross body movements), such as those in gluteal region and thigh, have very large motor units with an innervation ratio exceeding 1:500.

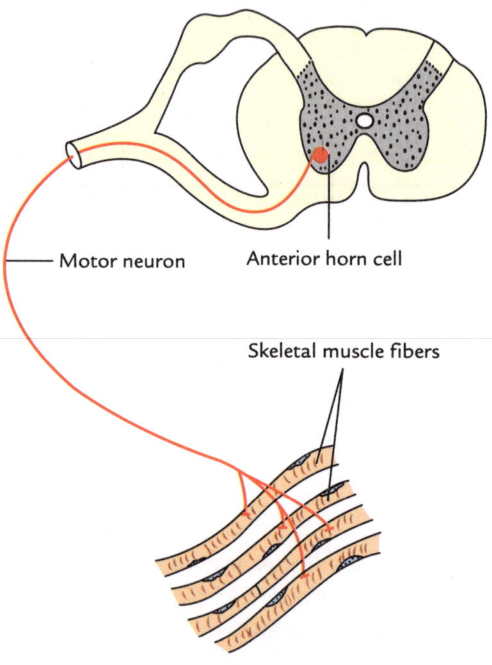

Fig. 9.13 Motor unit. It consists of a single motor neuron and all the muscle fibers that it innervates. Most muscles have an innervation ratio of one motor neuron per 100–150 muscle fibers. Muscles capable of precise movements have an innervation ratio of 1:10, whereas muscles responsible for gross body movement have an innervation ratio exceeding 1:500.

Neuromuscular Junction (Myoneural Junction, [Fig. 9.14])

The junction between the terminal end of axon (motor end plate) and sarcolemma of a muscle fiber (sole plate) is called **neuromuscular junction**.

When a motor nerve penetrates a muscle, it divides into number of branches or axons. The terminal end of axon contacts the sarcolemma of muscle fiber (the axon may branch to serve a number of muscle fibers).

Motor End Plate

It is the expanded terminal end of axon (also called presynaptic terminal). It is not covered by Schwann sheath as the terminal part of nerve fiber loses myelin sheath and Schwann sheath spreads over the surface of the sarcolemma.

The synaptic terminal contains numerous small synaptic vesicles containing neurotransmitter called **acetylcholine (Ach)**.

Sole Plate

The sarcoplasm underneath the sarcolemma (which is in contact with motor end plate) contains many muscle nuclei and mitochondria and forms the sole plate. The sarcolemma is thrown into numerous folds forming subneural clefts.

Synaptic Cleft (Neuromuscular Cleft)

It is a small gap between the plasma membrane of axon terminal (presynaptic membrane) and plasma membrane of sarcolemma (postsynaptic membrane).

Mechanism of Transmission of Impulse

As the nerve impulse reaches the axon terminal, it causes the release of acetylcholine into the synaptic cleft of the neuromuscular junction which soon binds with the receptors on the postsynaptic membrane leading to its depolarization (i.e. production of an action potential) and, consequently, the muscle contracts. As the action potential is produced, acetylcholine is immediately destroyed by an enzyme called acetylcholinesterase present in high concentration on the motor end plate.

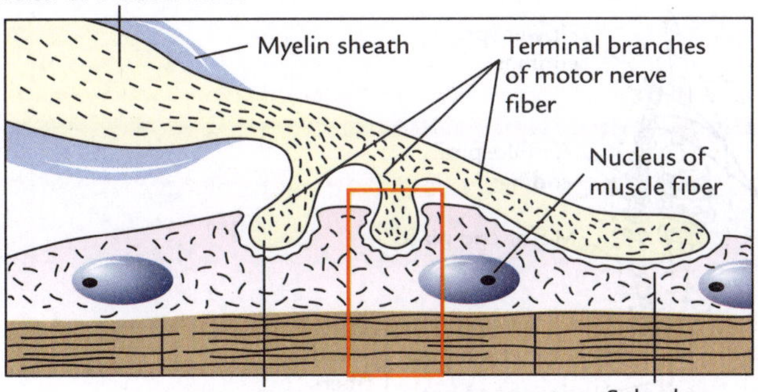

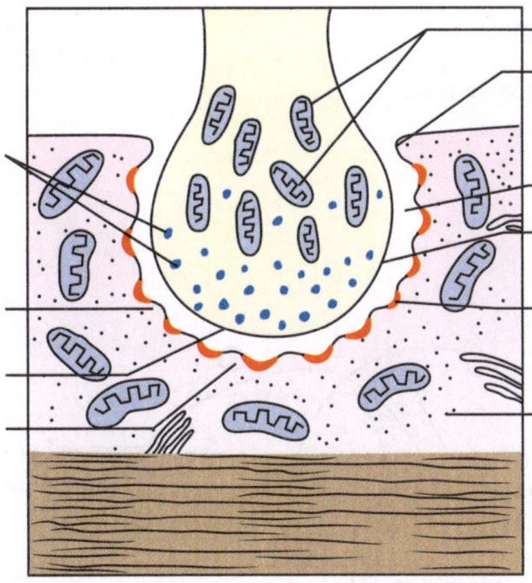

Fig. 9.14 Neuromuscular junction: **A,** site where nerve fiber and muscle fiber meet; **B,** showing motor end plate and sole plate (the motor end plate is the specialized portion of the terminal end of axon; the sole plate is the sarcolemma and underlying sarcoplasm).

Clinical correlation

- When a nerve fiber is cut, the nerve terminal degenerates but *sole plate* persists for a year or so. When the nerve fiber regenerates, a new *motor end plate* is formed.
- In *organophosphorus poisoning* (a commonly ingested poison to commit suicide), the organophosphates bind with and inhibit the action of AchE; as a result the Ach is not destroyed in the synaptic cleft, leading to continuous production of action potential and contraction of muscles, *viz.*, respiratory muscles. Consequently, there occurs spastic paralysis of respiratory muscles and death.
- *Myasthenia gravis* results from production of autoimmune antibodies that bind to acetylcholine receptors on postsynaptic membrane and destroy them, thus reducing their number. Therefore, when they are activated by the acetylcholine, the muscle cannot contract properly and exhibit a degree of flaccid paralysis.
- The acetylcholine receptors are also blocked by a poison called *curare*. Fortunately, curare is not a common poison to which people are exposed.

MUSCLE RECEPTORS

Neuromuscular Spindles (Muscle Spindles)

These are spindle-shaped sensory end organs within the skeletal muscles which provide sensory information to the CNS to control the tone of the muscle (Fig. 9.15).

Each spindle consists of a bundle of small specialized skeletal muscle fibers, surrounded by a fusiform connective tissue capsule. These fibers are called **intrafusal fibers.** The unspecialized muscle fibers outside the spindle are called **extrafusal fibers.**

The intrafusal muscle fibers are of two types: **nuclear chain fibers** and **nuclear bag fibers.** In nuclear chain fibers, the nuclei form a single longitudinal chain in the central unexpanded part, whereas in the nuclear bag fibers, nuclei are aggregated in the central expanded region.

The extrafusal fibers are supplied by large alpha (α) motor fibers, whereas intrafusal fibers are supplied by small gamma (γ) motor fibers.

The sensory innervation of the muscle spindle is by two types of sensory nerve endings:

1. Annulospiral
2. Flower spray

The **annulospiral nerve** endings wind spirally the central nuclear region of the intrafusal muscle fibers.

The **flower spray nerve endings** terminate at the ends of the intrafusal fibers away from the central nuclear region, resembling a spray of the flowers.

N.B.

The nuclear bag fibers are thicker and longer than the nuclear chain fibers and project beyond the spindle-shaped fibrous capsule to be attached with the extrafusal connective tissue.

Stretch Reflex

When the muscle is stretched, the intrafusal muscle fibers are elongated, thus stimulating the sensory nerve endings around them. The sensory nerve fibers carrying the information synapse with alpha (α) motor neuron, which in turn causes quick contraction of stretched muscle fibers (the stretch reflex) thus reducing tension in the intrafusal fibers (Fig. 9.16).

N.B.

- The muscle spindles regulate the degree and rate of contraction of extrafusal fibers.
- The stretch reflex is used by clinicians to elicit the tendon jerks.

Golgi Tendon Organs (Neurotendinous Spindles)

These are sensory organs located near the musculotendinous junctions. They monitor the tension produced on tendon during muscle contraction and prevents its damage from excessive stresses put on it.

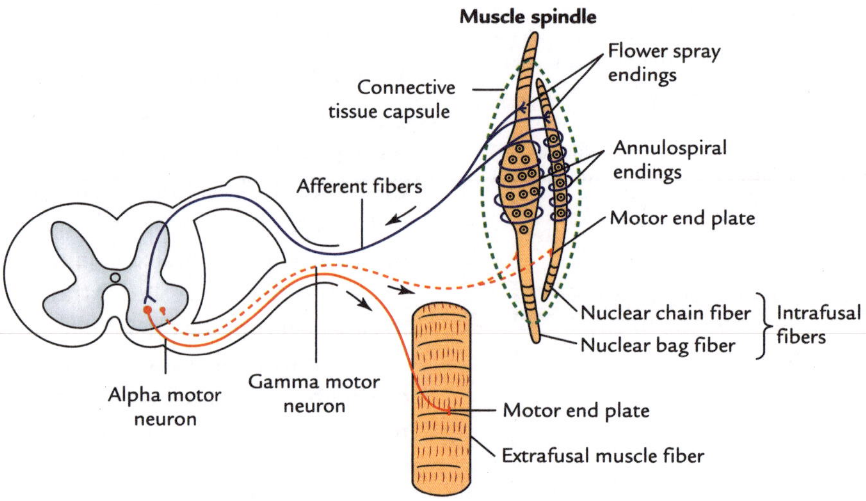

Fig. 9.15 Schematic structure of neuromuscular spindle and its nerve supply.

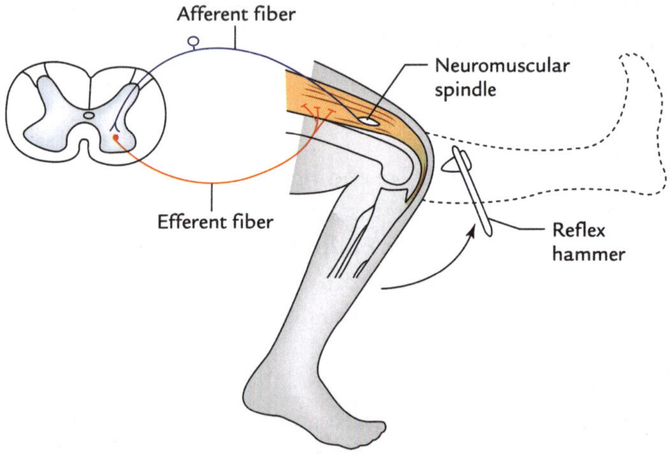

Fig. 9.16 Stretch reflex.

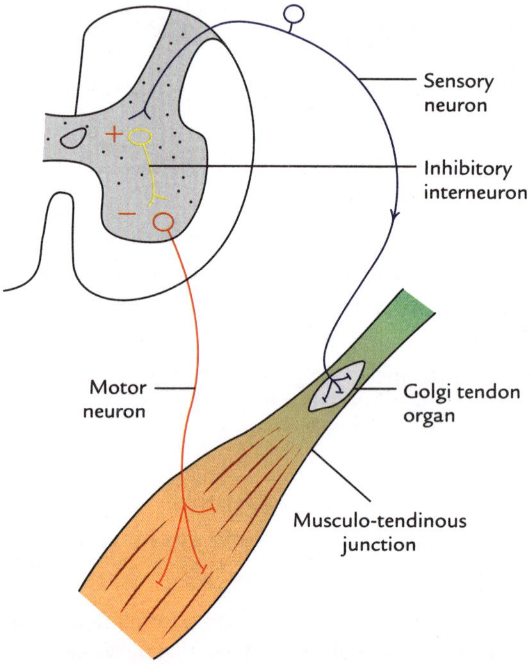

Fig. 9.17 Golgi tendon organ reflex. The Golgi tendon organ gives rise to afferents which end on an inhibitory interneuron. This reflex inhibits contraction in the same muscle.

The neurotendinous spindle is spindle-shaped, consisting of loosely arranged collagen fibers surrounded by a fibrous capsule. The collagen fibers (also called **intrafusal tendon fibers**) are innervated by myelinated nerve fibers which lose their myelin sheath before piercing the capsule of the spindle and terminate in club-shaped endings.

Clinical correlation

When the collagen fibers (intrafusal tendon fibers) within the neurotendinous spindle are stretched, the sensory fibers carrying this information stimulate inhibitory interneurons that synapse with Alpha-1 motor neurons, which in turn cause relaxation of muscles to which the particular tendon is attached. This is termed as *Golgi tendon organ reflex* (Fig. 9.17). The opposing actions of neuromuscular spindles (excitatory) and neurotendinous spindles (inhibitory) are in balance during stretch reflex activity.

SEGMENTAL INNERVATION OF MUSCLES

Most of the skeletal muscles are supplied by more than one spinal segments (hence more than one spinal nerves).

It is important to note the following facts regarding segmental innervations:

1. Most of muscles are supplied by two spinal segments (the intrinsic muscles of hand are unisegmental).
2. Muscles sharing a common primary action are supplied by the same spinal segments, and the antagonist muscles

(i.e. opposing primary action) are supplied by same number of spinal segments but one segment lower **en block**.

For example, the muscles flexing the elbow joint are supplied by C5 and C6 spinal segments, and muscles extending the elbow joint are supplied by C7 and C8 spinal segments.

It is neither necessary nor possible to remember the segmental innervation of all the muscles but students should remember the segmental innervation of muscles which are tested clinically by eliciting tendon jerks in patients.

The segmental innervation of these muscles is given in Table 9.4.

Clinical correlation

Paralysis of muscles: The loss of motor power, i.e. power to produce movements is called *paralysis*. It occurs due to damage of motor pathway consisting of upper and lower motor neurons. Damage of upper motor neurons causes *spastic paralysis* with exaggerated tendon jerks whereas damage of lower motor neurons causes *flaccid paralysis* with loss of tendon jerks.

ACTION OF MUSCLES

When muscle contracts, it brings about a movement. The range of movement depends on the length of fibers in the fleshy part and power generated during contraction.

Muscle Tone

It refers to the constant tension produced by muscles for long periods of time. Muscle tone is responsible for keeping our back and leg straight. The muscle tone is maintained by a small percentage of motor units. The motor units that are contracting are stimulated in such a way that tension produced in a muscle remains constant.

N.B.

The same motor units are not contracting all the time.

Length–Tension Relationship in Muscles

The tension refers to the force built-up within the muscle, which is necessary for a muscle to contract. Stretching a muscle builds up tension within the muscle which is released when the muscle contracts.

A muscle is capable of being shortened to one-half of its normal resting length. Also the muscle can be stretched twice as far as it can be shortened. The excursion of a muscle is the distance between maximum elongation and maximum shortening (Fig. 9.18). The action of muscle is strongest when it is slightly stretched.

Types of Muscle Contraction

Muscle contractions are of the following types:

1. **Isometric contractions:** In isometric contractions, the length of muscle does not change, but tension does increase, e.g. holding the arm outstretched.
2. **Isotonic contractions:** In isotonic contractions, the amount of tension produced by the muscle is constant during contraction, but the length of muscle changes. The length of muscle is reduced by one-third or more, e.g. movements of fingers and hands.
3. **Concentric contractions:** The muscle produces increasing tension as it shortens. A large percentage of movements produced by muscle contractions are concentric contractions.
4. **Eccentric contractions:** In eccentric contractions the tension is maintained in muscle while muscle increases in length, e.g. lowering the arm to the side of body.

Table 9.4 Segmental innervation of muscles commonly used for eliciting tendon jerks/reflexes

Muscle	Segmental innervation	Tendon jerk
Biceps brachii	C5, C6 (musculo-cutaneous nerve)	Biceps jerk (flexion of elbow by tapping the tendon of biceps brachii)
Triceps brachii	C7, C8 (radial nerve)	Triceps jerk (extension of elbow joint by tapping the tendon of triceps brachii)
Brachio-radialis (supinator longus)	C5, C6 (radial nerve)	Supinator jerk (flexion of elbow joint and supination of radio-ulnar joints by tapping the insertion of brachio-radialis tendon)
Quadriceps femoris	L2, L3, L4, ... (femoral nerve)	Knee jerk (extension of knee joint by tapping the tendon of quadriceps femoris)
Triceps surae	S1, S2 (tibial nerve)	Ankle jerk (plantar flexion of ankle joint by tapping the Achilles tendon)

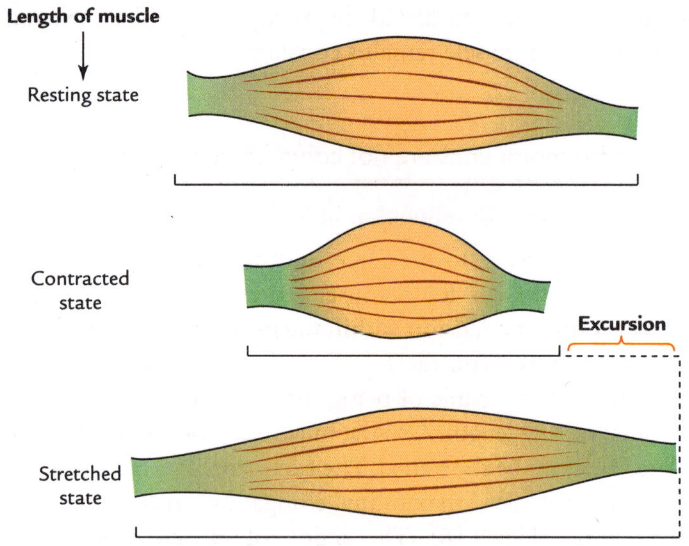

Fig. 9.18 Excursion of muscle.

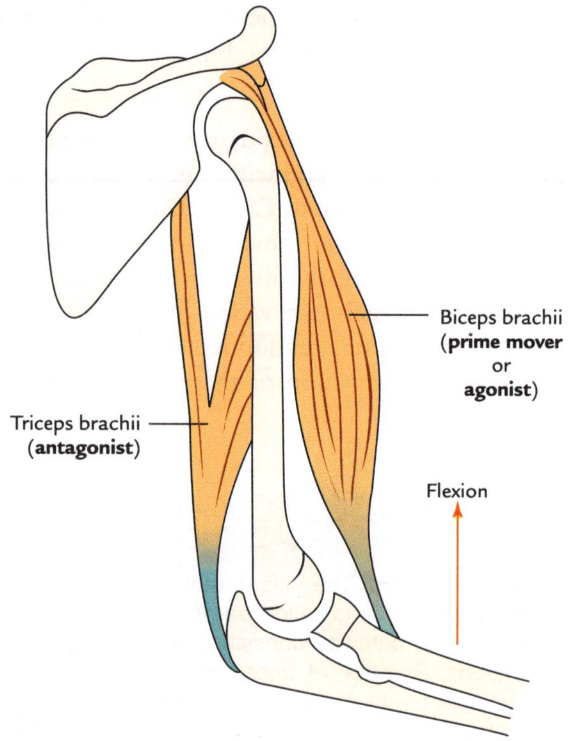

Fig. 9.19 Diagram to show prime mover and antagonist muscles. For flexion at elbow biceps brachii muscle acts as the prime mover, whereas triceps brachii acts as antagonist. (At the same joint, during extension, triceps acts as a prime mover and biceps acts as an antagonist.)

Active and Passive Insufficiency of Muscles

In muscles acting on one joint, the excursion of muscle will be greater than the range of motion allowed by the joint. However, for muscles acting on two or more joints, the muscle excursion is less than the combined range of motion allowed by the joints.

Active insufficiency: When muscle reaches a point where it cannot shorten further, it is termed as **active insufficiency**. It occurs in the agonist muscle that is contracting.

Passive insufficiency: When muscle cannot be elongated any farther without damage to its fibers, it is termed as **passive insufficiency**. It occurs in the antagonist muscle that is relaxed during a movement and is on the opposite side of a joint.

Think of how much you are hurt when slapped with a loose and stretched hand by a teacher.

Group Action of Muscles

With a few exceptions, a single muscle does not contract alone. Whole movement rather than individual muscles are represented in the cerebral cortex. Therefore, each movement requires contraction or relaxation of a whole group of muscles.

Further, each movement is brought about by a coordinated activity of different group of muscles. These muscle groups are classified according to the role played by them in the occurrence of a particular action:

1. **Prime movers (agonists):** These muscles are primarily responsible for producing a desired movement, e.g. biceps brachii is acting as a **prime mover** when it produces flexion at the elbow joint. Prime movers simply bring the insertion near its origin (Fig. 9.19).
2. **Antagonists:** An antagonist is the muscle which is able to produce movement opposite to a prime mover. Usually, however, the two muscles **agonist** and **antagonist** act in unison so that when the prime mover contracts, its antagonist undergoes a simultaneous relaxation. In this way, an accurate controlled movement is carried out, e.g. in flexion of elbow, the biceps acts as a prime mover while triceps 'pays out' and acts as an **antagonist** (Fig. 9.19). These muscles reverse role, of course, in extension of elbow.

N.B.

This is possible due to reciprocal innervation of opposite group of muscles regulated by the spinal cord through the stretch reflex.

3. **Fixators:** A muscle is said to act as a **fixator** when it contracts to stabilize the origin of the prime mover so that it can act efficiently, e.g. the muscles attaching the shoulder girdle to the trunk contract as fixators to allow the deltoid to act on the shoulder joint to produce abduction.
4. **Synergists:** When the prime mover crosses more than one joint to reach the joint where its main action takes

place, the undesired movement at the proximal joint is prevented by certain muscles known as **synergists**, e.g. the long flexors of fingers crossover the wrist joint and can flex it but this movement is disadvantageous if it is desired to clench the fist. The extensors of the wrist, therefore, contract as **synergists** to prevent wrist flexion (Fig. 9.20).

These terms are applied for a particular muscle during a particular movement. Many muscles can act as prime mover, an antagonist, a fixator or a synergist depending upon the movement to be accomplished.

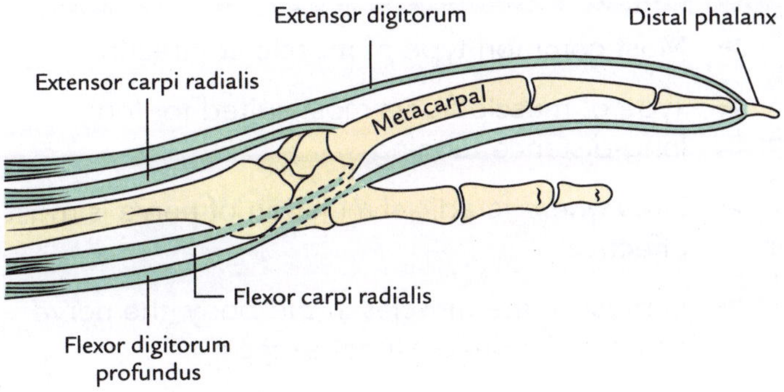

Fig. 9.20 The flexor and extensor muscles of corpus act as synergists to stabilize corpus so that long flexor and extensor of hand can flex and extend fingers.

Golden Facts to Remember

➢ Total number of muscles in the body	About 400
➢ All the muscles of body develop from mesenchyme *except*	Arrector pili, muscles of iris and myoepithelial cells which develop from ectoderm
➢ Largest muscle in the body	Gluteus maximus
➢ Longest muscle in the body	Sartorius
➢ Smallest muscle in the body	Stapedius
➢ Most important property of a muscle	Contractility
➢ Most abundant muscles type in the body	Skeletal muscles
➢ Functional contractile unit of a muscle	Motor unit
➢ Functional unit of a muscle fiber	Sarcomere
➢ Most variable muscle in the body	Palmaris longus (in the forearm)
➢ Longest tendon in the body	Plantaris (in the leg)
➢ Largest tendon in the body	Achilles tendon (tendo-calcaneus)
➢ Most important reflex for maintaining the health of a muscle	Stretch reflex
➢ Most commonly used muscle for intramuscular injection	Deltoid (in shoulder region)
➢ Muscles with smallest motor unit	Extraocular muscles
➢ Muscles with largest motor unit	Muscles of lower limb; e.g. gluteus maximus
➢ Most common involuntary movements of skeletal muscles	Myokymia
➢ Most commonly ruptured tendon in the body	Tendo-calcaneus
➢ Most differentiated muscle in the body	Cardiac muscle
➢ All the muscle need nerve stimulus to contract *except*	Cardiac muscle which can contract without nerve stimulus (myogenic contraction)

Continued

➢ Most common type of muscle contraction	Concentric contractions
➢ Type of muscle fibers most suited for long long-distance running	Slow-twitch fibers (red-fibers)
➢ Sites where faradic stimulation of nerve is most effective	Nerve points
➢ In most of the muscles in the body, the nerve enters in its deep aspect except	Serratus anterior in which the nerve enters in its superficial aspect
➢ Skeletal muscle can repair themselves to some extent	Due to proliferation of satellite cells which fuse to form new skeletal muscle fibers
➢ Damaged cardiac muscle (e.g. myocardial infarction) is replaced by fibrous tissue, because	Cardiac muscle repair (regeneration) is nonexistent for it does not contain satellite cells
➢ Type of muscle with highest regenerative capacity	Smooth muscle

Multiple Choice Questions

1. **The skeletal muscle presents all of the following features *except:***
   (a) Its fibers present cross-striations
   (b) Its fibers are unbranched and multinucleated
   (c) Its actions are involuntary
   (d) It possesses stretch receptors

2. **All of the following muscles have pennate fasciculi *except:***
   (a) Flexor pollicis longus
   (b) Flexor hallucis longus
   (c) Deltoid
   (d) Trapezius

3. **Regarding stretch reflex, all of the following statements are true *except:***
   (a) It is monosynaptic reflex
   (b) It involves alpha (α) motor neuron
   (c) It is used to elicit tendon jerks
   (d) It regulates the rate of contraction of intrafusal fibers

4. **In the movement of flexing the elbow joint, the biceps brachii acts as:**
   (a) Synergist
   (b) Antagonist
   (c) Fixator
   (d) Prime mover

5. **All of the following features, regarding red muscle fibers, are true *except:***
   (a) Speed of contraction is slow
   (b) Are fatigue resistant
   (c) Have few mitochondria
   (d) Have high glycogen content

6. **The muscles capable of highly dextrous movements contain:**
   (a) One motor unit per muscles fiber
   (b) Many muscle fibers per motor unit
   (c) Few muscle fibers per motor unit
   (d) Many motor units per muscle fiber

7. **Select the *incorrect statement* about the tendon:**
   (a) It attaches the muscle belly to the periosteum of bone
   (b) It is made of dense regular connective tissue
   (c) It serves to support the weight
   (d) It heals quickly if ruptured

8. **In clenching the fist, which of the following muscles acts as synergists:**
   (a) Flexors of the wrist
   (b) Extensors of the wrist
   (c) Adductors of the wrist
   (d) Abductors of the wrist

Answers

1. c, **2.** d, **3.** d, **4.** d, **5.** c, **6.** a, **7.** d, **8.** b

CHAPTER 10

Cardiovascular System

Learning Objectives

After studying this chapter, the student should be able to:

- define cardiovascular system and enumerate its functions
- write about blood and its components
- elucidate the structure of the heart and its position within the thorax
- describe the structure and functions of arteries, veins and capillaries
- explain the relationship between different types of blood vessels
- outline the differences between the arteries and veins, and capillaries and sinusoids
- outline the various types of portal circulation and discuss each type of portal circulation in detail
- discuss arteriovenous anastomosis and its functional significance
- describe fetal circulation and tell how it is different from adult circulation

INTRODUCTION

The cardiovascular system consists of heart and blood vessels. The system supplies nutrients to and removes waste products from various tissues of the body. The conveying medium is blood which flows through tubular channels called *blood vessels*. It is thus a closed system and blood in it serves as medium for transportation of various agents such as nutrients, O_2, CO_2, etc.

The heart pumps the blood and provides the major force that causes the blood to circulate, whereas blood vessels carry blood to all the tissues of the body and back to the heart. In addition, the blood vessels participate in the regulation of the blood pressure. The vessels which carry the blood away from the heart are called **arteries** (Fig. 10.1), while the vessels which bring back the blood to the heart are called **veins** (Fig. 10.2).

The microscopic vessels connecting the arteries and veins are called **capillaries**. These vessels allow easy exchange of nutrients, metabolites and respiratory gases (O_2 and CO_2).

FUNCTIONS OF CARDIOVASCULAR SYSTEM

The cardiovascular system perform the following functions:

1. Transports nutrients to different parts of the body.
2. Removes waste products of metabolism from organs and tissues of the body.
3. Is responsible for gaseous exchange in the lungs, i.e. intake of O_2 and elimination of CO_2.
4. Carries hormones and other regulatory molecules from their site of origin to distant target tissues.
5. Helps to protect (by leukocytes and their products) the body from infection.

COMPONENTS OF CARDIOVASCULAR SYSTEM

The cardiovascular system comprises:

1. Blood
2. Heart
3. Blood vessels

BLOOD

Blood is taught in detail in physiology; at the same time, it is important to have some knowledge of blood before discussing the other components of cardiovascular system.

The blood is a highly specialized connective tissue consisting of blood cells and plasma.

Blood Cells

The blood cells are of three types:

1. Erythrocytes
2. Leukocytes
3. Thrombocytes (platelets)

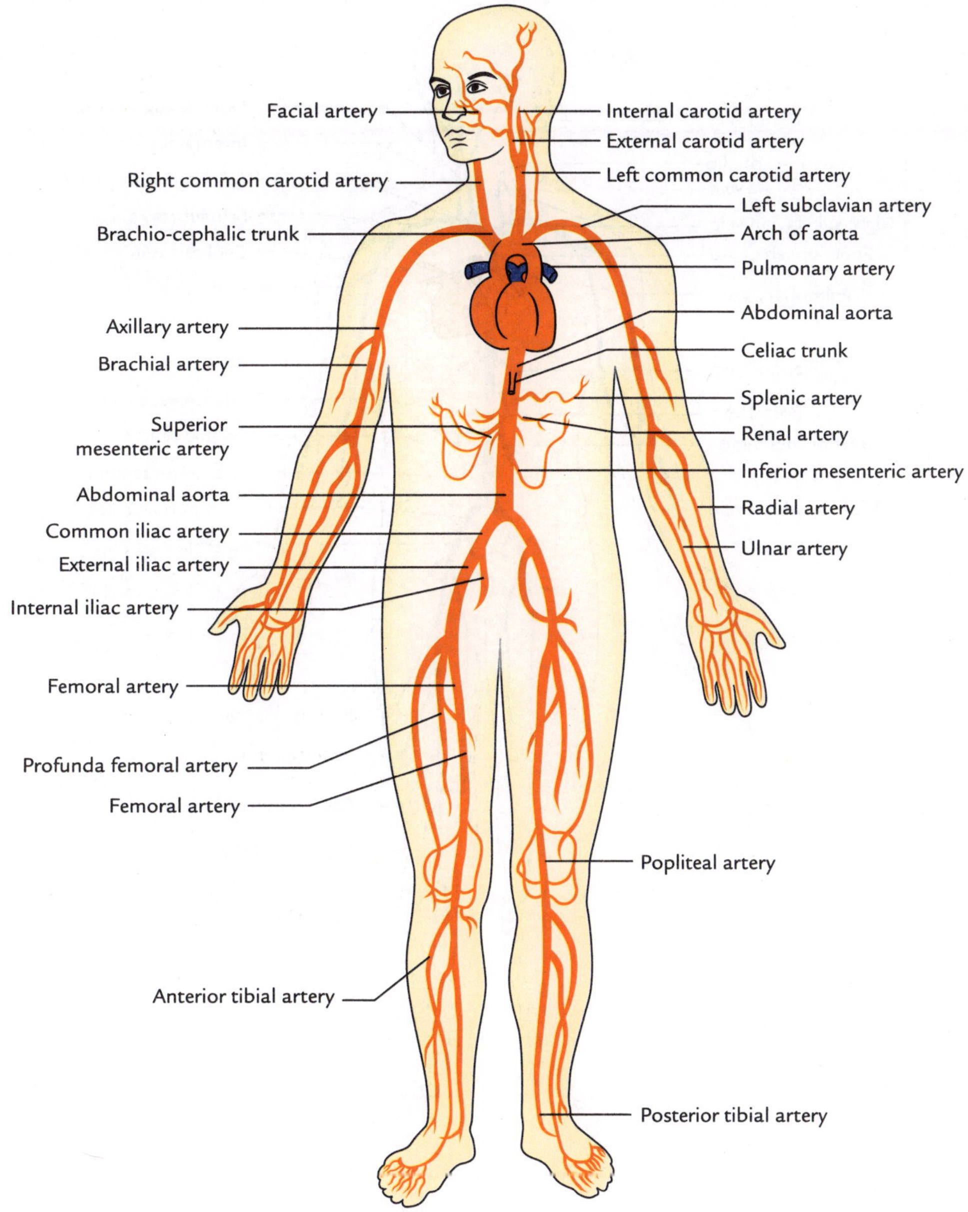

Fig. 10.1 Arteries of the body.

Erythrocytes: The erythrocytes (red blood cells, RBCs) are disc-shaped cells that lack nuclei and mitochondria. They get energy from anaerobic respiration and transport O_2 and CO_2.

Leukocytes: The leukocytes (white blood cells) are of two types:

1. Granulocytes, i.e. they have granules in their cytoplasm.
2. Agranulocytes, i.e. they do not have granules in their cytoplasm.

Types of granulocytes

1. **Neutrophils:** They are called *neutrophils* because their granules have no affinity either to eosin (pink to red) stain or hematoxylin (blue to purple) stain. They have multi-lobed nucleus and play an important role in phagocytosis of bacteria and dead cells; they thus impart natural (innate) immunity. Neutrophils are the first to arrive at an area of tissue damage.
2. **Eosinophils**: They are so called because their granules stain with eosin. They have bilobed nucleus. They play a role in reducing the severity of allergic reaction by secreting **histaminase.** Their level in blood increases in allergic reactions (e.g. eosinophilia).
3. **Basophils**: They are so named because their granules stain blue with hematoxylin. They release anticoagulant heparin, histamine, and 5-hydroxytryptamine. Basophils play a role in the immediate (type I) hypersensitivity reaction (*anaphylactic reactions*) causing allergic rhinitis, asthma, urticaria and anaphylaxis.

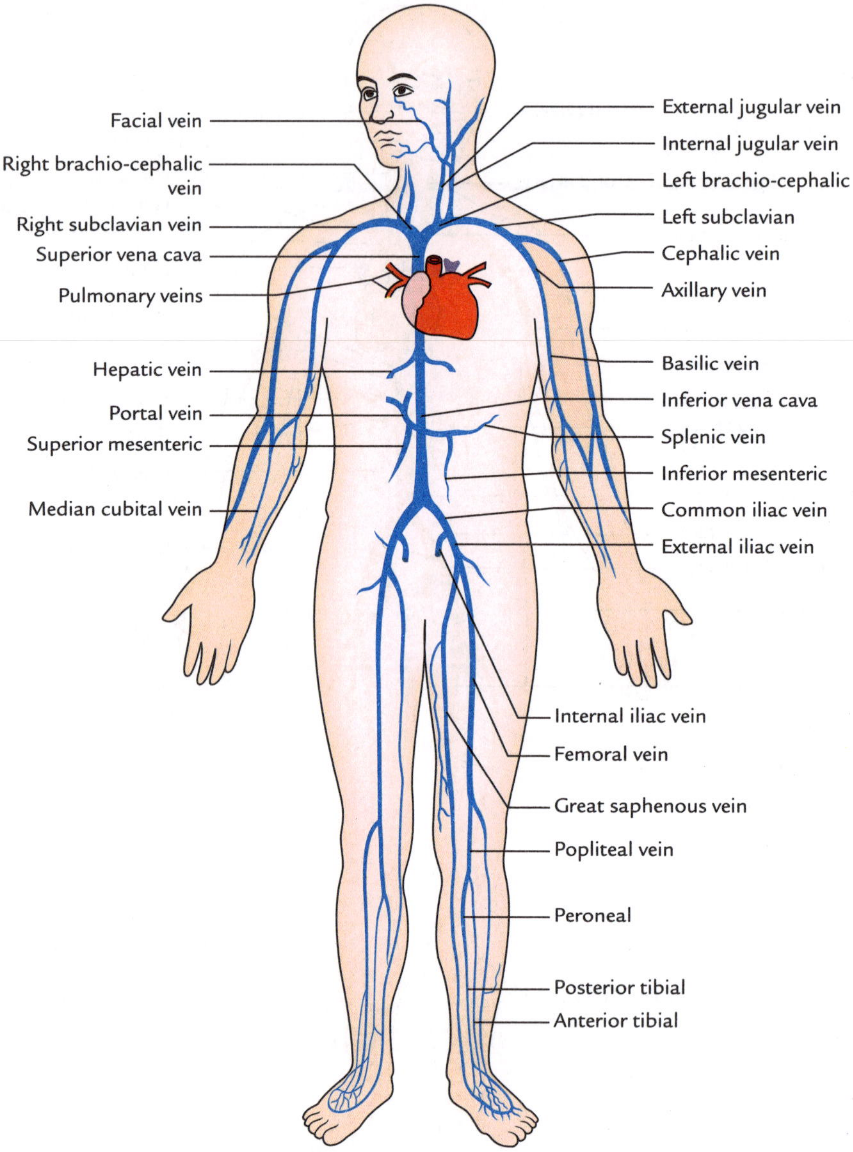

Fig. 10.2 Veins of the body.

Types of agranulocytes

1. **Monocytes:** They are phagocytic cells and member of monocyte macrophage system. They respond to inflammation by leaving the peripheral blood to enter the tissue and are called **macrophages.**
2. **Lymphocytes:** They are only slightly larger than RBCs. The nucleus nearly fills the cells. Lymphocytes are of two types:
   (a) B lymphocytes
   (b) T lymphocytes

B lymphocytes differentiate in bone marrow. In response to antigen, they proliferate and produce plasma cells that secrete immunoglobulins (IgM and IgD). The B cells plasma cells and immunoglobulins are the basis of **humoral response.**

T lymphocytes are the lymphocytes which mature and become immunocompetent in the thymus and then enter the blood to reach the lymph nodes and spleen.

Clinical correlation

Basis of immunization: During fetal development, B lymphocytes differentiate in the bone marrow. Mature (or virgin) cells express antigen specific IgM and IgD on the cell surface. Mature B cells migrate to the spleen, lymph nodes and gut associated lymph tissue and wait for antigen exposure. When exposed to antigens, they differentiate into plasma cells which produce antibodies (immunoglobulins). B cells, plasma cells and immunoglobulins together constitute the *humoral response*.

B memory cells are programmed to react to the same antigen. Upon re-exposure to that antigen, it results in faster immune response called *secondary immune response*.

The immunoglobulins secreted by a B memory cells have higher affinity for antigen than that produced during the initial exposure. This is the basis for *immunization*.

Thrombocytes (platelets): These are in fact the fragments of large cells called **megakaryocytes** found in the bone marrow. The platelets play an important role in blood clotting. They constitute the major portion of the mass of the clot. Platelets that attach together in the blood clot also release a chemical called **serotonin** which causes constriction of blood vessels, thus reducing the flow of blood to the injured area.

Plasma

The plasma is the fluid portion of the blood. Ninety percent of it is made up of water and the remaining is made up of proteins, inorganic salts, lipids, etc.

There are three types of plasma proteins:

1. Albumins
2. Globulins
3. Fibrinogen

Albumins are produced in the liver and provide necessary viscosity to the blood to maintain and regulate the blood pressure.

Globulins are of three types: (a) alpha globulin, (b) beta globulin and (c) gamma globulin. The alpha and beta globulins are synthesized within liver and transport fat- and lipid-soluble vitamins. The gamma globulins are produced in lymphoid tissue and are called **antibodies**. They play an important role in immunity.

Fibrinogen is synthesized in liver and plays an important role along with thrombocytes in clotting of blood.

N.B

If fibrinogen is removed from plasma, it is called *serum*.

Clinical correlation

The blood can also serve to transport disease-causing bacteria, viruses and other toxins. However, drugs given to treat the diseases are also transported through blood.

HEART

The heart is a four-chambered, hollow muscular organ, roughly of the size of a clenched fist. It is situated in the thoracic cavity between the lungs.

About two-third of the heart is located on the left of the midline and one-third on the right of the midline. The heart is enclosed in a serous sac (*serous pericardium*) which in turn is enclosed in a dense fibrous connective tissue called **fibrous pericardium**. The serous pericardium consists of inner visceral and outer parietal layer with a potential cavity between the two layers called **pericardial cavity**. The heart acts as a central muscular pump about 5 L of blood/min. It takes about 1 min for the blood to reach the most distal parts of the body and back to the heart.

Weight of the Heart

- 310 g in adult males
- 255 g in adult females

Wall of the Heart

The wall of the heart consists of three distinct layers. From superficial to deep, these are:

1. **Epicardium**—made up of visceral pericardium.
2. **Myocardium**—made up of cardiac muscle.
3. **Endocardium**—made up of endothelial cells. It is continuous with the endothelial lining of blood vessels.

Chambers of the Heart

The interior of the heart is divided into four chambers: right and left atria and right and left ventricles (Fig. 10.3):

Right and left atria are above and **right and left ventricles** are below. Each atrium has an ear-shaped appendage called an *auricle*.

The atria are separated from each other by interatrial septum while ventricles are separated from each other by interventricular septum.

Base of the Heart

It lies opposite to middle, four thoracic vertebra (i.e. T5 to T8) in supine position. Right one-third of base is formed by right

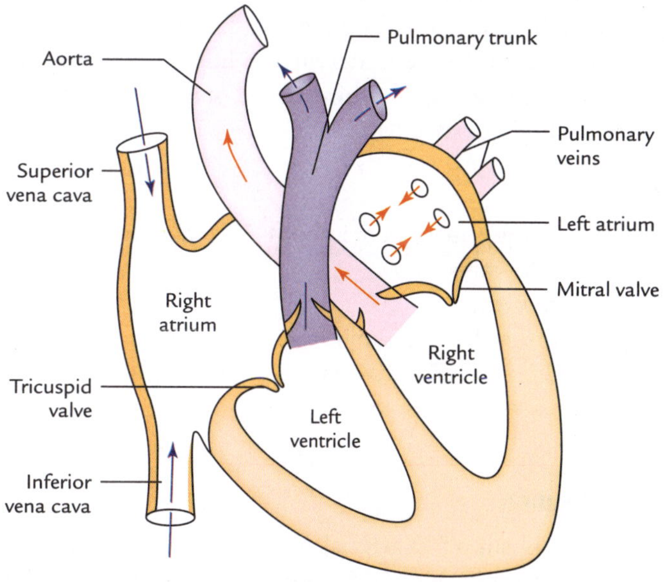

Fig. 10.3 Chambers of the heart.

atrium and left two-third by left atrium. The atria are receiving chambers whereas the ventricles are pumping chambers.

The **right atrium receives the deoxygenated blood** from systemic circulation through the superior and inferior vena cavae. Blood from right atrium passes through right atrioventricular valve (*tricuspid valve*) into the right ventricle. The **left atrium receives the oxygenated blood** from pulmonary circulation through four pulmonary veins. Blood from left atrium passes through left atrio-ventricular valve (mitral valve or bicuspid valve) into the left ventricle.

Right ventricle contracts to pump blood into the lungs through pulmonary trunk and pulmonary arteries. Left ventricle contracts to pump blood into the rest of the body through aorta and its branches.

Apex of the Heart

It is cone-shaped lower and outer end of the heart formed by the left ventricle.

Functions of the Heart

The heart functions as a **double pump** (Fig. 10.4):

1. The right half of the heart receives deoxygenated blood, i.e. blood is low in oxygen and pumps it to the lungs through pulmonary trunk and pulmonary arteries.
2. The left half of the heart receives oxygenated blood, i.e. oxygen-rich blood from the lungs and pumps it to the rest of the body through aorta and its branches.

Thus, heart regulates two circuits of blood flow: pulmonary and systemic.

Apex Beat

When the heart contracts, the thrust of the heart is felt in the left precordium. The outermost and the lowermost thrust on the front of the left half of the chest felt by flat hand is called **apex beat**. In adults, it is felt in the left fifth intercostal space, half inch medial to the midclavicular line. In children, it is felt in the left second or third intercostal space, half inch lateral to the midclavicular line.

N.B.

On an average, heart beats about 70 times in males and 75 times in females.

Normal heart rate

(a) In infants = 130–150/min
(b) In children = 100–130/min
(c) In adults = 60–90/min

Arterial Supply

The heart is supplied arterial blood by the right and left coronary arteries (Fig. 10.5), which arise from ascending aorta immediately above the aortic orifice in the heart. The coronary arteries receive about 5% of blood pumped from the heart, although the heart comprises only a small proportion of body weight. The large blood supply, especially to the left ventricle, is in keeping with the importance of the heart to the body function.

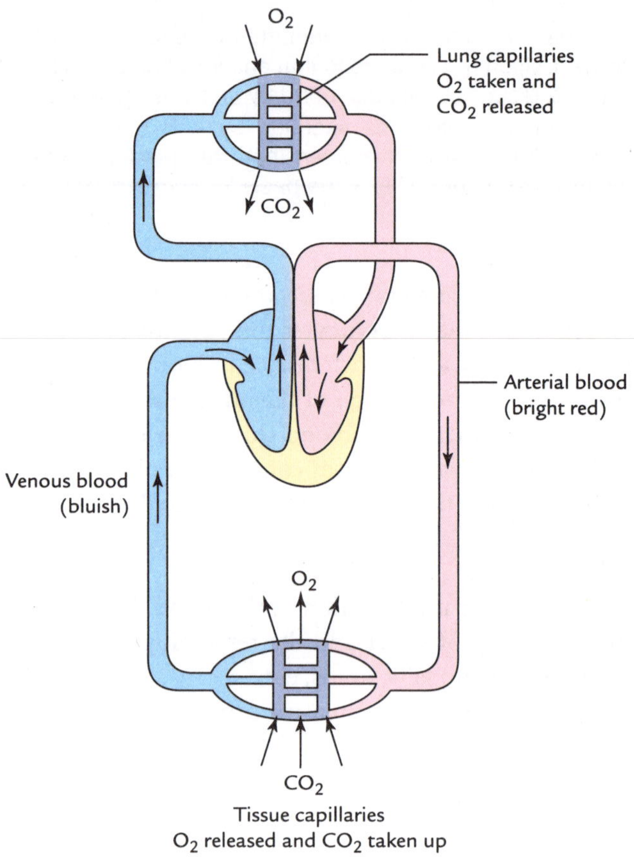

Fig. 10.4 Transport of gases through circulatory system.

N.B.

The coronary arteries are unique in the sense that they are filled during diastole.

Clinical correlation

- **Angina pectoris:** If coronary arteries are narrowed, there will be reduced blood and O_2 supply to cardiac muscle. As a result, individual feels pain in his/her left precordium, medial side of arm and forearm. The pain typically occurs on exertion and relieved by rest. This clinical condition is called *angina pectoris*.
- **Myocardial infarction:** If coronary arteries are blocked, there will be myocardiac ischemia leading to cellular necrosis. This clinical condition is called *myocardial infarction* or *heart attack*. It typically occurs at rest and the pain lasts longer than 10 minutes.
- **Heart attacks:** These are one of the most common cause of death these days. The risk of attack can be minimized by: (a) reducing excess weight, (b) avoiding high blood pressure (hypertension), (c) taking low cholesterol diet, (d) avoiding smoking and (e) doing regular exercises.

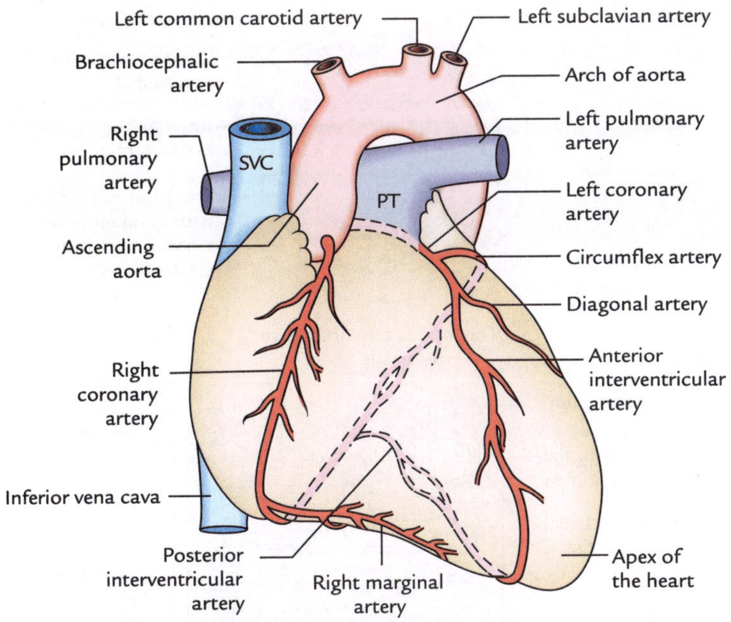

Fig. 10.5 Arterial supply of the heart.

Venous Drainagae

The venous blood from heart is drained into the coronary sinus through great, middle and small cardiac veins, posterior vein of left ventricle, oblique vein of left atrium and right marginal vein. The coronary sinus in turn opens into the right atrium. The other small veins (also called *venae chordae minimae* or *Thebesian veins*) directly drain into the chambers of the heart.

Nerve Supply

The heart is supplied by both sympathetic and parasympathetic fibers. The stimulation of sympathetic fibers results in increase in heart rate and force of contraction of heart rate.

The stimulation of parasympathetic fibers (vagus nerve) results in decrease in heart rate and force of contraction of the heart.

N.B.

All the cardiac branches of sympathetic chain and vagus nerve contain both sensory and motor fibers *except the cardiac branch* from superior cervical sympathetic ganglion, which contain only postganglionic motor nerves.

CONDUCTING SYSTEM OF THE HEART

The cardiac muscle has property of being stimulated automatically by its own conducting system formed of cardiac fibers which are specialized for initiation and conduction of cardiac impulse. This phenomenon is known as automaticity. The automaticity of heart is further regulated by nerve impulses from brain or circulating metabolites and hormones either increase or decrease the heart rate.

Conducting system of the heart consists of following components (Fig. 10.6):

1. **Sinoatrial (SA) node.** It is located in the right atrium in the upper part of the sulcus terminalis. It initiates impulses; hence it is also called as a *pacemaker of the heart.*
2. **Atrioventricular (AV) node.** It is located in the lower part of interatrial septum. It also generates impulses but at a slower rate than SA node.
3. **Atrioventricular bundle.** It connects atrial and ventricular musculature.
4. **Right and left bundle branches.** They are located in the muscular part of interventricular septum.
5. **Purkinje fibers.** They are the terminal branches of bundle branches.

N.B.

Cardiac muscle can contract without nerve stimulus (myogenic contraction) whereas other muscles of the body need nerve stimulus to contract.

BLOOD VESSELS

The blood vessels form a closed system of tubes that carry blood away from the heart to the tissues of the body and then return it back to the heart.

The blood vessels include:

1. Arteries
2. Capillaries
3. Veins

Arteries (distributing channels) are thick-walled tubes that carry blood away from the heart. The blood leaving the heart passes through the vessels of progressively smaller diameters referred to as arteries and arterioles (Fig. 10.1).

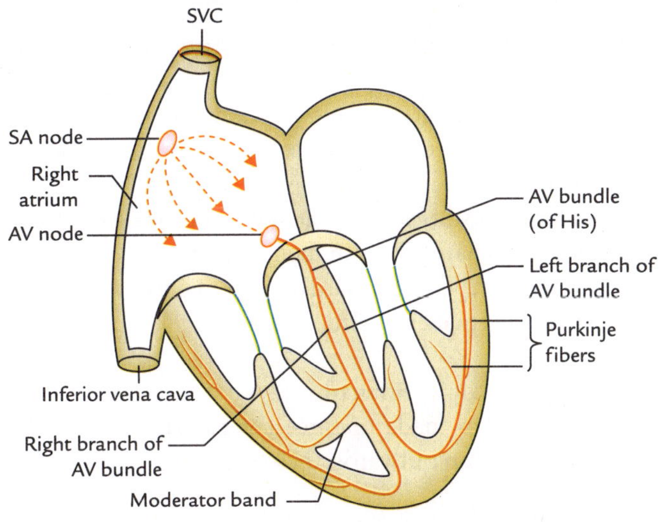

Fig. 10.6 Conducting system of the heart. (*Source:* Fig. 20.20, Page 272, *Textbook of Anatomy: Upper Limb and Thorax, 2e*, Vishram Singh. Copyright Elsevier 2014, All rights reserved.)

N.B.

The word 'artery', meaning air tube, was first used by Aristotle because after death when rigor mortis passes over, the liquid blood is collected in the dilated veins and arteries become empty. Sometimes air bubbles appear within arteries due to decomposition

Capillaries are microscopic vessels that connect arterioles and venules.

Veins (draining channels) are thin-walled tubes that carry blood from tissues of different parts of the body back to the heart. The blood returning to the heart from the capillaries passes through the vessels of progressively larger diameters, termed as veins and venules (Fig. 10.2).

N.B.

Except for the capillaries and the venules, the blood vessel walls consist of three layers.

Classification of Blood Vessels

Functionally the blood vessels are classified into five types:

1. **Conducting vessels**, e.g. large arteries (for details, see arteries).
2. **Distributing vessels**, e.g. small arteries (for details, see arteries).
3. **Resistance vessels**, e.g. arterioles (for details, see arteries).
4. **Exchange vessels**, e.g. capillaries, sinusoids and postcapillary venules.
5. **Capacitance or reservoir vessels**, e.g. large venules and veins. These are low pressure, large volume vessels. The high capacitance of these vessels is due to the fact that they are thin walled and have the capacity to dilate.

Arteries

Characteristic Features

The salient features of arteries are as follows:

1. They are thick-walled vessels and carry blood from the heart to capillaries.
2. They are often accompanied by vein/veins and nerve/nerves; and three of them together form the neurovascular bundle.
3. Their lumen is smaller than that of accompanying vein/veins.
4. They do not have valves in their lumen.
5. They divide repeatedly like a branch of a tree and gradually become smaller in size.

General (Microscopic) Structure

The arterial wall is made of three layers/coats (Fig. 10.7 A and B). From within outwards, these are:

1. Tunica intima
2. Tunica media
3. Tunica adventitia

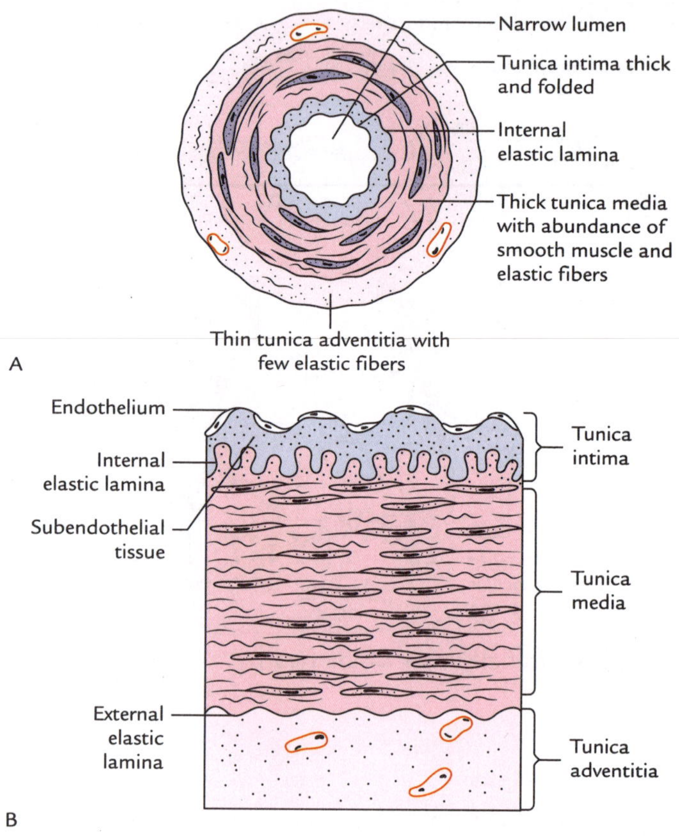

Fig. 10.7 Microscopic structure of a medium-sized artery: **A**, cross section showing different wall layers and the lumen; **B**, magnified view of the wall layers.

Tunica intima is made of endothelium, consisting of flattened cells and basal lamina. Externally, the endothelium is supported by subendothelial loose connective tissue and fenestrated membrane of elastic tissue called **internal elastic lamina.**

Tunica media is the thickest layer and made of alternate layers of circularly arranged smooth muscle fibers and elastic fibers. The tunica media is limited externally by fenestrated membrane of elastic tissue called **external elastic lamina.**

Tunica adventitia is thin but strongest of all coats. The tunica adventitia is made of longitudinally arranged connective tissue fibers (both elastic and collagen) and connective tissue cells. It merges with the perivascular sheath.

The structure of artery is summarized in Table 10.1.

Clinical correlation

- **Arteriosclerosis (or hardening of the arteries):** It is the age-related progressive generalized degenerative disorder of arterial walls usually seen after the middle age. There is generally a slow loss of elasticity and thickening of tunica intima due to increase in collagen and accumulation of lipid. Consequently, it leads to diffuse narrowing of lumen of blood vessels. Ischemia of the tissue supplied by affected arteries occurs. In lower limb, it is seen in the form

Table 10.1 Structure of artery

Name of the layer	Composition
Inner layer (*Tunica intima*)	Endothelium Subendothelial tissue Internal elastic lamina
Intermediate layer (*Tunica media*)	Circular smooth muscle fibers Elastic fibers External elastic lamina
Outer layer (*Tunica adventitia*)	Fibroelastic tissue

of *intermittent claudication,* characterized by pain, weakness in muscle at work especially during walking that is almost immediately relieved by rest. In the brain, it is seen in the form of mental function.

- **Atherosclerosis**: It is an arteriosclerosis in which plaques (patchy accumulation) of lipid, fibrous tissue and macrophages called *atheroma* accumulate in the tunica intima, which make the luminal surface of the artery uneven that can initiate the formation of a blood clot called a *thrombus* which may occlude the lumen, e.g. if it occurs in coronary artery it may lead to *myocardial infarction (heart attack).*

N.B.

An embolus is a thrombus that has dislodged from the wall of the vessel and moves in the bloodstream. Both thrombus and embolus can occlude flow. An embolus lodged in the coronary artery (coronary embolism) is called *coronary thrombus* in a vessel of *lung*, it is called *pulmonary thrombus* and in a vessel of *brain it is called cerebral thrombus.*

Classification

Functionally, arteries are classified into three types:

1. Elastic (conducting) arteries
2. Muscular (distributing) arteries
3. Arterioles (resistance vessels)

N.B.

There is a gradual change in diameter, thickness of wall, amount of elastic tissues and muscular tissues in the wall from larger size elastic arteries to muscular arteries, to arterioles.

Elastic arteries (conducting vessels) are large arteries arising from the heart and their main branches, e.g. aorta, brachiocephalic trunk, common carotid artery and the subclavian artery. They are called *elastic arteries* because tunica media of these arteries is predominantly made up of elastic fibers. They are also called **conducting vessels** as their main function is to conduct blood from the heart to the muscular arteries.

Muscular arteries (distributing vessels) are medium-sized arteries supplying individual organs and various parts of the limbs, e.g. renal, testicular, uterine, radial, posterior and anterior tibial arteries, etc. They are also called **distributing vessels.** There is gradual change from elastic to muscular arteries; the elastic material decreases and muscular tissue becomes the main constituent of tunica media (75%). These arteries regulate the flow of blood to an organ or part, as the smooth muscle of tunica media can alter the size of its lumen by contraction or relaxation.

Arterioles are smallest divisions of the muscular arteries with 100 mm or less in diameter. Their narrow lumen is surrounded by abundant muscle tissue. They are the main source of peripheral resistance to the blood flow; hence they are also called **resistance vessels.** They play an important role in regulating the **diastolic blood pressure.**

As the arterioles progressively divide into smaller branches, their walls become thinner and form successively **terminal arterioles** and **meta-arterioles:**

1. The large arterioles (i.e. arterioles at their arterial end) have all the three coats.
2. The **terminal arterioles** (15–20 mm in diameter) are devoid of internal elastic lamina and have continuous coat of muscle, cells arranged in one or two layers.
3. In **meta-arterioles**, the smooth muscles are replaced by discontinuous noncontractile cells called pericytes or Rouget cells. The meta-arterioles terminate into capillaries.
4. In some vascular beds, a meta-arteriole is directly connected with a venule by a **thoroughfare channel** or **preferred channel**, and the capillaries take origin as side branches of the thoroughfare channel to form capillary network (Fig. 10.8). The entry of blood through capillary is regulated by precapillary sphincters.

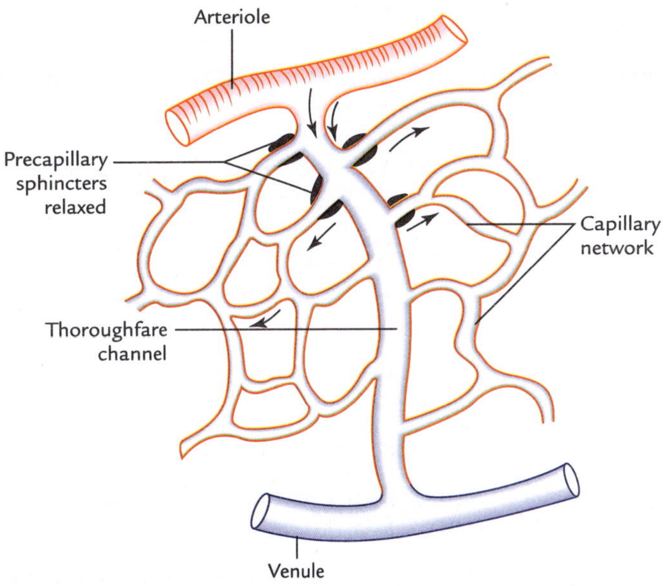

Fig. 10.8 Thoroughfare channels.

N.B.

Blood flowing through the 'thoroughfare channels' bypasses the capillary bed.

Blood Supply of the Arteries

Tunica adventitia and outer two-third of tunica media are supplied by **vasa vasorum.**

Tunica intima and inner one-third of tunica media are supplied by **luminal blood through diffusion.**

Minute veins accompanying arteries drain the blood from the arterial wall.

Lymphatics are also present in the tunica adventitia.

N.B.

Vasa vasorum (nutrient vessels) supply only large arteries and some medium-sized arteries (more than 1 mm in diameter). They form dense capillary plexus in the tunica adventitia and may penetrate up to the middle of tunica media.

Clinical correlation

Syphilitic aneurysm: The vasa vasorum are involved in *tertiary syphilis*, leading to poor blood supply of the tunica adventitia and outer two-third of tunica media. As a result, these layers undergo ischemic degeneration. Consequently, weakness of these layers leads to *syphilitic aneurysm*.

Nerve Supply

The arteries are mostly supplied by nonmyelinated *sympathetic nerve fibers* called **nervi vasorum/nervi vascularis.**

The sympathetic fibers supplying arteries generally cause vasoconstriction (i.e. constriction of smooth muscles in the wall of arteries) *except* in heart, brain and skeletal muscles where they cause vasodilatation.

N.B.

A few myelinated sympathetic fibers also supply the arteries. They are said to be sensory in nature (pain sensations).

Filling of the Arteries

All the arteries are filled with blood during systole *except* coronary arteries (supplying heart) which are filled during diastole.

Arterial Pulse

The force exerted by blood against the wall of vessels is called **blood pressure.** Normal blood pressure of an adult is about 120/80 mmHg (120 stands for systolic pressure and 80 stands for diastolic pressure). The systolic pressure results due to contraction of heart during ventricular systole, whereas diastolic pressure results due to contraction of smooth muscle of the arterial wall. The difference between the systolic and diastolic pressure is called **pulse pressure.**

A pulse is a palpable impulse of pressure wave of blood flow initiated by ventricular systole.

Clinical correlation

Sites where arterial pulse is routinely palpated: A pulse is a palpable impulse of pressure wave of blood flow initiated by ventricular systole. The student must know the sites where arterial pulse is routinely palpated by the clinicians. These seven sites are listed in Table 10.2 and illustrated in Figure 10.9.

Table 10.2 Seven routinely palpated sites of arterial pulses

Pulse	Site	Assessment criteria
Carotid	Along the anterior border of sterno-cleidomastoid muscle in neck at the level of cricoid cartilage	Most reliable pulse in physiological shock or cardiac arrest, when pulses at other sites are not palpable
Brachial	Medial to the tendon of biceps brachii in front of elbow	To auscultate the blood pressure
Radial	Radial side of front of forearm at wrist lateral to the tendon of flexor carpi radialis	Most commonly felt pulse to assess the character and rate of the pulse
Femoral	Below the inguinal ligament midway between pubic symphysis and anterior superior iliac spine	To locate femoral vein for venepuncture, which lies just medial to it
Popliteal	Behind the knee in the popliteal fossa	To assess the status of circulation in the lower limb
Posterior tibial	Medial side of ankle midway between medial malleolus and tendo-calcaneous	To assess the status of circulation in the foot
Dorsalis pedis	Over the dorsum of foot just medial to the tendon of extensor hallucis longus	To assess the status of circulation in the foot

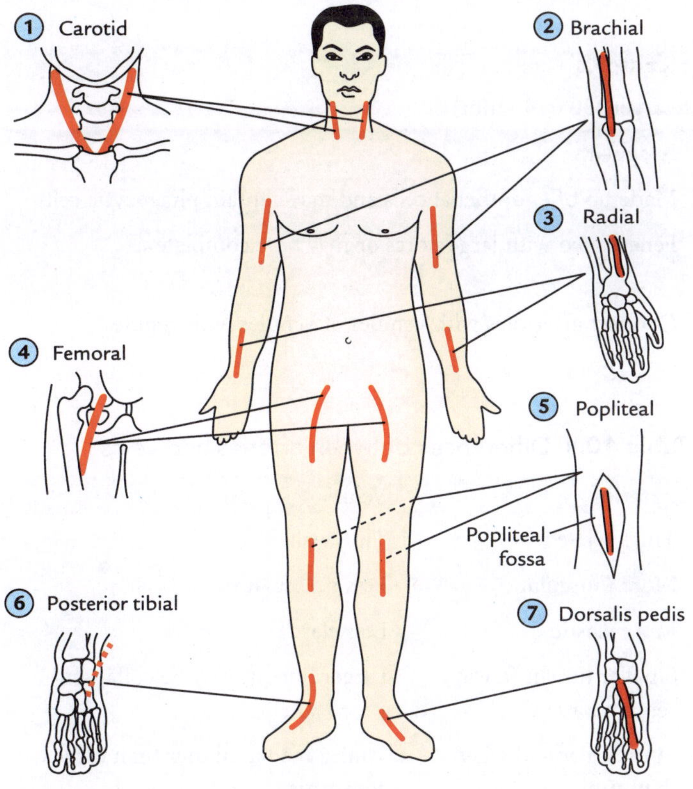

Fig. 10.9 Seven sites where arterial pulses are routinely palpated.

Capillaries

The capillaries are thin-walled and endothelium lined thin microscopic vessels that connect arterioles and venules. There are over 40 billion capillaries in the body with extensive network of vessels almost in every tissue of the body. The fact that the capillaries provide a total surface area of 1000 sq miles for exchange between blood and tissue fluid. The average diameter of capillary is 6 to 8 mm. As the diameter of erythrocytes is about 7 mm, only one erythrocyte passes at a time. Thus RBCs pass through a capillary in a single 'file'.

Unlike the vessels of the arterial and venous system, the walls of capillaries are made up of only one cell layer of squamous epithelium called **endothelium**.

N.B.

The flow of blood through capillaries is called *microcirculation.*

Types

According to the nature of endothelial lining, the capillaries can be classified into the following two types:

1. Continuous capillaries
2. Fenestrated capillaries

In **continuous capillaries,** the endothelial cells form a continuous tube. The cells are held together by tight junctions. The main feature of continuous capillaries is the pinocytic vesicles in endothelial cells. This indicates that transport of material takes place through the cytoplasm of endothelial cells and may account for selective nature of transport.

Sites: Continuous capillaries are found in skin, muscle, lung and brain.

Fenestrated capillaries are characterized by the wide pores between the endothelial cells. These pores are closed by a layer of mucoprotein called **diaphragm**. The diffusion of substance takes place through these diaphragms.

Sites: Fenestrated capillaries are found in pancreas, endocrine glands, intestinal villi, choroid plexus, ciliary processes of eye, etc.

N.B.

The renal glomeruli also have fenestrated (discontinuous) capillaries but pores are not closed by diaphragms.

Sinusoids

The sinusoids are large irregular vascular spaces which connect arteriole with venule or venule with venule. They replace capillaries in certain organs such as liver, spleen, bone marrow, suprarenal glands, parathyroid glands, etc.

The lumen of sinusoids is irregular and wide (about 30 to 40 mm in diameter). The walls of sinusoids are thin and made up of endothelial cells with large pores or slits which are not closed by diaphragms. The wall of sinusoid may be incomplete and contain phagocytic cells; *viz.* sinusoids in liver contain Kupffer cells which remove bacteria and other foreign particles from the blood. The sinusoids are closely surrounded by the parenchyma of the organ.

Functions

Due to irregular lumen, the flow of blood is sluggish in sinusoids that allow sufficient time for exchange of substances between blood and tissue fluid. The differences between capillaries and sinusoids are highlighted in Table 10.3.

Veins

Characteristic Features

The salient features of veins are as follows:

1. They are thin-walled vessels that carry blood from capillaries to the heart.
2. The large veins are formed by the union of smaller veins like tributaries of a river.
3. They have larger lumen as compared to arteries and less amount of muscular and elastic tissue in their walls.
4. Their lumen is often provided with valves, which prevent the reflex of the blood and thus maintain unidirectional flow of blood even against gravity.

Table 10.3 Difference between capillaries and sinusoids

Features	Capillaries	Sinusoids
Lumen	Smaller (5 to 8 mm)	Larger (30 to 40 mm)
	Regular	Irregular
Wall	Made up of endothelial cells	Made up of endothelial cells and may contain phagocytic cells
	Continuous or fenestrated with small pores closed by diaphragms	Fenestrated with large pores or may be incomplete
Location in circulatory system	Connect arterioles and venules	Connect arterioles with venules or venules with venules

5. Large veins have **dead space** around them for their dilation during increased venous return.

General Structure

The general structural features of the veins are similar to those of arteries, i.e. their wall is also made up of three layers that are ill-defined (Fig. 10.10). The tunica adventitia is the thickest and the best developed layer. It contains collagen, elastic and muscle fibers. The tunica media is poorly developed. The proper internal elastic lamina in tunica intima is absent.

The differences between arteries and veins are enumerated in Table 10.4.

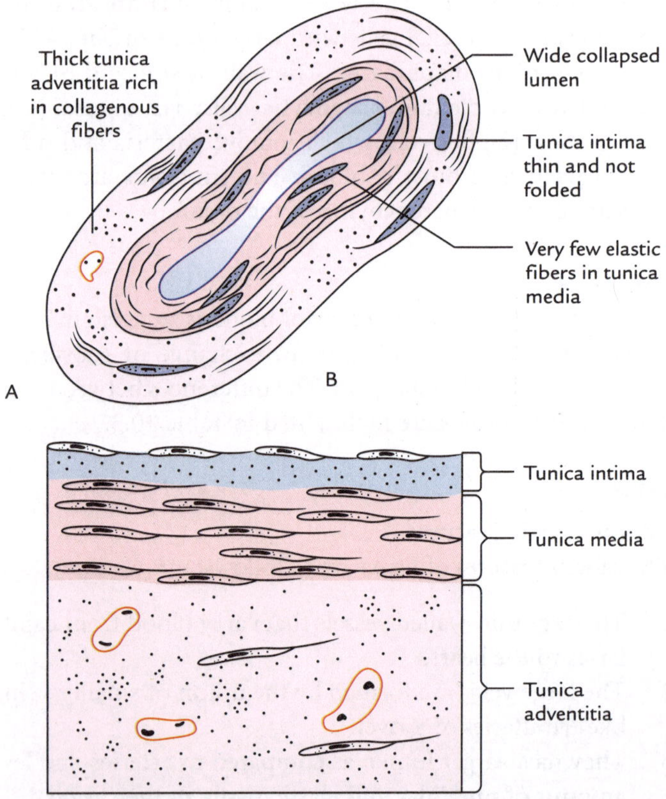

Fig. 10.10 Microscopic structure of a medium-sized vein: **A**, cross section showing different wall layers and the lumen; **B**, magnified view of the wall layers.

Table 10.4 Differences between arteries and veins

Arteries	Veins
Thick walled	Thin walled
More muscular	Less muscular
More elastic	Less elastic
Smaller lumen (always remain patent)	Larger lumen (may be collapsed)
Tunica media thicker than tunica adventitia	Tunica media thinner than tunica adventitia
No valves in the lumen	Valves mostly present in the lumen

N.B.

Thickest coat in arteries is tunica media, whereas thickest coat in veins is tunica adventitia.

Classification

The veins are classified into following three types:

1. Large
2. Medium-sized
3. Small (also called venules)

Large veins: All three layers of wall, i.e. tunica intima, tunica media and tunica adventitia are well differentiated. The tunica adventitia is always thicker than tunica media.

The walls of large veins have some elastic tissue which resists the pressure of the right atrial systole, e.g. inferior vena cava (IVC) and superior vena cava.

Medium-sized veins: These veins also have all three layers in their wall but it becomes gradually difficult to distinguish the three layers with decreasing size of medium-sized veins, splenic vein, testicular vein, etc.

Small veins or venules: These veins are of two types:

1. **Postcapillary venules:** They are the smallest veins and receive blood from capillaries. Their wall is made up of endothelium. These veins have special permeability, i.e. diffusion of fluid and white blood cells into the surrounding tissue and absorption of intercellular fluid from the tissue into the venules.

2. **Muscular venules:** They are so called because of the presence of one or two layers of smooth muscle cells outside the endothelium.

N.B.

The veins are *capacitance vessels* because they return varying quantities of venous blood towards the heart and have the capacity to distend or collapse.

Blood Supply

The larger veins-like arteries are also supplied by nutrient vessels called **vasa vasorum**, but in the veins they penetrate up to the tunica intima.

Nerve Supply

It is the same as arteries, but nerve fibers innervating the veins are fewer in number than arteries.

Pattern of Distribution of Arteries and Veins

The venous patterns are far more variable than arterial patterns, e.g.

1. Large veins are usually single.
2. Medium-sized veins are usually double, lying on either side of a medium-sized artery, *viz.* deep veins distal to elbow and knee, hence they are called **venae comitantes.**
   These veins are united to each other by short channels which form a network around the artery.
3. In several regions, the venous patterns are quite different than those of arterial patterns, *viz.* in brain, liver and lungs.

Venous Valves

The inner lining of most medium- and small-sized veins are thrown at intervals into delicate semilunar folds called **cusps.** With the wall of the vein, each cusp forms a bulging pocket or **sinus.**

The cusps are arranged in pairs facing each other to form **valves** (Figure. 10.11). The valves open only in one direction, i.e. towards the heart.

N.B.

Venous valves are bicuspid and consist of two valves.

The valves present near the termination of internal jugular, subclavian and femoral veins prevent the venous blood from being forced back into head, neck and limbs during increased intrathoracic pressure (e.g. during deep inspiration) and during increased intraabdominal pressure (e.g. during defecation; Fig. 10.12).

N.B.

- The valves are most numerous in the veins of the limbs, and they are commonly placed just before the mouth of a tributary.

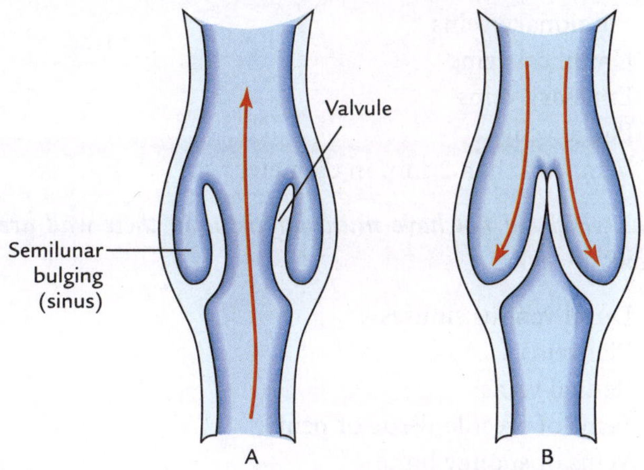

Fig. 10.11 Opening and closing of venous valves: **A**, the valve opens by forward pressure towards the heart; **B**, the valve closes by backward pressure.

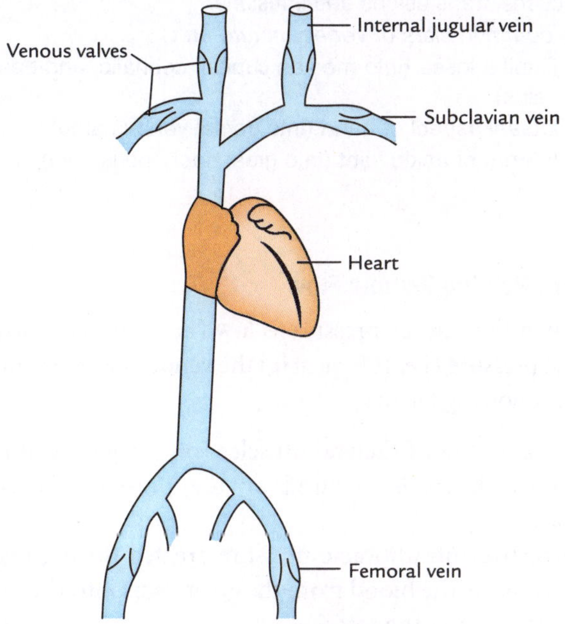

Fig. 10.12 Venous valves near the heart.

- The muscle fibers in venous wall tend to arrange in a loop near the point of drainage of a tributary to act as *sluice gate.*

Veins which do not have valves in their lumen are as follows:

1. Superior vena cava
2. Inferior vena cava
3. Hepatic veins
4. Renal veins
5. Uterine veins
6. Ovarian veins
7. Facial veins

8. Pulmonary veins
9. Umbilical veins
10. Emissary veins
11. Portal veins
12. Veins less than 2 mm in diameter

Veins which do not have muscular tissue in their wall are as follows:

1. Dural venous sinuses
2. Pial veins
3. Retinal veins
4. Veins of erectile tissue of penis
5. Veins of spongy bone

Clinical correlation

Sites of venepuncture: The superficial veins are commonly used for obtaining blood samples or giving intravenous injections, transfusions and infusions.

The common sites of venepuncture are:

(a) Cubital fossa (into median cubital, cephalic, and basilic veins)
(b) Dorsal aspect of hand (into dorsal venous arch)
(c) In front of ankle joint (into great saphenous vein)

Factors Helping Venous Flow

Although the venous pressure is low (i.e. 2 mmHg) than the arterial pressure (i.e. 100 mmHg) the venous blood is pumped by the following factors:

1. Mass action of skeletal muscles (one way flow of blood to the heart is ensured by the presence of *venous* valves).
2. Negative intrathoracic pressure created during inspiration sucks the blood from the great veins into the thorax.
3. Pulsations of the arteries.

N.B.

The effect of the massaging action of skeletal muscles on the venous blood flow is often described as the *skeletal muscle pump*.

Clinical correlation

Varicose veins: The accumulation of blood in the veins of the legs over a long period of time, as may occur in people whose profession requires standing still all the day, can cause the veins to stretch to the point where the venous valves are no longer efficient. Consequently, due to backflow of blood the superficial veins become dilated and tortuous, a condition called *varicosity of veins*. The great saphenous vein of lower limb is most commonly affected.

ANASTOMOSIS

Anastomosis is the communication between the blood vessels forming collateral channels.

ARTERIAL ANASTOMOSIS

The arteries do not always end in capillaries rather their branches join/unite with branches of the other arteries forming **anastomosis** (Fig. 10.13). The anastomosis provides *collateral channel for circulation* when one of these arteries is blocked.

Different Types of Anastomosis:

The anastomosis are of two types (Fig. 10.13):

1. **Actual anastomosis:** It may occur in the following ways:
   (a) *End to end anastomosis*: when arteries join end to end, e.g. labial arteries, facial arteries, arterial arches in palms and soles.

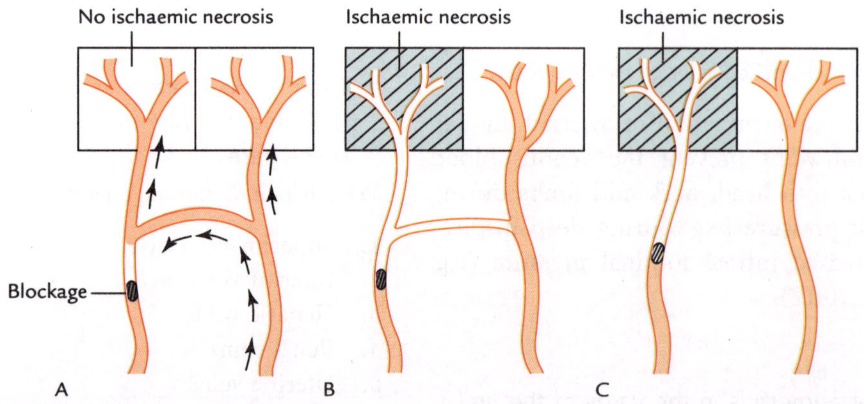

Fig. 10.13 Arterial anastomosis and end arteries: **A**, functional anastomosis; **B**, functional end artery (nonfunctional anastomosis); **C**, anatomical end artery.

(b) *Convergent anastomosis*: When two arteries converge and join each other to form a larger artery, e.g. two **vertebral arteries** unite to form a larger **basilar artery.**

2. **Potential anastomosis:** The potential anastomosis takes place between terminal arterioles. In such type of anastomosis, collateral circulation cannot take place if one of the artery is suddenly blocked. However, if sufficient time is given, the arterioles can dilate and establish collateral circulation, e.g. coronary arteries (for details see N.B. given below).

End Arteries

These are the arteries whose branches do not anastomose with branches of other adjacent arteries, e.g. (a) central artery of retina, (b) arteries of spleen, liver, kidneys, metaphyses of long bones and (c) central (medullary) branches of cerebral arteries.

If these arteries are blocked, the area supplied suffers from ischemia that may lead to cell necrosis.

N.B.

Functional end arteries are not the actual (anatomical) end arteries because they anastomose at the level of arterioles (potential anastomosis) but if they are blocked, the tissues supplied become ischemic, e.g. coronary arteries, and cortical branches of cerebral arteries.

ARTERIOVENOUS ANASTOMOSES

The direct connections between the arteries and veins without the intervention of capillaries are termed as **arteriovenous anastomoses** or **shunts**. The terminal arteriole or its side branch joins the venule. The *AV (arteriovenous) shunts* have thick muscular wall and are abundantly supplied with vasomotor sympathetic nerves, and thereby may act as sphincter.

Sites

Arteriovenous anastomoses are found at the following sites:

1. Skin of nose, lips and external ear
2. Mucous membrane of alimentary canal and nose
3. Erectile tissue of sex organs
4. Thyroid gland
5. Tongue

Functions

Arteriovenous anastomoses permit direct transfer of blood from arterial to venous channels, bypassing the capillary bed when sphincters are relaxed (Fig. 10.14). The functions of arteriovenous anastomoses include:

1. Regulation of temperature
2. Regulation of regional blood flow
3. Regulation of blood pressure

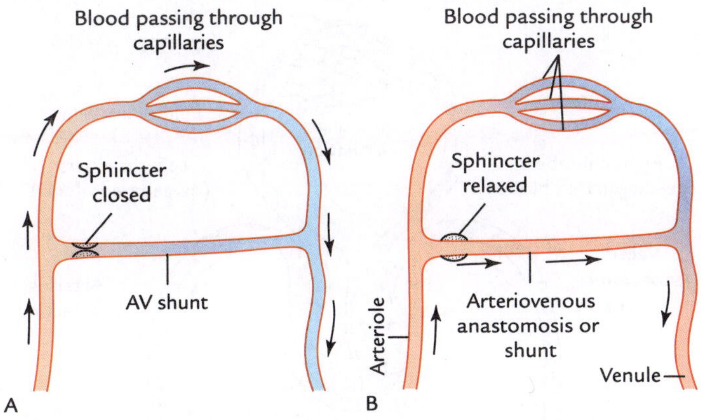

Fig. 10.14 Functioning of arteriovenous anastomoses (or shunt): **A**, blood not passing through shunt because sphincter is closed, hence it is passing through capillaries (when tissue or organ is active); **B**, blood passing through shunt because sphincter is relaxed, hence little or no blood is passing through capillaries (when tissue or organ is at rest).

Clinical correlation

In organs like kidney and intestine, the arteriovenous anastomoses open up following massive hemorrhage during road accidents or war injuries. This allows the blood to bypass the capillary bed of kidney and intestine, thus making blood available to vital organs like heart and brain. For this reason, anuria often occurs after accidents but once the volume of blood in general circulation improves, the AV shunts gradually close, allowing the blood to pass through the glomerular capillaries. Consequently, the output of urine improves, which is good clinical sign after the accident.

CIRCULATION OF BLOOD

In adult individuals, the blood circulates through an estimated 60,000 miles of vessels through the body to provide food and oxygen to trillions of living cells in the body. At the same time, it removes the waste products of their metabolism.

TYPES OF BLOOD CIRCULATION

Blood circulation in the body can be categorized into the following three types (Fig. 10.15):

1. **Pulmonary circulation:** The deoxygenated blood entering the right atrium passes to the right ventricle which pumps it through pulmonary trunk and pulmonary arteries to the capillaries of the lungs (where it is oxygenated), then through the pulmonary veins it returns to the left atrium.

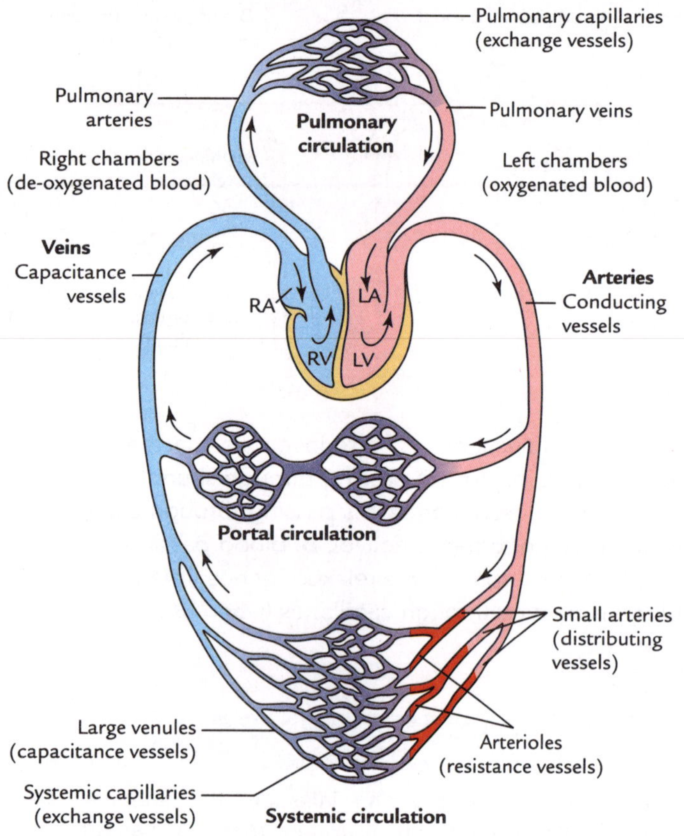

Fig. 10.15 Types of circulation: pulmonary, systemic and portal.

2. **Systemic circulation:** The oxygenated blood from left atrium passes to the left ventricle which pumps it through aorta and its branches to the capillaries of the rest of the body.

   The capillaries join to form veins which become increasingly larger till finally the superior and inferior vena cavae and cardiac veins return the deoxygenated blood to right atrium.

   The right atrium receives the same amount of deoxygenated blood which was pumped by the left ventricle, and at the same rate.

N.B

Students must note that blood appears red when oxygen content is high and appears blue when oxygen content is low. Therefore, blood is 'red' in pulmonary veins, left side of the heart and systemic arteries, whereas the blood is 'blue' in systemic veins, right side of the heart and pulmonary arteries. These structures, therefore, should be colored red and blue accordingly in anatomical illustrations.

3. **Portal circulation:** It is in fact a part of systemic circulation. It begins with capillaries and ends with capillaries, i.e. blood passes through two sets of capillaries before draining into systemic vein.

   The **portal vessels** are the vessels which connect the two sets of capillaries at their two ends.

   The vessel draining the first capillary network is known as portal vessel, which branches like an artery to form the second set of capillaries or sinusoids. Such type of circulation is seen in liver **(hepatic portal circulation)**, hypophysis cerebri **(hypothalamo-hypophyseal portal circulation)** and kidney **(renal portal circulation):**

   (a) *Hepatic portal circulation* (Fig. 10.16): The venous blood passes from capillary bed of GIT, spleen and pancreas through portal vein to the liver. In the liver, it passes through a secondary capillary bed, the hepatic sinusoids, before entering the general circulation via the inferior vena cava.

   In this way, blood with high concentration of nutrients absorbed from the stomach and intestines goes to the liver first, where certain modifications take place before it is supplied to the other parts of the body

N.B.

Hepatic portal system is essentially concerned with the transport of absorbed nutrient from food to the liver and their subsequent metabolism.

   (b) *Hypothalamo-hypophyseal portal circulation* (Fig. 10.17): The blood passes from capillary network in the hypothalamus through portal vessels into capillary network in the anterior pituitary. The vein/veins arising from capillary network in anterior pituitary then merges with the general circulation.

   The neurohormones produced and secreted by the hypothalamus enter the capillary network within the hypothalamus to reach the anterior pituitary where they act on the

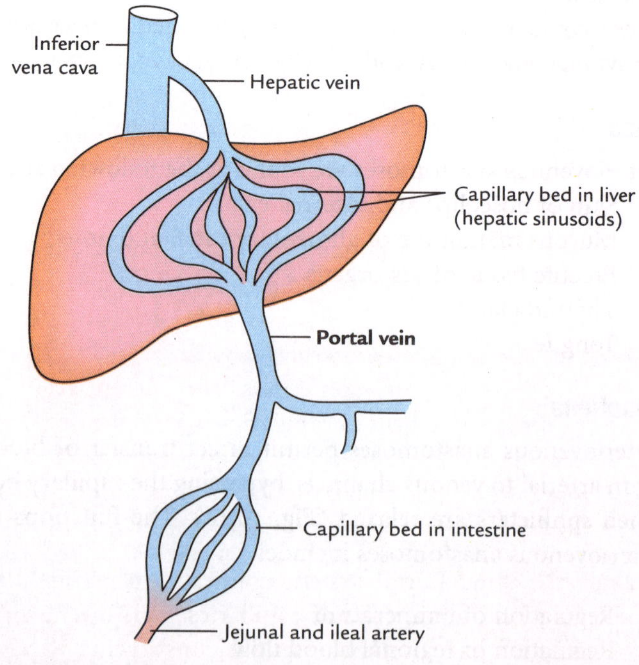

Fig. 10.16 Hepatic portal circulation.

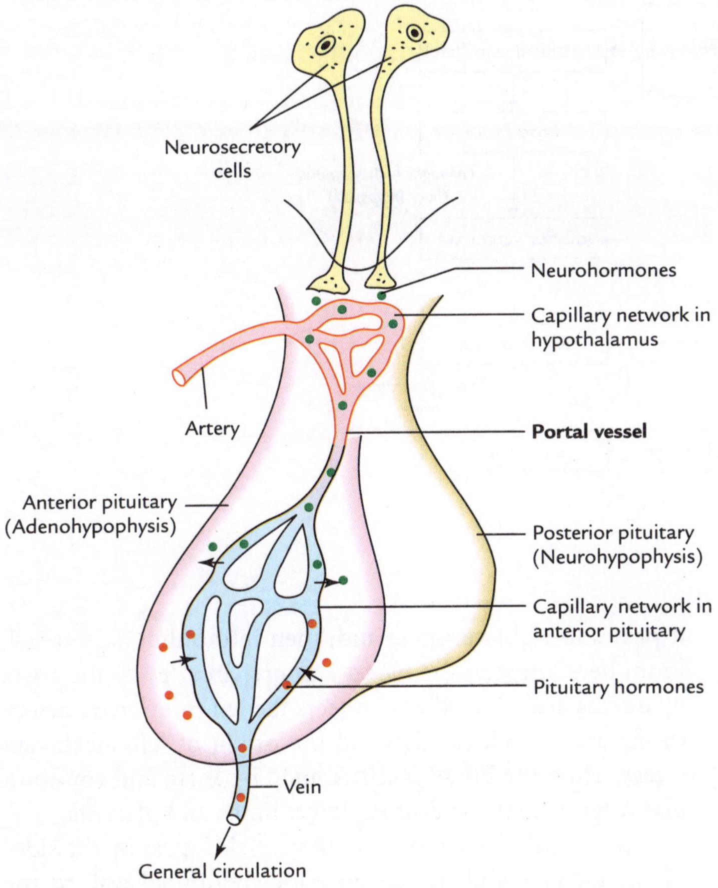

Fig. 10.17 Hypothalamo-hypophyseal portal system.

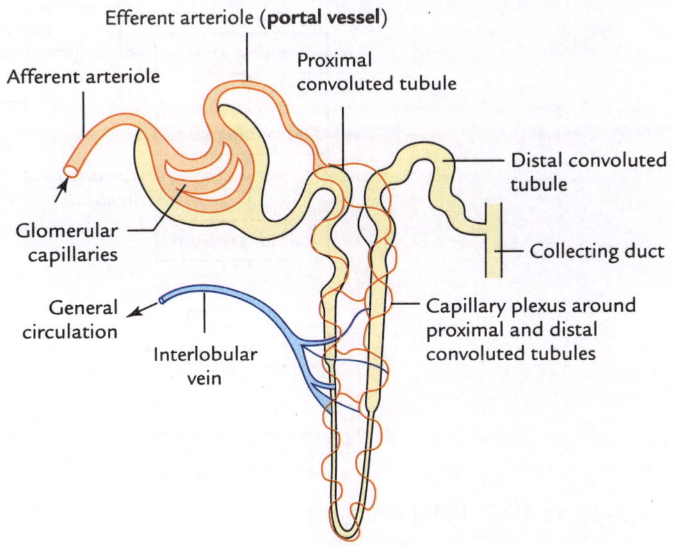

Fig. 10.18 Renal portal circulation.

cells of anterior pituitary to either increase or decrease their secretion. The hormones secreted by anterior pituitary enter the capillary network within the anterior pituitary and then carried by the general circulation to the target tissue.

N.B.

Through hypothalamo-hypophyseal portal system, the hypothalamus regulates the activities of adenohypophysis (anterior pituitary) by means of neurohormone (releasing or inhibiting hormones).

(c) *Renal portal circulation* (Fig. 10.18): The afferent arterioles supply blood to the glomerular capillaries of the renal corpuscle. Efferent arterioles (portal vessels) arise from glomerular capillaries and carry the blood away from glomerulus. The efferent arteriole gives rise to plexus of capillaries around the proximal and distal convoluted tubules (peritubular capillaries). The peritubular capillaries drain into general circulation through interlobular vein.

Thus the renal portal system connects the glomerular capillaries with the peritubular capillaries. This mechanism helps reabsorption of some essential constituents of glomerular filtrate back to the blood.

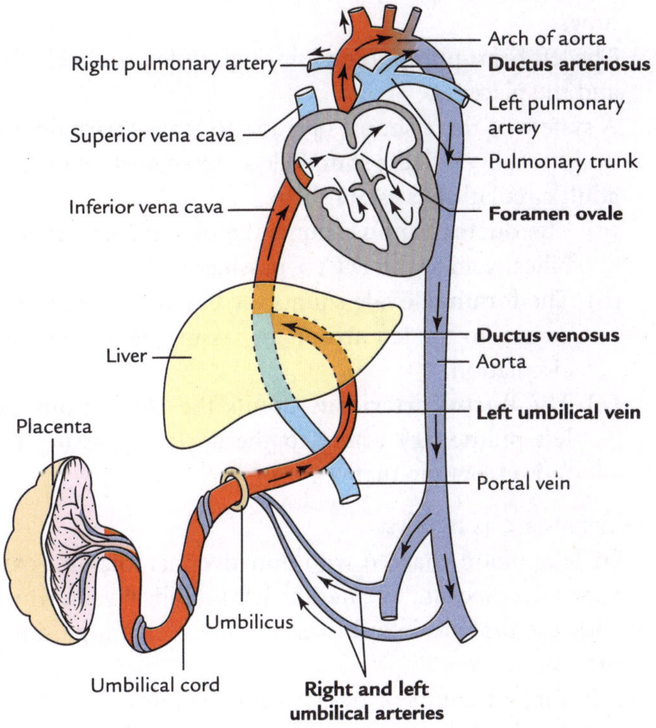

Fig. 10.19 Fetal circulation.

FETAL CIRCULATION

The fetal circulation is different from circulation in the adult (Fig. 10.19). This is because of the following reasons:

1. The collapsed fetal lungs are nonfunctional.
2. The portal circulation is of little significance.
3. The oxygenation of blood occurs in placenta.

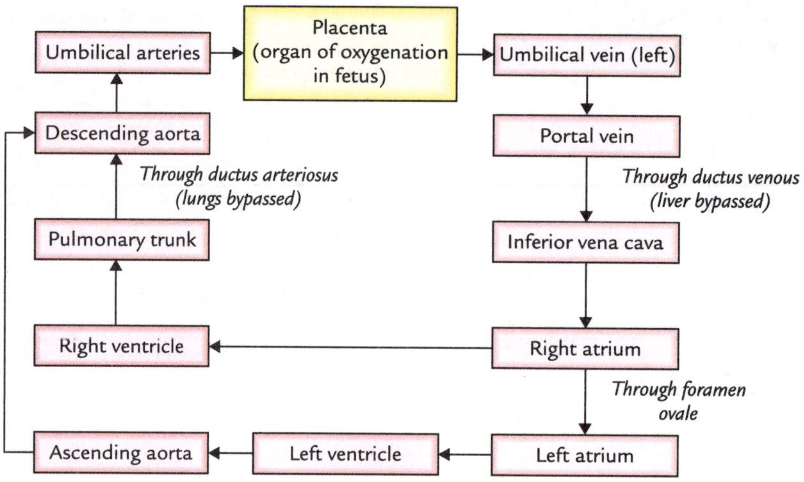

Flowchart 10.1 Fetal circulation.

The three cardinal features of fetal circulation are:

1. The right heart pumps very little blood to the collapsed lungs.
2. The left heart pumps blood through systemic circulation and the placenta.
3. A system of three shunts operates to bypass partially the lungs and liver. These shunts close down postnatally and adult circulation is established:
   (a) The **ductus venous** shunts the blood from the umbilical vein to the IVC, bypassing the liver.
   (b) The **foramen ovale** shunts the blood from the right atrium to the left atrium, bypassing the pulmonary circulation.
   (c) The **ductus arteriosus** shunts the blood from the left pulmonary artery to the aorta, bypassing the pulmonary circulation.

The details are as follows:

The fetal blood charged with nutritive material and oxygen leaves the placenta to enter the left umbilical vein, which traverses the umbilical cord to end in the remaining branch of portal vein.

Only some amount of blood from left portal vein flows through the liver; however, most of the blood bypasses the liver via **ductus venosus** to the inferior vena cava which opens into right atrium.

Most of the blood brought in the right atrium by the IVC is shunted through foramen ovale (opening in the interatrial septum) into left atrium, thereby short circuiting pulmonary circuit. It then passes through the left ventricle into the ascending aorta and aortic arch, and by their branches it is distributed to the heart, head and neck and upper limbs. The blood from head and neck and upper limbs returns to the right atrium through superior vena cava. From right atrium it passes to right ventricle and, then into pulmonary trunk. From here, most of the blood is short-circuited to the aorta by ductus arteriosus that connects the left pulmonary artery to the aortic arch just beyond the origin of left subclavian artery. Then the blood is distributed by aorta and common iliac arteries to the abdomen, lower limbs and placenta.

The umbilical arteries, one on each side, pass by the sides of the bladder and up the anterior abdominal wall to the umbilicus and then through the umbilical cord to the placenta.

The fetal circulation is summarized in Flowchart 10.1.

The remnants formed by the closure of fetal circulatory structures after birth, following the start of neonatal circulation are presented in Table 10.5.

N.B.

- Since the functions of placenta are concerned with (a) nutrition, (b) excretion and (c) respiration in fetus, the portal, renal and pulmonary circulations are of little significance. The placental circulation is paramount.
- The placenta is the organ of oxygenation in fetus.

Table 10.5 Remnants that result from the closure of fetal circulatory structures

Fetal structure	Adult remnants
Ductus venosus	Ligamentum venosum
Foramen ovale	Fossa ovalis
Ductus arteriosus	Ligamentum arteriosum
Left umbilical vein	Ligamentum teres hepatis
Right and left umbilical arteries	Medial umbilical ligaments

Golden Facts to Remember

➢ First organ in the body to start functioning	Heart
➢ Largest artery in the body	Aorta
➢ Largest vein in the body	Inferior vena cava (IVC)
➢ Longest vein in the body	Great saphenous vein
➢ Largest portal vessel in the body	Portal vein
➢ Most commonly used artery for measuring blood pressure	Brachial artery
➢ Most commonly felt arterial pulse in the body	Radial pulse
➢ Most reliable pulse in the body	Carotid pulse
➢ Best example of an end artery in the body	Central artery of retina of the eye
➢ Best example of functional end arteries	Coronary arteries
➢ Most commonly used vein for intravenous injection	Median cubital vein (in the cubital fossa)
➢ Total length of all capillaries joined end to end	60,000 miles
➢ Total amount of blood in the vascular system	5 L
➢ Most abundant leucocytes in peripheral circulation	Neutrophils
➢ All the cells of the blood are nucleated *except*	Mature red blood cells (RBCs)
➢ All the arteries in the body contain oxygenated blood *except*	Pulmonary arteries in adults and umbilical arteries in fetus, which contain deoxygenated blood
➢ All veins in the body contain deoxygenated blood *except*	Pulmonary veins in adults and umbilical vein in fetus, which contain oxygenated blood
➢ All the arteries in the body are filled during systole *except*	Coronary arteries which are filled during diastole
➢ Vessels responsible for maximum peripheral vascular resistance	Arterioles

Multiple Choice Questions

1. **All of the following are examples of elastic arteries *except:***
   (a) Aorta
   (b) Common carotid artery
   (c) Subclavian artery
   (d) Radial artery

2. **All of the following are examples of distributing vessels *except:***
   (a) Common carotid artery
   (b) Renal artery
   (c) Testicular artery
   (d) Uterine artery

3. **Arterioles are the examples of:**
   (a) Distributing vessels
   (b) Conducting vessels
   (c) Resistance vessels
   (d) Capacitance vessels

4. **Fenestrated capillaries are found in all of the following sites *except:***
   (a) Pancreas
   (b) Lung
   (c) Intestinal villi
   (d) Ciliary processes of the eye

5. **Veins are an example of:**
   (a) Conducting vessels
   (b) Distributing vessels
   (c) Capacitance vessels
   (d) Resistance vessels

6. **All of the following are examples of end arteries *except:***
   (a) Central branches of cerebral arteries
   (b) Central artery of retina
   (c) Facial artery
   (d) Splenic artery

7. **All of the following are veins without valves in their lumen *except:***
   (a) Inferior vena cava
   (b) Saphenous veins
   (c) Emissary veins
   (d) Veins less than 2 mm in diameter

8. **All of the following veins do not have muscular tissue in their wall *except:***
   (a) Retinal veins
   (b) Veins of spongy bone
   (c) Venules
   (d) Veins of erectile tissue of penis

9. **Which of the following arteries are examples of functional end arteries:**
   (a) Central branches of cerebral arteries
   (b) Coronary arteries
   (c) Arteries of spleen, liver and kidneys
   (d) Arteries supplying metaphyses of long bones

10. **Arteriovenous anastomoses are found at all of the following sites *except:***
    (a) Skin of lips
    (b) Erectile tissue of sex organs
    (c) Thyroid gland
    (d) Liver

11. **All of the following are features of veins *except:***
    (a) Thin walls
    (b) Thin tunica adventitia
    (c) Thin tunica media
    (d) Wider lumen

12. **Stimulation of sympathetic fibers causes vasodilatation of all of the following arteries *except:***
    (a) Arteries of heart
    (b) Arteries of GIT
    (c) Arteries of brain
    (d) Arteries of skeletal muscles

13. **Nerve supply of arteries is mostly derived from:**
    (a) Myelinated sympathetic nerve fibers
    (b) Nonmyelinated sympathetic nerve fibers
    (c) Myelinated parasympathetic nerve fibers
    (d) Nonmyelinated parasympathetic nerve fibers

14. **All of the following are examples of portal circulation *except:***
    (a) Pulmonary circulation
    (b) Hepatic circulation
    (c) Renal circulation
    (d) Circulation in hypophysis cerebri

15. **Which of the following arteries are filled mainly during diastole:**
    (a) Common carotid arteries
    (b) Hepatic arteries
    (c) Coronary arteries
    (d) Renal arteries

Answers

1. ***d*****, 2.** ***a*****, 3.** ***c*****, 4.** ***b*****, 5.** ***c*****, 6.** ***c*****, 7.** ***b*****, 8.** ***c*****, 9.** ***b*****, 10.** ***d*****, 11.** ***b*****, 12.** ***b*****, 13.** ***b*****, 14.** ***a*****, 15.** ***c***

CHAPTER 11

Lymphatic System

Learning Objectives

After studying this chapter, the student should be able to:
- define lymphatic system and discuss its functions
- elucidate the components of lymphatic system
- outline the structure and functions of lymph nodes
- describe the location, structure and functions of spleen
- describe the location and functions of thymus gland
- describe the location and functions of mucosa-associated lymphoid tissue **MALT**
- discuss the roles of the different types of T lymphocytes in providing cell-mediated immunity
- explain the process of antibody-mediated immunity
- correctly solve the review questions given at the end of the chapter

INTRODUCTION

The lymphatic system consists of an extensive network of extremely variable lymph vessels and lymph nodes through which lymph circulates (Fig. 11.1). The lymphatic system defends the body from bacteria, viruses and other harmful agents.

The lymphatic system is essentially a drainage system which is accessory to the venous system (Fig. 11.2). Most of the tissue fluid formed at the arterial ends of the capillaries is absorbed back into the blood by the venous ends of the capillaries. The remaining tissue fluid is absorbed by lymph capillaries which begins blindly in the tissue spaces and is sent back to the blood.

In addition to lymph vessels and lymph nodes, the lymphatic system consists of large amount of lymphatic tissue present in the body in different forms.

The functions of the lymphatic system are as follows:

1. Drains excess tissue fluid to the venous system, i.e. tissue fluid which could not be drained by the venous system.
2. Absorbs fat from the intestine and transports it to the blood.
3. Helps to provide immunological defences against disease-causing agents.

COMPONENTS OF THE LYMPHATIC SYSTEM

The lymphatic system consists of:

1. Lymph
2. Lymph capillaries
3. Lymph vessels
4. Lymphoid organs
   (a) Lymph nodes
   (b) Spleen
   (c) Thymus
5. Epithelio-lymphoid system
6. Bone marrow

LYMPH

The tissue fluid that enters the lymph capillaries is called **lymph**. Generally, it is clear watery fluid similar in composition to plasma, with the important exception of plasma proteins. However, the lymph from small intestine is milky white (called **chyle**) because it contains large droplets of fat absorbed from intestine. The lymph transports the plasma proteins that seep out of the capillary beds back to the blood stream. It also carries away larger particles, e.g. bacteria and cell debris which is then filtered out and destroyed by the lymph nodes. Thus, the lymph contains lymphocytes, macromolecules of protein, fat droplets and particulate matter such as dust particles, carbon particles,

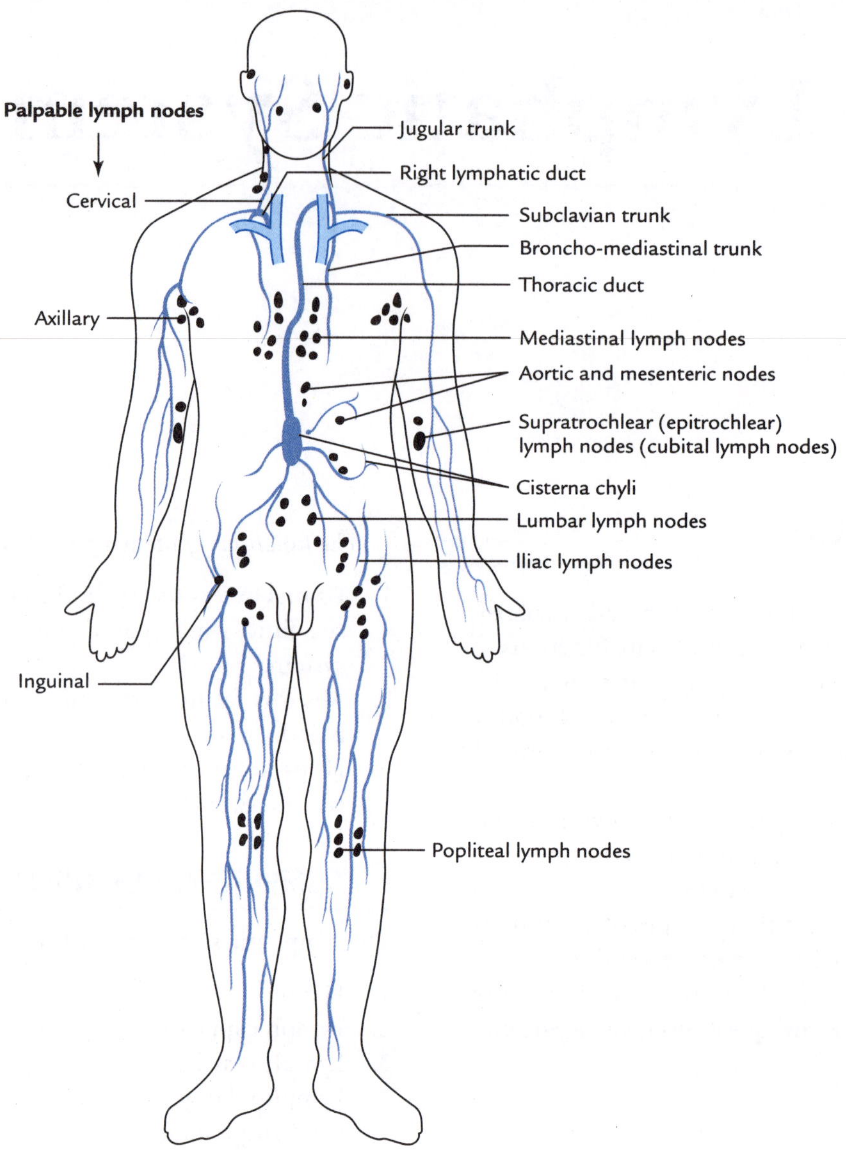

Fig. 11.1 Schematic diagram of a human being showing major locations of lymph nodes, thoracic duct, right lymphatic duct and other lymph vessels.

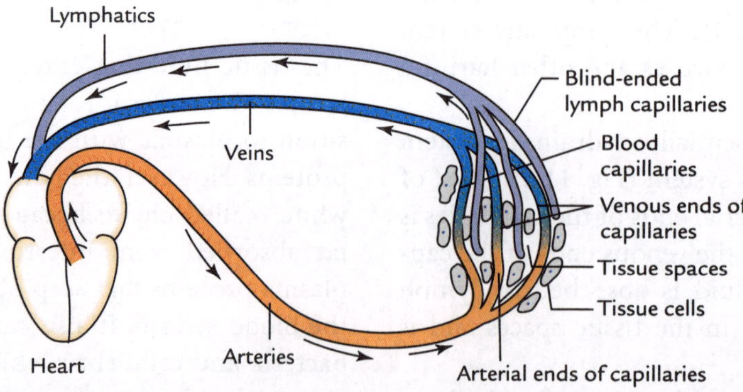

Fig. 11.2 Schematic diagram showing the relationship between lymphatic system and cardiovascular system.

bacteria, etc. To an extent the constitution of lymph is similar to that of plasma.

Clinical correlation

Lymphoedema: About 30 L of fluid passes from the arterial ends of capillaries into the intercellular space every day. Out of this, about 27 L of fluid consisting of micromolecules are absorbed back by venous ends of the capillaries. The remaining 3 L of fluid consisting of macromolecules of protein, fat droplets and particulate matter such as a bacteria is absorbed by lymph capillaries. For this reason, the lymphatic system is regarded as '**drainage system of the coarse type**' and venous system as '**drainage system of the fine type**'. If extra 3 L of fluid is not drained by the lymphatic system, the accumulation of this fluid in the tissue will cause edema (swelling).

LYMPH CAPILLARIES

The lymph capillaries are microscopic blind-ended lymph vessels which begin in the intercellular spaces. They form vast network in intercellular spaces of most of the tissues of the body (Fig. 11.2). The walls of the lymph capillaries like those of blood capillaries are made up of single layer of endothelial cells but they are more permeable to tissue fluid containing large molecules such as proteins, particulate matter and colloidal material.

N.B.

- Lymph capillaries are most numerous in *skin, glands, mucous and serous membranes.*
- Lymph capillaries within the villi of small intestine are called *lacteals*. They absorb fat and transport it to the blood.

The lymph capillaries differ from blood capillaries in following respects:

1. Begin blindly in intercellular spaces.
2. Have bigger lumen which is less regular.
3. Are permeable to bigger molecules hence absorb tissue fluid containing particulate matter and colloid material.

The sites where lymph capillaries are absent are:

1. Epidermis
2. Hair
3. Nails
4. Cornea
5. Articular cartilage
6. Brain and spinal cord
7. Bone marrow
8. Splenic pulp

LYMPH VESSELS

The lymph capillaries unite to form lymphatic vessels. They are thin-walled vessels, 0.5 to 1.0 mm in diameter, and have beaded appearance due to the presence of numerous valves within their lumen. The flow of lymph in lymphatic vessels is unidirectional towards the large veins at the root of the neck due to the presence of these valves. The lymphatic vessels pass through a series of lymph nodes before the lymph is drained into the venous system (Fig. 11.3). The lymph nodes filter the lymph to make it free from pathogens and harmful agents.

In fact, once the vessels are formed, they converge on a lymph node. The lymph passes through this lymph node and leaves it through another lymph vessel which enters another lymph node. The lymph leaves this node through yet another vessel. This process is repeated. The smaller lymph vessels merge to form progressively larger lymph vessels called **lymph ducts** which empty into subclavian veins.

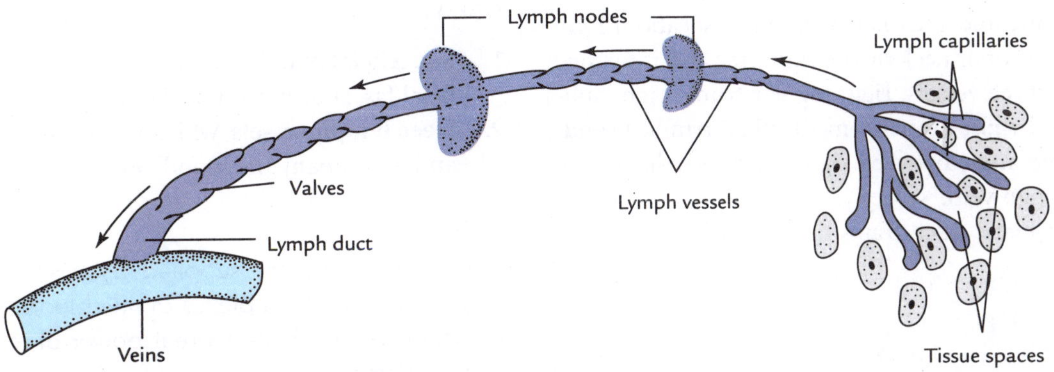

Fig. 11.3 Schematic diagram showing origin of lymph vessels form lymph capillaries present in the tissue spaces and drain into lymph nodes. Lymph trunk opens into the vein. Note the beaded appearance of lymph vessels due to the presence of valves in their lumen.

Clinical correlation

- **Lymphangitis:** Sometimes lymph vessels become inflamed leading to lymphangitis. This often results in visible red streaks in the skin extending from the site of infection to the group of lymph nodes where the lymph vessels drain, e.g. in infection of red streaks on the hand may be seen spreading from the hand to the axilla.
- **Elephantiasis:** If lymph vessels draining the lower limb are blocked by long slender worms of filaria, the accumulation of fluid in the interstitial spaces and lymph vessels may cause permanent swelling and enlargement of lower limb resembling an elephant's leg producing a clinical condition called *'elephantiasis'*.

There are two types of principal lymph ducts:

1. Thoracic duct
2. Right lymphatic duct

Thoracic Duct

The **thoracic duct** is the largest lymphatic duct (about 45 cm long) in the body. This begins as the large sack-like dilated lymph channel called **cysterna chyli** lying in front of the bodies of L1 and L2 vertebrae and ends in the angle between the left internal jugular vein and left subclavian vein (Fig. 11.4).

It drains lymph from whole of the body *except* right upper quadrant (Fig. 11.4) from which the lymph is drained by right lymphatic duct.

The thoracic duct drains the lymph from:

1. Lower extremities
2. Abdomen
3. Left thoracic region
4. Left upper limb
5. Left side of head and neck

Right Lymphatic Duct

The right lymphatic duct is a dilated lymph vessel about 1 cm long. It lies in the root of neck on the right side and is formed by the union of three vessels: right jugular trunk, right subclavian trunk and right broncho-mediastinal trunk. It ends by opening in the angle between right brachiocephalic vein and right subclavian vein.

The right lymphatic duct drains the lymph from:

1. Right upper limb
2. Right thoracic region
3. Right side of head and neck

Structure of a lymphatic duct: Like the wall of veins, the wall of lymphatic ducts have same three layers, i.e. tunica adventitia, tunica media and tunica intima.

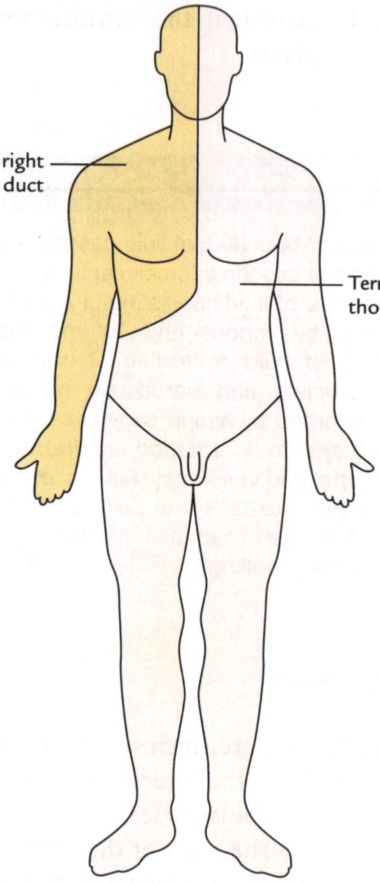

Fig. 11.4 Lymphatic drainage of the body: upper right quadrant of the body drains into the right lymphatic duct. The remaining body drains into the thoracic duct.

The lumen of lymphatic ducts contains valves which are more numerous and closely packed than veins. The lumen of vessel proximal to the valve is expanded into a sinus. The valves are so closely placed that lymph vessels when filled with lymph has a **beaded appearance** (Fig. 11.3).

Superficial and Deep Lymph Vessels

According to the location, the lymph vessels are divided into two types:

1. **Superficial lymph vessels,** which are found in the superficial fascia deep to skin. They join deep lymph vessels.
2. **Deep lymph vessels,** which are found deep to deep fascia and accompany the blood vessels.

N.B.

- Lymph vessels are supplied by vasa vasorum and are accompanied by a plexus of fine blood vessels.
- Lymph vessels have a great power of regeneration after their damage.
- The valves in lymph vessels permit the flow of lymph only in one direction, i.e. from periphery to the center and prevent the backflow.

Drainage of Lymph

The factors responsible for the drainage of lymph through the lymph vessels and lymphatic ducts are as follows:

1. Contraction of smooth muscle in the wall of the lymph vessel.
2. Pulsation of arteries lying near the lymph vessels.
3. Massaging action from contraction of surrounding muscles.
4. Filtration pressure in tissue spaces generated by filtration of fluid from blood capillaries.
5. Respiratory movements.
6. Negative pressure in brachio-cephalic veins.
7. Valves within the lumen of the lymph vessels.

N.B.

There is no *pump*, like the heart, involved in the onward movement of lymph but the muscle tissue in the walls of large lymph vessels has an intrinsic ability to contract rhythmically, the so-called '*lymphatic pump*'.

LYMPHOID ORGANS

The lymphoid organs are made up of lymphatic tissues. The lymphatic tissue is a specialized connective tissue and consists of:

(a) framework of reticular fibers and reticular cells;
(b) lymphocytes (mainly) and related plasma cells and macrophages.

A circumscribed concentration of lymphatic tissue are called **lymph nodules**, which are found both in scattered lymphatic tissue and encapsulated lymphoid organs.

The lymphatic nodules may show lightly stained area in its center called **germinal center**, which contains large euchromatic lymphoblasts and plasmoblasts which produce lymphocytes and plasma cells. In the lymph nodule, the germinal center develops only when the nodule is exposed to the antigen. The germinal centers are absent in embryonic life and in old age. The germinal center is surrounded by darkly stained zone of densely packed small lymphocytes.

The lymphoid organs are classified into the following two types:

1. **Primary lymphoid organs**, which are involved in the production of lymphocytes, *viz.* bone marrow, thymus.
2. **Secondary lymphoid organs**, which are involved in activation of lymphocytes and initiation of an immune response, *viz.* lymph nodes, spleen.

N.B.

- Lymphocytes are capable of identifying foreign antigens at molecular level and responding to them immunologically.
- Macrophages phagocytose foreign agents such as bacteria, viruses and cancer cells.

Lymph Nodes

The lymph nodes are oval or bean-shaped bodies, 0.1–2.5 cm long that lie along the course of lymph vessels. The lymph passes through a number of lymph nodes, usually 8–10 before reaching the large lymphatic ducts. The size of lymph nodes varies from pinhead to a large bean and are somewhat flattened. The lymph nodes are pink in living body and brownish in cadaver (embalmed dead bodies).

N.B.

The lymph nodes draining the lymph from lungs are black due to retention of inhaled carbon particles whereas those draining the small intestine are creamy white due to retention of emulsified fat.

The lymph nodes tend to occur in clusters/groups in specific regions of the body (Fig. 11.4). Some of the body's principal groups of lymph nodes are:

1. Cervical lymph nodes in the neck.
2. Axillary nodes in the upper limb.
3. Mediastinal lymph nodes in the thorax.
4. Aortic and mesenteric lymph nodes in the abdomen.
5. Iliac nodes in the pelvis.
6. Popliteal and inguinal nodes in the lower limb.

The superficial lymph nodes are arranged along the veins, and deep along the arteries.

The superficial lymph nodes are present in the superficial fascia, deep to skin whereas deep lymph nodes are located deep to deep fascia. The superficial lymph nodes drain into deep lymph nodes.

N.B.

There are about 450 lymph nodes in the body of a young individual; out of which 60–70 are found in the region of head–neck, 100 in the thorax and 250 in the abdomen and pelvis.

Structure of Lymph Nodes (Fig. 11.5)

The lymph nodes are oval or reniform and slightly flattened. They present a slight depression on the side called **hilum**. Many afferent lymph vessels enter the gland at periphery and a single efferent lymphatic vessel leaves the gland through hilum. The artery enters and vein leaves the gland at the hilum. Each lymph node consists of **fibrous capsule** and **gland substance** (parenchyma).

Capsule

The fibrous capsule invests the entire node and is separated from the gland substance by subcapsular space called **subcapsular sinus**.

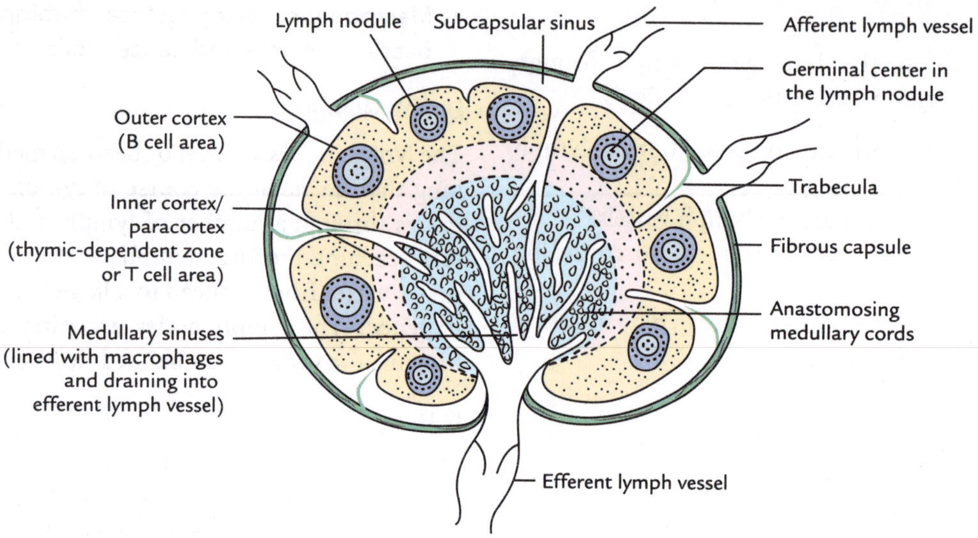

Fig. 11.5 Structure of a lymph node.

A number of trabeculae extended from capsule at variable distances into the substance of the gland. The trabeculae are accompanied by paratrabecular spaces which are continuous with the subcapsular sinus.

The afferent lymph vessels pierce the capsule and drain into subcapsular sinus. From subcapsular sinus, the lymph drains via a series of interconnected channels, the cortical and medullary sinuses, into the hilum of the node from which arises single efferent lymph vessel.

Gland Substance (Parenchyma)

The gland substance is divided into two portions:

1. An outer portion called **cortex**
2. An inner portion called **medulla**

The outer portion of cortex, the superficial cortex, contains B lymphocytes which form variable number of densely packed **lymphoid follicles/nodules.** Many of these nodules show less dense central regions called **germinal centers.** The lymphoid follicles without germinal centers are called **primary nodules** and those with germinal centers are called **secondary nodules.**

The germinal centers are the areas of rapid lymphocyte division and occupied by lymphoblasts and plasmoblasts. The peripheral portion of the nodule consists of small lymphocytes and plasma cells.

The inner portion of cortex (paracortex) contains T lymphocytes (*thymic-dependent zone*). The T lymphocytes do not organize themselves to form lymphoid nodules.

The medulla contains network of anastomosing cords of cells called **medullary cords.** The cells within medullary cords are: B lymphocytes, plasma cells and macrophages.

N.B.

Both cortex and medulla in addition to lymphocytes contain:

- *Reticular cells*, which along with reticular fibers form the framework of lymph node.
- *Plasma cells*, B lymphocytes mature into plasma cells and are mainly located into the medullary cords.
- *Macrophages*, mainly present in the medulla but also common in germinal centers. These cells present the antigens to lymphocytes for immunological response.
- The parenchyma of both cortex and medulla is traversed by blood vessels and lymph sinuses.

Circulation of Lymph and Blood in Lymph Nodes (Fig. 11.6)

Circulation of Lymph

Afferent lymph vessels bring the lymph to the lymph node, where it flows through *subcapsular*, *cortical* and *medullar sinuses* and finally leaves the gland through efferent lymph vessels. The sinuses are lined with phagocytic macrophages that remove bacteria and other foreign material from lymph.

N.B.

- Lymph nodes are the only structures which filter the lymph.
- Lymph nodes are the only lymphoid organs which have both afferent and efferent lymph vessels.

Flow of Blood (Fig. 11.6)

The blood reaches the lymph node through arteries that enter through hilum. These arteries branch in medulla and form capillary plexuses within the cortex. The lymphocytes

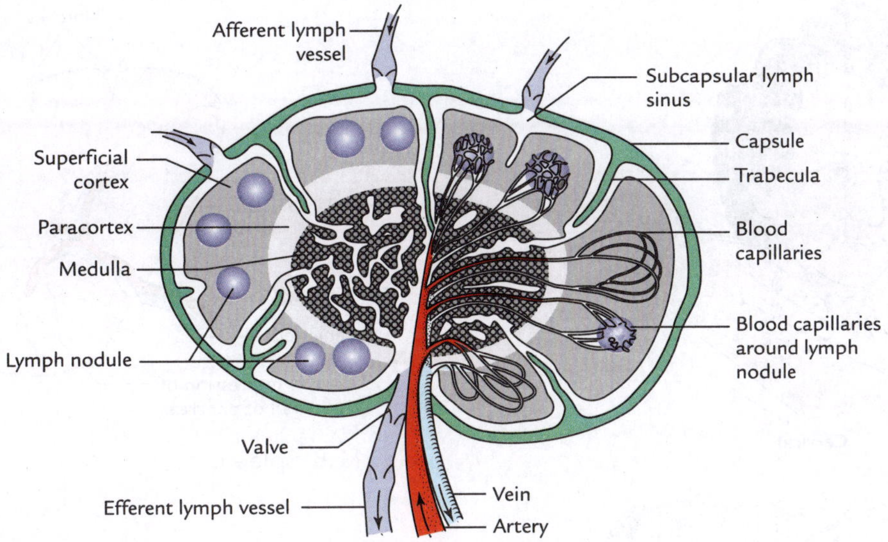

Fig. 11.6 Schematic diagram of a lymph node showing blood and lymph circulation. Note that lymph enters through the convex side of the lymph node and leaves through the hilum while blood enters and leaves the lymph node through the hilum.

enter lymph nodes mainly via the arteries. They leave the blood by migrating across the walls of postcapillary venules.

The arteries enter the lymph nodes through its hilum and give straight branches which traverse the medulla. In the cortex, arteries form dense arcades of arterioles and capillaries in numerous anastomosing loops eventually forming venules and veins. The capillaries are profuse around the lymph nodules. Postcapillary high endothelial venules (HEV) are abundant in paracortex and are the important sites of blood-borne lymphocyte extravasation into lymphoid tissue. The veins leave the lymph node through its hilum.

N.B.

Most of the lymphocytes enter the lymph node through blood while only few enter through lymph of afferent lymph vessel.

Functions of Lymph Nodes

1. Filter the lymph (i.e. when lymph passes through the lymph node, foreign particles, injurious substances, including pathogens are removed by phagocytic activities of macrophages of the lymph nodes).
2. Evoke immunological response. (The plasma cells of lymph node produce antibodies in response to infection.)
3. Produce various types of lymphocytes. (The germinal centers of lymphatic nodules within the node are sites of lymphocyte production.)
4. Provide portal of entry for lymphocytes into lymphatic channels.

Clinical correlation

- **Lymphoid nodules:** They are circumscribed structures made up of compact lymphoid tissue. Its lightly stained central portion is called *germinal center*. It is made up of lymphoblasts which give rise to lymphocytes. Its darkly stained peripheral portion contains lymphocytes.
- **Germinal centers are absent in embryonic life and in old age:** In lymphoid nodules, germinal center develops only after birth when it is exposed to antigens. The germinal center regresses when infection subsides. The lymphoid nodules atrophy with increasing age and may be absent in old age.
- **Spread of cancer:** The lymph vessels are the most convenient routes of spread of the cancer cells, i.e. they are major routes by which carcinoma metastasizes. When cancer cells enter the lymph vessels, they are trapped in the lymph nodes. If cancer cells escape from the lymph nodes, they may pass through lymph vessels to the blood and eventually reach to the other parts of the body. Therefore, during cancer surgery, malignant (cancerous) lymph nodes are often removed and their vessels are tied off and cut to prevent the spread of cancer.
- **Lymphadenitis:** The acute lymphadenitis (acute infection of lymph nodes) is often caused by microbes transported in it, through lymph from the area of infection. The lymph nodes become inflamed and enlarged; and then can be palpated by the clinician. The commonly palpated lymph nodes are cervical, axillary and inguinal (Fig. 11.1). Figure 11.7 shows the method of palpating cervical, axillary and epitrochlear nodes.

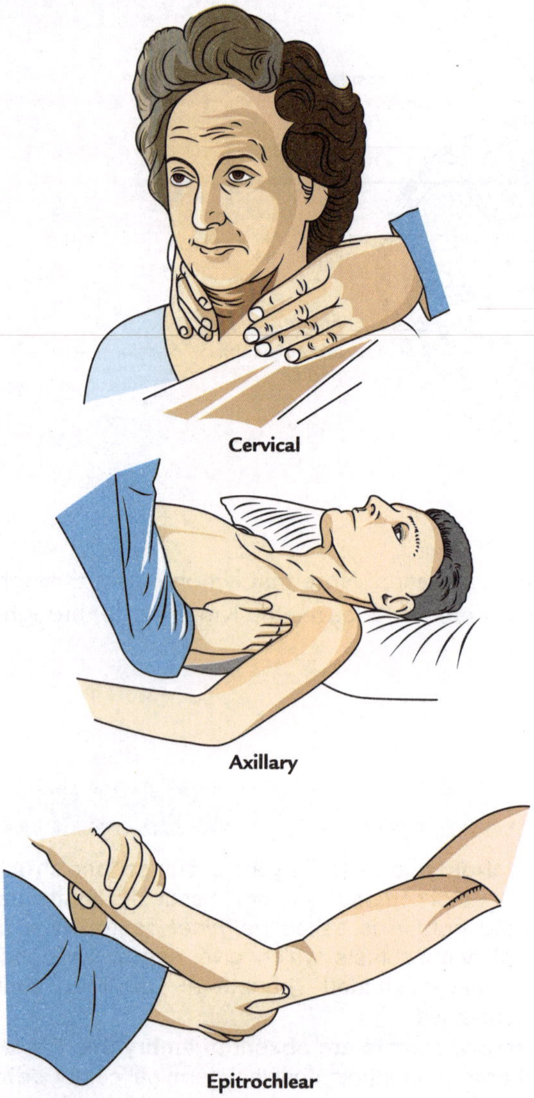

Fig. 11.7 Palpation of lymph nodes.

Spleen

The spleen (Fig. 11.8) is the largest lymphoid organ in the body. It is located deep in the left hypochondrium of abdominal cavity between fundus of stomach and the diaphragm. It is purplish and varies in size in different individuals. Usually it is of the size of a closed fist of that individual.

Structure

It consists of red and white pulp—the spleen thus represents the **hemolymph node** in the human body. The **white pulp** is the **lymphatic tissue sheath** that surrounds the central artery. This periarterial lymphatic tissue sheath possesses nodules with or without centers. These nodules are called **splenic nodules** or **Malphigian corpuscles**. The **red pulp** consists of network of anastomosing splenic cords (cords of Billroth). The splenic cords are made up of lymphocytes (both B and T type), macrophages and plasma cells. The spaces between

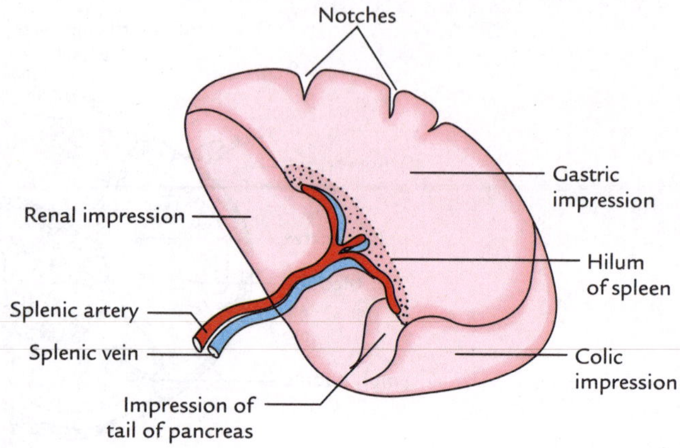

Fig. 11.8 Spleen.

the cords are occupied by blood sinusoids. The spleen is covered by a connective tissue capsule which sends trabeculae within the substance of the organ where they are repeatedly divided to form the network. The blood-borne antigens are removed in the spleen.

N.B.

Hemal nodes: These are found along the course of blood vessels in relation to thoracic and abdominal viscera. Their sinuses are filled with blood rather than lymph. The hemal nodes represent an intermediate stage between lymph node and spleen

Functions

1. Filters the blood from antigens and microorganisms.
2. Evokes immunological response against the antigens circulating in the blood.
3. Produces B and T lymphocytes.
4. Removes old and abnormal RBCs.
5. Removes bacteria by phagocytosis.
6. Stores blood.
7. Forms blood cells during fetal life.

Clinical correlation

Splenomegaly: The enlargement of spleen (splenomegaly) is usually secondary to other conditions, e.g. infections, circulatory disorders, blood diseases, malignant neoplasms:

(a) Spleen may be infected by blood-borne microbes, e.g. malaria, typhoid fever.
(b) Circulatory disorder like portal obstruction due to cirrhosis of liver leads to congestion of blood in spleen.
(c) In blood diseases like chronic myeloid leukemia, the spleen enlarges to extra workload associated with removing abnormal blood cells.
(d) Malignant neoplasms, e.g. lymphomas may cause metastatic tumors in spleen.

N.B.

The most common causes of enlargement of spleen are portal hypertension, malaria, chronic myeloid leukemia and typhoid fever.

Thymus

The thymus is an asymmetrical bilobed organ/gland located in the superior mediastinum of thoracic cavity behind the manubrium of sternum. This extends upwards into the root of the neck (Fig. 11.9). The thymus is devoid of lymph capillaries and lymphoid nodules.

The thymus is the central lymphoid organ and essential for development of other lymphoid organs. It is large and well developed in fetus and in early childhood. It attains its peak development at puberty and thereafter it starts involuting and is replaced by fibrofatty tissue. It weighs about 12–15 g at birth , 30–40 g at puberty and 10–15 g at 60 years.

Structure

The thymus consists of supporting framework made by epithelial reticular cells and parenchymal cells, *viz.* lymphocytes and macrophages. Thus thymus contains the following three main types of cells:

1. Epitheliocytes (thymic epithelial cells)
2. Lymphocytes
3. Macrophages

Thymus has dual origin, its epitheliocytes (epithelial reticular cells) arise from endoderm of third pharyngeal pouch whereas its lymphocytes and macrophages arise from mesoderm. Each lobe of thymus is divided into incomplete lobules. Each lobule has a darkly stained cortex at periphery and a lightly stained medulla in the center. The cortex is densely packed with lymphocytes (thymocytes). The outer part of the cortex contains immature large lymphocytes (lymphoblasts) which divide by mitosis to produce clones of small T lymphocytes which are pushed into deep part of the cortex. The epitheliocytes help in maturation of T lymphocytes through the hormone (**thymosin**) secreted by them. Immunocompetent T-cells leave the thymus and through circulation reach the peripheral lymphoid tissue. The medulla mainly consists of epitheliocytes and few lymphocytes. The most important feature of medulla is the presence of **Hassall's corpuscles.** These are made up of concentrically arranged flattened cells which are the degenerating epitheliocytes. The center of corpuscle contains homogeneous hyaline material produced by degenerating cells of the corpuscle.

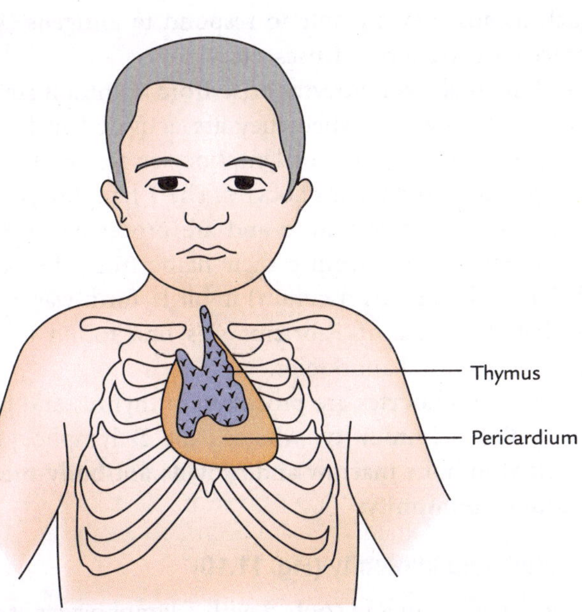

Fig. 11.9 Location of thymus.

N.B.

The reticulum of all the lymphoid organs is made of reticular cells and reticular fibers except thymus where the reticulum is formed by epitheliocytes.

Functions

The thymus is the site of production of T lymphocytes. It receives immunologically incompetent stem cells from bone marrow. In the thymus, these cells divide and mature into **T lymphocytes**, the specialized group of lymphocytes (thymus-dependent cells). These cells leave the thymus via blood to the lymph nodes, spleen and other lymphatic tissues. The T lymphocytes are important for both cellular and humoral immunological responses.

The thymus secretes a hormone called **thymosin** which supports the activity of T lymphocytes throughout the body

The production of T lymphocytes is most prolific in youth, an essential requisite to the development of protective immune function. For this reason, the thymus weighs about 10–15 g at birth and about 20–30 g at puberty. Therefore, it regresses and is converted into fibrofatty tissue.

Clinical correlation

Enlargement of thymus gland: It is associated with some autoimmune diseases e.g. thyrotoxicosis, Addison's disease and myasthenia gravis. Autoimmune conditions are those in which the immune system treats normal body cells or secretions as antigens and destroy them.

EPITHELIO-LYMPHOID SYSTEM

It consists of mucosa-associated lymphoid tissue (MALT). The large amount of unencapsulated lymphatic tissue exist in the walls of alimentary, respiratory and genitourinary tracts. It is collectively termed as mucosa-associated lymphoid tissue (MALT). The mucosa-associated lymphoid tissue is generally subdivided into the following two types:

1. Gut-associated lymphoid tissue (GALT)
2. Bronchus-associated lymphoid tissue (BALT)

The important collections or aggregations of mucosa-associated lymphoid tissue are as follows:

1. Pharyngeal tonsil
2. Tubal tonsil
3. Palatine tonsil
4. Lingual tonsil
5. Peyer's patches
6. Abdominal tonsil

Pharyngeal tonsil: It is the aggregation of lymphoid tissue underneath the mucous lining of the roof and posterior wall of the pharynx. When enlarged due to infection, it is termed as **adenoid** which obstructs nasal respiration and makes breathing through mouth obligatory.

Tubal tonsil: It is the aggregation of lymphoid tissue around the upper and posterior margin of the opening of the pharyngo-tympanic tube in the nasopharynx.

Palatine tonsil: It is a large aggregation of lymphoid tissue, one on each side, in the lateral wall of oropharynx in the triangular fossa called **tonsillar fossa.** They are commonly infected in children causing **tonsillitis.**

Lingual tonsil: The dorsal surface of posterior one-third of tongue (pharyngeal part) contains numerous lymphoid follicles underneath the mucosa, which together form the lingual tonsil.

Peyer's patches: These are aggregated lymphoid follicles varying from 2 to 10 cm in length, underneath the mucous membrane of small intestine, being largest and most numerous in the ilium and placed lengthwise along the antimesenteric border. The Peyer's patches are ulcerated in typhoid fever forming ulcers (typhoid ulcers) having long axis perpendicular to the long axis of the bowel.

Abdominal tonsil: There is a huge amount of lymphoid tissue underneath the mucous membrane of appendix in the form of rounded aggregations of lymphoid follicles which form a ring and together constitute the abdominal tonsil.

Reticulo-Endothelial System

The cells of this system are concerned with phagocytosis. They pick up, ingest and store foreign substances. Thus cells of this system are important for general and local defense mechanisms.

Different types of cells in reticulo-endothelial system are enumerated in Table 11.1.

Table 11.1 Different types of cells in reticulo-endothelial system and their sites of location

Cells	Sites of location
Macrophages	Connective tissue, bone marrow, suprarenal gland
Pericytes (Rouget cells)	Capillaries
Monocytes	Blood
Dust cells (alveolar macrophages)	Lungs
Reticular cells	Spleen and lymphoid tissue
Kupffer cells	Liver
Microglia	Central nervous system

LYMPHOCYTES AND IMMUNITY

Immunity is the defense mechanism of the body, i.e. the ability of the body to resist damage from foreign substances such as microorganisms and harmful toxins (antigens) released by them. The defense mechanism of the body includes **phagocytosis**, which is a nonspecific engulfing process and **immune response**, which is a specific reaction to microorganisms and antigens. The cell type involved in immune response is lymphocytes. The lymphocytes are smaller than monocytes and have large nuclei.

The lymphocytes circulate in blood and are present in large numbers in lymphatic organs and tissues. They develop from pluripotent stem cells in red bone marrow and then travel in blood to lymphoid tissues elsewhere in the body where they are activated, i.e. becoming immunocompetent which means they are able to respond to antigens (foreign material, e.g. bacteria, viruses, etc.)

Although all lymphocytes arise from common stem cells in bone marrow but when they are activated in lymphoid tissue, two distinct types of lymphocytes are produced, *viz.* T lymphocytes and B lymphocytes. The T lymphocytes are so named because they mature and are processed in thymus. The B lymphocytes acquire their name from the bursa of Fabricius (cloacal diverticulum) in birds, for it was in chickens that the bursa of Fabricius was first found to be the source of humoral antibodies.

The T lymphocytes are processed in thymus and provide **cell-mediated immunity**, whereas the B lymphocytes are processed in bone marrow and provide **antibody-mediated (humoral) immunity**.

Cell-Mediated Immunity (Fig. 11.10)

When antigen comes in contact with T lymphocytes, it stimulates the division and proliferation of the T lymphocytes,

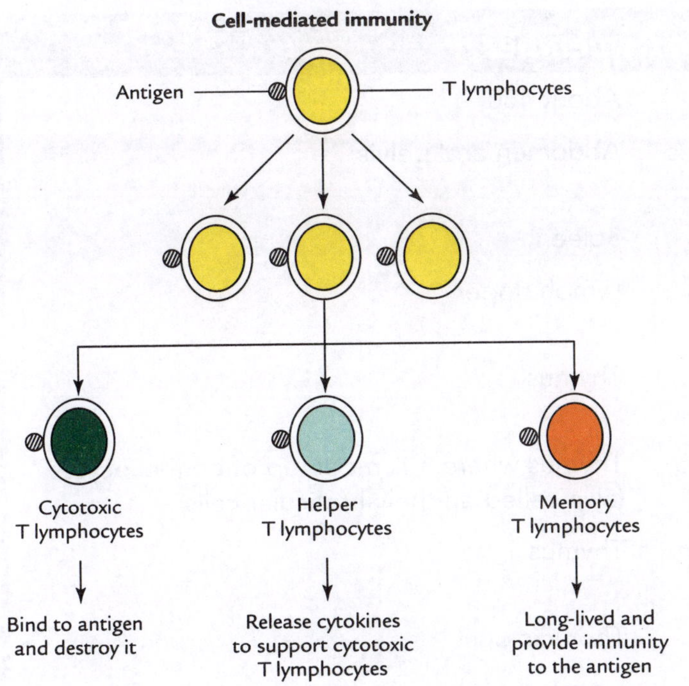

Fig. 11.10 Proliferation of T lymphocytes in cell-mediated immunity.

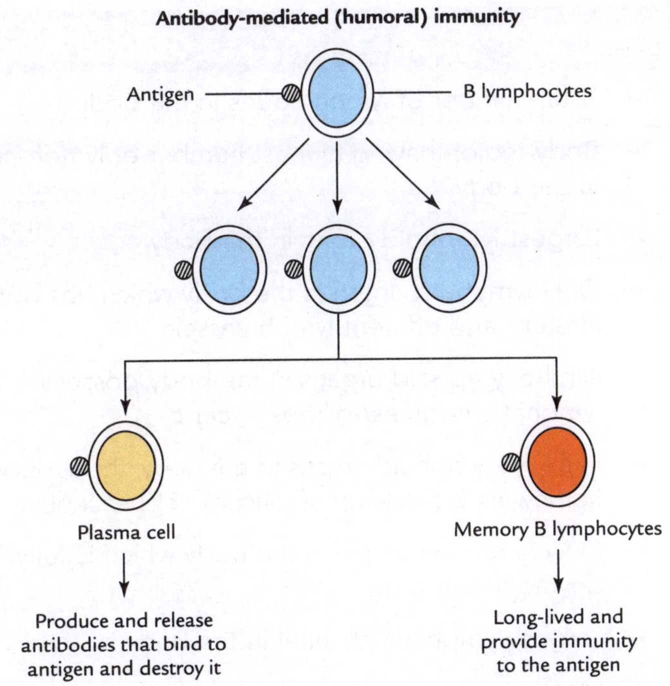

Fig. 11.11 Proliferation of B lymphocytes in antibody-mediated (humoral) immunity.

leading to production of three main types of specialized T lymphocytes:

1. Cytotoxic T lymphocytes
2. Helper T lymphocytes
3. Memory T lymphocytes

All these cells tackle the same antigen in different ways (Fig. 11.10), e.g. the cytotoxic T lymphocytes bind to antigen and destroy it. The helper T lymphocytes release cytokines to support cytotoxic T lymphocytes. The memory T lymphocytes are long lived and provide immunity to the antigen.

N.B.

One of the primary causes of acquired immunodeficiency syndrome (AIDS) is the killing of helper T lymphocytes by human immunodeficiency virus.

Antibody-Mediated (Humoral) Immunity

The B lymphocytes, unlike T lymphocytes, which are free to circulate around the body are fixed with lymphoid tissue. When B lymphocytes come in contact with an antigen, they enlarge and begin to divide (Fig. 11.11). It produces two functionally distinct types of cells—plasma cells and memory B lymphocytes. The plasma cells produce and release antibodies (i.e. immunoglobulins—IgG, IgA, IgM, IgE and IgD) that bind to antigen and destroy it. The memory B lymphocytes are long lived and provide immunity to the antigen.

BONE MARROW

The bone marrow is soft pulpy vascular tissue. It consists of a delicate network of reticular tissue stroma and clusters of hemopoietic cells. For details see Chapter 6, page 73.

Golden Facts to Remember

➢ Total number of lymph nodes in the body	About 450
➢ Body region having highest number of lymph nodes in the body	Abdomen and pelvis
➢ Largest lymphoid organ in the body	Spleen
➢ Only lymphoid organ in the body which has both afferent and efferent lymph vessels	Lymph node
➢ All the lymphoid organs in the body possess lymphatic nodules/follicles *except*	Thymus
➢ In all the lymphoid organs of the body, the supporting framework is made up of reticular cells *except* in	Thymus where it is made up of epitheliocytes (also called epithelial reticular cells)
➢ Only lymphoid organ in the body which is fully developed at birth	Thymus
➢ Largest lymphatic channel in the body	Thoracic duct
➢ Most common route for spread of cancer (metastasis)	Lymph vessels
➢ All lymphocytes arise from common stem cells in bone marrow *except*	During embryonic life when they arise from yolk sac, liver, and spleen
➢ Most abundant cell types present in the lymphoid organs	Lymphocytes
➢ Largest lymphatic sac in the body	Cisterna chyli
➢ Most abundant immunoglobulin (antibody) in the body	IgG

Multiple Choice Questions

1. **All are true statements, regarding lymphatic system *except*:**
   (a) Return all the tissue fluid to the venous system
   (b) Lymph is filtered by lymph nodes
   (c) Spleen and thymus are lymphoid organs
   (d) Lymph capillaries begin blindly in intercellular spaces

2. **Thoracic duct drains lymph from all of the following regions *except*:**
   (a) Right lower limb
   (b) Right side of the head and neck
   (c) Left lower limb
   (d) Left side of the head and neck

3. **All the lymphoid organs have lymphoid nodules *except*:**
   (a) Spleen
   (b) Lymph node
   (c) Thymus
   (d) Palatine tonsil

4. **Lymphoid organ having both afferent and efferent lymph vessels is:**
   (a) Spleen
   (b) Thymus
   (c) Lymph node
   (d) Tonsil

5. **All are true regarding thymus *except that it*:**
   (a) Is located in the superior mediastinum
   (b) Secretes a hormone called '*thymosin*'
   (c) Filters blood to remove blood-borne antigens
   (d) Receives immunologically incompetent cells from bone marrow

6. **All of the following factors help in lymphatic drainage *except*:**
   (a) Respiratory movements
   (b) Filtration pressure in tissue spaces
   (c) Positive pressure in brachio-cephalic veins
   (d) Presence of valves within the lumen of lymph vessels

7. **All of the following sites are devoid of lymph capillaries *except*:**
   (a) Epidermis
   (b) Dermis
   (c) Hair
   (d) Nails

8. **Lymph vessels are present in all *except*:**
   (a) Brain
   (b) Liver
   (c) Lungs
   (d) Vagina

9. **Which of the following is primary lymphoid tissue?**
   (a) Lymph node
   (b) Spleen
   (c) Thymus
   (d) Palatine tonsil

10. **Epithelial reticulum is a feature of:**
    (a) Spleen
    (b) Lymph node
    (c) Thymus
    (d) All of the above

Answers

1. *a*, **2.** *b*, **3.** *c*, **4.** *c*, **5.** *c*, **6.** *c*, **7.** *b*, **8.** *a*, **9.** *c*, **10.** *c*

CHAPTER

12

Nervous System

Learning Objectives

After studying this chapter, the student should be able to:

- define the nervous system and list its functions
- outline the subdivisions of the nervous system
- outline the main morphological types of neurons and describe the structure of a typical neuron
- describe the various types of neuroglia and discuss their function
- describe the structure and functions of a synapse and elucidate the various types of synapses
- classify the nerves and discuss the reflex action
- describe the typical spinal nerve and list the spinal nerves that form nerve plexuses
- present a brief account of a 'dermatome'
- identify two divisions of autonomic nervous system
- compare and contrast the effects of sympathetic and parasympathetic stimulation
- explain how referred pain occurs
- enumerate the neurotransmitters liberated by pre- and postganglionic fibers of parasympathetic and sympathetic nervous system
- correctly solve the review questions given at the end of the chapter

INTRODUCTION

The nervous system integrates and controls the activities of all other systems of the body, hence it is also termed as '**master system**' of the body. The functions of nervous system include:

1. Reception of stimuli from within and outside the body.
2. Integration of sensory information.
3. Initiation and execution of motor responses.
4. Assimilation of experience, an essential requisite to memory, learning and intelligence.

Due to these functions, an individual is able to maintain the internal environment of the body and react to the changes in the external environment.

All activities of nervous system whether simple or complex involve three neural factors or elements: (a) reception, (b) integration and (c) response.

In human beings, the integrative element shows maximum degree of development and they are the most intellectual animals in the animal kingdom.

SUBDIVISIONS OF THE NERVOUS SYSTEM

ANATOMICAL SUBDIVISION (Fig. 12.1)

1. **Central nervous system (CNS):** It includes brain and spinal cord.
2. **Peripheral nervous system (PNS):** It includes all neural structures outside the CNS, *viz.*
   (a) Peripheral nerves
   - 12 pairs of cranial nerves
   - 31 pairs of spinal nerves

   (b) Ganglia (autonomic and sensory)
   (c) Autonomic nervous system (sympathetic and parasympathetic nervous systems).

FUNCTIONAL SUBDIVISION (Fig. 12.2)

1. **Afferent (sensory) division:** It brings information to the CNS.
2. **Efferent (motor) division:** It gives appropriate motor command to muscles and glands. The efferent division is further divided into components:
   (a) *Somatic nervous system:* It innervates somatic structures like skeletal muscles and responsible for voluntary motor activities.
   (b) *Autonomic nervous system:* It innervates visceral structures like cardiac muscle, smooth muscle and glands. The activities of viscera are mostly involuntary, i.e. not under voluntary control.

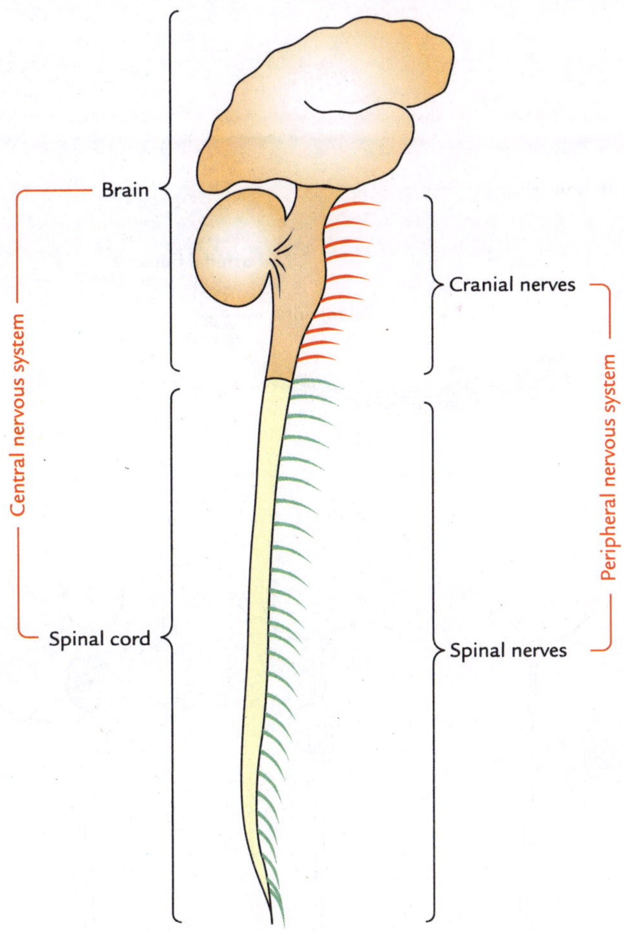

Fig. 12.1 Anatomical subdivision of the nervous system.

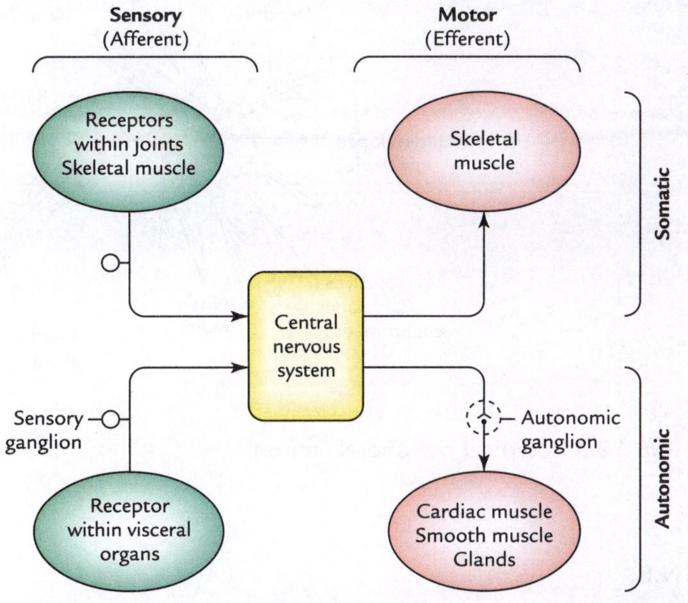

Fig. 12.2 Functional subdivision of the nervous system.

STRUCTURAL ORGANIZATION OF THE NERVOUS SYSTEM

The structural organization of the nervous system is very simple as it consists of only two principal types of cells: (a) neurons and (b) neuroglia

The neurons are the structural and functional units of the nervous system whereas neuroglia provides structural and functional support to the neurons.

NEURONS

The neurons are the *structural and functional units* of the nervous system. The number of neurons in the nervous system is estimated to be in the range of 100 billion. The two main properties of neurons are excitability and conductivity. The neurons are specialized for reception, integration, transformation, and transmission of impulses. The neurons are highly differentiated cells and have lost their power of division.

Structure of a Neuron (Fig. 12.3)

A neuron consists of a cell body (perikaryon or soma) and has two processes.

Cell Body

The cell body consists of a mass of cytoplasm surrounded by a plasma membrane. It contains a large vesicular nucleus with prominent nucleolus.

The two main characteristic features of the cytoplasm of the neuron are:

1. Presence of a basophilic **Nissl substance** (Nissl bodies)
2. **Neurofibrils**

The *Nissl substance* is composed of the large aggregations of rough endoplasmic reticulum, which contain ribonucleic acid concerned with protein synthesis, *viz.* neurotransmitters. The *neurofibrils* are filamentous strands of proteins.

N.B.

There are no centrioles and centrosome in the nerve cell body, which indicates that the highly specialized nerve cell has lost its power of division. Consequently, once the nerve cell is destroyed it is replaced by neuroglia.

Process

The processes are of two types:

1. Numerous short processes called **dendrites** (*dendron* = tree).
2. A single long process called **axon.**

The dendrites bring impulses towards the cell body, hence they often branch profusely to increase the reception area of the neuron.

The axon is a single long process. It does not branch except at its termination to form **telodendria** which possess terminal **boutons** (*presynaptic knobs*).

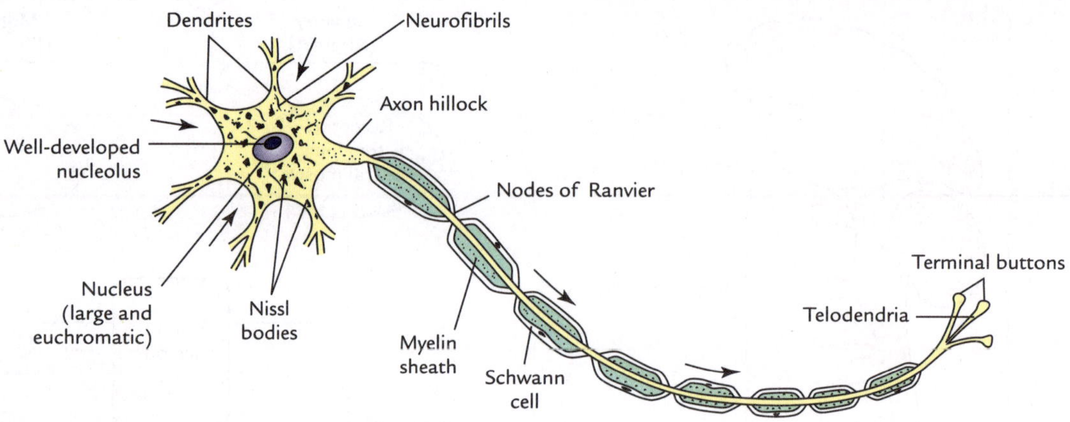

Fig. 12.3 A typical peripheral neuron.

N.B.

- Collection of nerve cell bodies within the CNS is called nucleus, whereas the collection of nerve cell bodies outside the CNS is called ganglion.
- Axon is termed as *nerve fiber.*
- Bundles of nerve fibers within the CNS form *tracts* while outside the CNS they form *peripheral nerves.*
- *Gray matter* consists of mainly nerve cell bodies and dendrites while *white matter* consists of mainly nerve fibers.

Classification of Neurons

A. According to polarity (Fig. 12.4)

1. **Pseudo-unipolar neurons:** They appear to have only one process which soon divides into a central branch that functions as axon and a peripheral branch that serves as a dendrite. Most sensory neurons of the nervous system are pseudo-unipolar type.

N.B.

Pseudo-unipolar neurons are so called because originally two processes emerge at the same pole. But during the course of development, two processes fuse to form a single process that bifurcates at a little distance from the cell body.

Sites of Location:
(a) Posterior (dorsal) root ganglia of spinal nerves
(b) Sensory ganglia of cranial nerves

2. **Bipolar neurons:** They have two processes one on each pole, one process acts as the dendrite and the other process acts as an axon.
Sites of Location:
(a) Retina of the eye
(b) Olfactory epithelium
(c) Vestibulocochlear ganglia

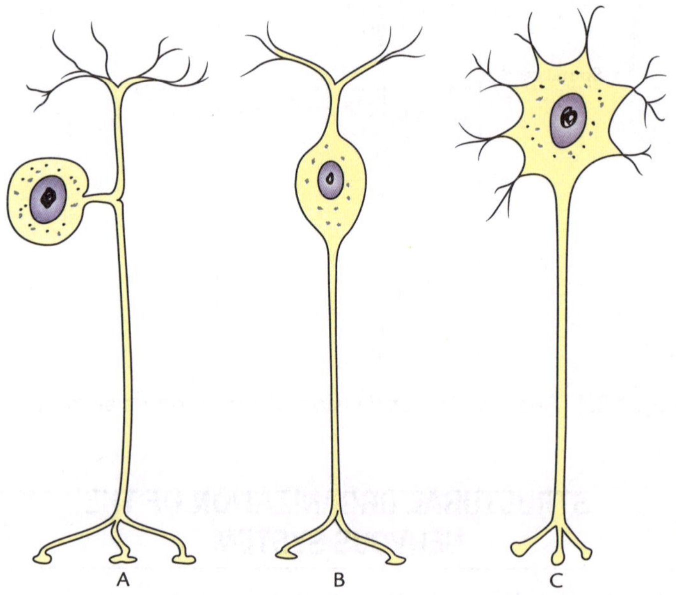

Fig. 12.4 Three main types of neurons, based on their morphology: **A**, pseudo-unipolar; **B**, bipolar; **C**, multipolar.

3. **Multipolar neurons:** They have several dendrites and only one axon extending form the cell body. They are the most common type of neurons in the nervous system.
Sites of Location:
(a) Motor neurons forming tracts of brain and spinal cord.
(b) Motor neurons of anterior horn cells forming peripheral nerves.
(c) Motor neurons of autonomic ganglia.

B. According to relative length of axons and dendrites

1. **Golgi type I neurons:** These neurons have long axons which may be up to 1 m long, e.g. *pyramidal cells* of

cerebral cortex, *anterior horn cells* of spinal cord and *Purkinje cells* of cerebellum.

2. **Golgi type II neurons (microneurons):** The axons of these neurons are short and morphologically similar to dendrites, giving these neurons a star-shaped appearance.

C. According to the shape of the cell body

1. **Pyramidal cells:** The cell body is cone/pyramidal shaped and dendrites arise from the angles of the cone, e.g. pyramidal cells of motor cortex of cerebral hemisphere.
2. **Fusiform cells:** The cell body is spindle shaped and processes emerge at the both ends, e.g. fusiform cells of motor cortex of cerebral hemisphere.
3. **Pyriform cells:** The cell body is flask shaped. A thick dendrite arises from the upper end and divides repeatedly, whereas the axon arises from the base, e.g. Purkinje cells of cerebellum.

Other types

1. **Stellate cells:** Dendrites extend in all directions from the cell body, e.g. stellate cells of cerebellar cortex and sympathetic ganglia.
2. **Glomerular cells:** Dendrites at their tip are highly coiled, granule cells of cerebellar cortex.
3. **Amacrine cells:** They lack an obvious axon and a single process permit conduction in either direction, e.g. amacrine cells of retina of the eye.

GANGLION

These are collections of cell bodies of neurons outside the central nervous system. They can be classified into two types:

1. **Cerebrospinal ganglia:** They are connected with sensory afferent nerve fibers of the cranial and spinal nerves, hence they are called **sensory ganglia.**
2. **Autonomic ganglia:** They are connected with autonomic outflow and consist of cell bodies of multipolar motor neurons, hence they are called **motor ganglia**. They are relay stations of preganglionic sympathetic and parasympathetic fibers.

The sympathetic ganglia lie away from the viscera they supply whereas parasympathetic ganglia lie near the viscera they supply.

NEUROGLIA (Fig. 12.5)

They provide structural and functional support to the axons. The neuroglia play no important role in propagation of impulses or processing of perceived information.

The neuroglia are far more numerous (about 5–10 times more) than neurons and account for more than half of the brain's weight.

Structure of Neuroglia

Neuroglia are highly branched cells and occupy the spaces between the neurons to provide a microenvironment suitable

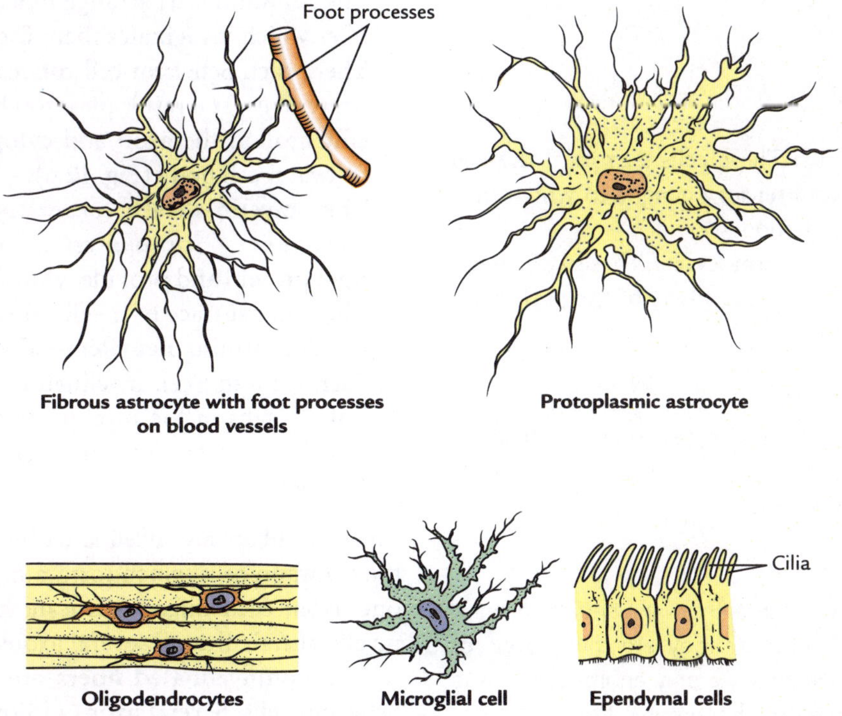

Fig. 12.5 Different types of neuroglia.

for neuronal activity. (Remember that nervous tissue has no intercellular matrix.)

Classification of Neuroglia

According to their location, origin and function

[A] Neuroglia in CNS

1. **Astrocytes:** These are the largest and most numerous. The astrocytes are star-shaped with many dendrite-like processes whose ends possess small swellings called **foot processes.** The foot processes form sleeve around the capillaries. The sleeve along with endothelial wall of the capillary forms the **blood–brain barrier.** The astrocytes are of two types: (a) protoplasmic found in gray matter and (b) fibrous found in white matter.
2. **Oligodendrocytes:** These are smaller than astrocytes and as the name implies, have fewer processes. Oligodendrocytes form myelin sheath around the fibers of CNS.
3. **Ependymal cells:** These cells line the ventricles of brain and the central canal of spinal cord.
4. **Microglia:** These are the smallest glial cells. These are phagocytic cells derived from mesoderm.

Clinical correlation

Gliosis: The microglia migrate to areas damaged by infection, trauma or stroke and perform phagocytosis. The damaged neurons are replaced by the proliferation of astrocytes, a process called '*gliosis*'.
Glioblastoma multiforme: It is the most fatal brain tumor with life expectancy of 2–3 months only. It arises from astrocytes.

[B] Neuroglia in PNS

1. **Satellite (capsular) cells:** These cells surround the cell bodies of autonomic and sensory ganglia to which they provide support and nutrition.
2. **Schwann cells or neurolemmocytes:** These cells form myelin sheath around the nerve fibers of the peripheral nervous system.

According to their structure

1. **Macroglia:** They include astrocytes, oligodendrocytes and ependymal cells.
2. **Microglia:** (already described.)

N.B.

- Schwann cells form neurolemma (Schwann sheath) around all nerve fibers of PNS whether they are myelinated or nonmyelinated. The Schwann cells play an important role in the regeneration of the peripheral nerve fiber.
- All the neuroglia develop from neural crest except microglia which develops from mesoderm (bone marrow).

Functions of Neuroglia

The functions performed by neuroglial cells are as follows:

1. Provide structural and functional support to neurons.
2. Help to form blood–brain barrier.
3. Phagocytose foreign substances.
4. Produce cerebrospinal fluid (CSF).
5. Form myelin sheaths around axons.

NERVE FIBERS

The axon of nerve cell is called **nerve fiber.** The bundles of nerve fibers within the central nervous system are called tracts, whereas the bundles of nerve fibers in the peripheral nervous system are called **peripheral nerves** or simply **nerves.**

The following two types of nerve fibers are found in the nervous system:

1. Myelinated nerve fibers
2. Nonmyelinated nerve fibers

MYELINATION OF NERVE FIBERS

The fibers of the CNS are myelinated by oligodendrocytes while those of PNS by Schwann cells.

The myelination of a peripheral nerve fiber occurs in the following way:

- The Schwann cells arrange in a sequence along the nerve fiber which invaginates them forming **mesaxons.**
- Then, each Schwann cell rotates many times around the nerve fiber; as a result mesaxon becomes wrapped repeatedly around the axon and cytoplasm is extruded in the Schwann cell body (Fig. 12.6).
- Thus **myelin sheath** *consists of many layers of plasma membrane of Schwann cell*, which is made up of white lipid protein and provide whitish appearance to the fiber. The outer surface of myelin sheath is encased in a glycoprotein forming **neurilemmal sheath.**
- Each Schwann cell myelinates only 1 mm of axon, thus leaving gaps in the myelin sheath where the axon is exposed to the exterior. These gaps are called the **nodes of Ranvier.**

The CNS fibers are myelinated by oligodendrocytes. Unlike the Schwann cells which form a myelin sheath around only one axon, each oligodendrocyte has extensions that form myelin sheath around several axons.

The **nonmyelinated fibers** are also surrounded by the Schwann cells. Several axons (15 or more) become longitudinally invaginated into the cytoplasm of Schwann cell and are sealed by plasma membrane (Fig. 12.7).

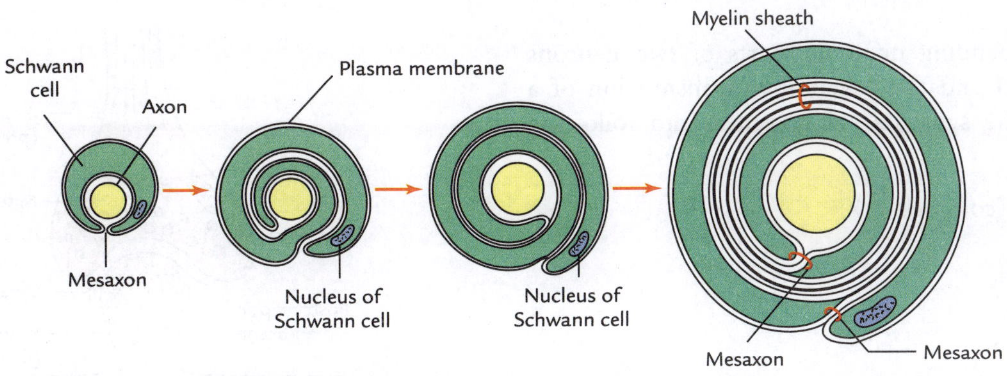

Fig. 12.6 Stages in the formation of myelin sheath around a peripheral nerve fiber.

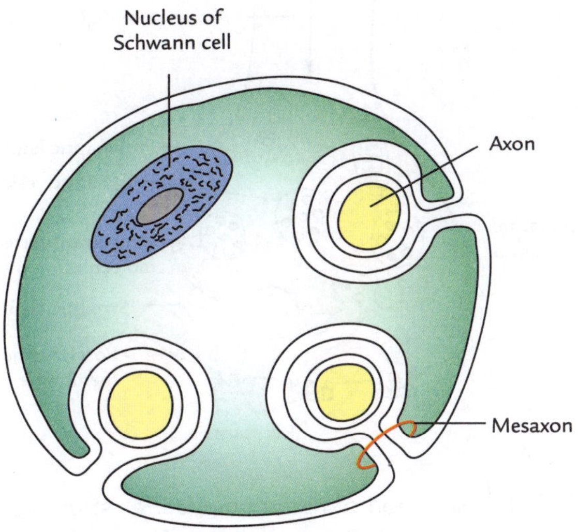

Fig. 12.7 Relationship of several nonmyelinated axons to a Schwann cell.

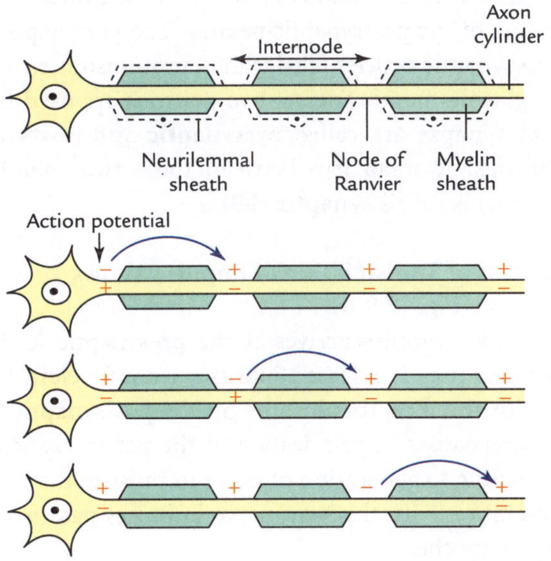

Fig. 12.8 Conduction of action potential along an axon.

The examples of myelinated fibers are:

1. Nerve fibers of the somatic nervous system more than 1 μm in diameter.
2. All preganglionic fibers of autonomic nervous system (ANS).

The examples of nonmyelinated nerve fibers are:

1. Nerve fibers of somatic nervous system less than 1 μm in diameter.
2. All postganglionic fibers of autonomic nervous system.

CONDUCTION OF ACTION POTENTIAL ALONG AN AXON (Fig. 12.8)

When the nerve is stimulated, the plasma membrane becomes depolarized and an **action potential** (tiny electrical charge) is generated. This action potential then spreads along the plasma membrane.

The speed of conduction of action potential is faster along the myelinated nerve fibers as it jumps from one node to the other and is called **saltatory conduction** (*saltase* = to leap/jump). The speed of conduction is slower in nonmyelinated fibers, as advancement of the action potential is consistent and at a moderate pace. Thus the conduction of action potential in myelinated fibers is like a **grasshopper jumping** whereas in nonmyelinated fibers it is like a **grasshopper walking**.

Transmission of Impulses

In nervous system, the information passes from one place to the other in the form of an **action potential or nerve impulse**. The nerve impulse is akin to a tiny electrical charge generated due to exchange of sodium (Na^+) and potassium (K^+) ions across the plasma membrane following a stimulus.

The nerve impulse travels progressively along a nerve fiber and then passes on to another neuron across the *synapse*.

Synapse

The junction at which the nerve impulse passes from one neuron to another is called **synapse**. The synapse is the contact between two neurons by contiguity and not by continuity.

Types of Synapses

Anatomically, depending upon the parts of two neurons coming in contact and the direction of transmission of a nerve impulse, the synapses are classified into following types:

1. Axodendritic (commonest)
2. Axosomatic
3. Dendrosomatic
4. Dendroaxonic
5. Dendrodendritic
6. Axoaxonic

Structure of Synapse (Fig. 12.9 A)

It consists of a synaptic knob of presynaptic neuron and plasma membrane of the postsynaptic neuron. The presynaptic knob contains synaptic vesicles filled with neurotransmitter.

The plasma membranes of two neurons apposed to each other at synapse are called **presynaptic and postsynaptic membranes**. A small gap between these two membranes (20–30 nm) is called **synaptic cleft.**

Mechanism of Transmission of Impulse Across the Synapse (Fig. 12.9 B)

As the nerve impulse arrives at the presynaptic knob, the neurotransmitter is released into the synaptic cleft. Here it binds with the receptors located on the postsynaptic membrane. This causes depolarization of the postsynaptic membrane, leading to generation of nerve impulse in the postsynaptic membrane. In this way, nerve impulses pass from one neuron to another.

Neurotransmitter

It is a chemical substance involved in transmission of nerve impulse across the synapse. There are number of neurotransmitters but the most common of them is **acetylcholine**. The acetylcholine once liberated in the synaptic cleft, binds with the receptors of the postsynaptic membrane to depolarize it. The remaining acetylcholine in the synaptic cleft is broken down into **acetate** and **choline** by an enzyme called **acetylcholine esterase.**

N.B.

The nerve impulse causing depolarization of postsynaptic membrane is called *excitatory nerve impulse*, whereas nerve impulse causing hyperpolarization of postsynaptic membrane is called *inhibitory nerve impulse* (Fig. 12.10).

Clinical correlation

The synaptic transmission may be affected by various drugs, e.g. *caffeine* is a stimulant that increases the rate of transmission across the synapse. That is why office workers are very fond of taking tea and coffee.

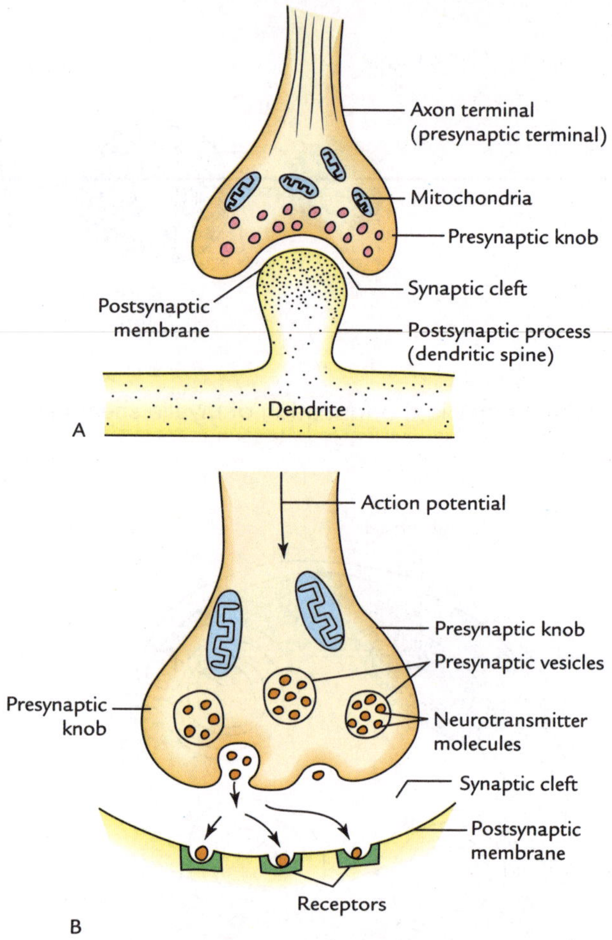

Fig. 12.9 Transmission of nerve impulse: **A**, structure of synapse (axodendritic); **B**, mechanism of transmission of nerve impulse at synapse.

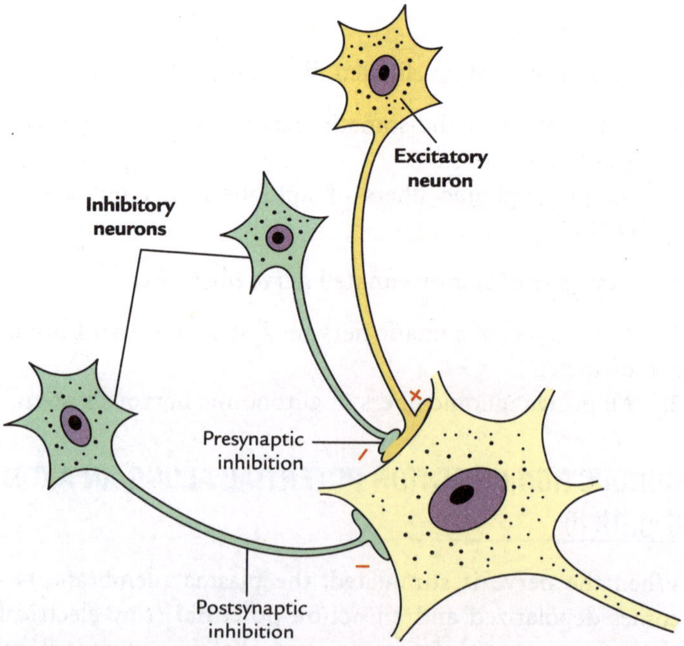

Fig. 12.10 Excitatory and inhibitory synapses in a motor neuron.

NERVES

The term 'nerve' refers to the peripheral nerve. The peripheral nerve consists of bundles of nerve fibers.

STRUCTURE OF A NERVE/PERIPHERAL NERVE

Each nerve consists of bundles or fasciculi of nerve fibers and connective tissue.

Each nerve fiber is enclosed in a delicate connective tissue sheath called **endoneurium.**

Each group of nerve fibers (fasciculus) is surrounded by a connective tissue sheath called **perineurium.**

The entire nerve is surrounded by a dense connective tissue sheath called **epineurium** which contains blood vessels (Fig. 12.11).

N.B.

The three connective tissue sheaths provide a considerable mechanical strength to the peripheral nerve and form half of the bulk of the nerve.

CLASSIFICATION OF NERVES

The nerves are classified into following three types:

1. Motor nerves
2. Sensory nerves
3. Mixed nerves

The **sensory nerves** transmit impulses from receptors in the periphery to the CNS.

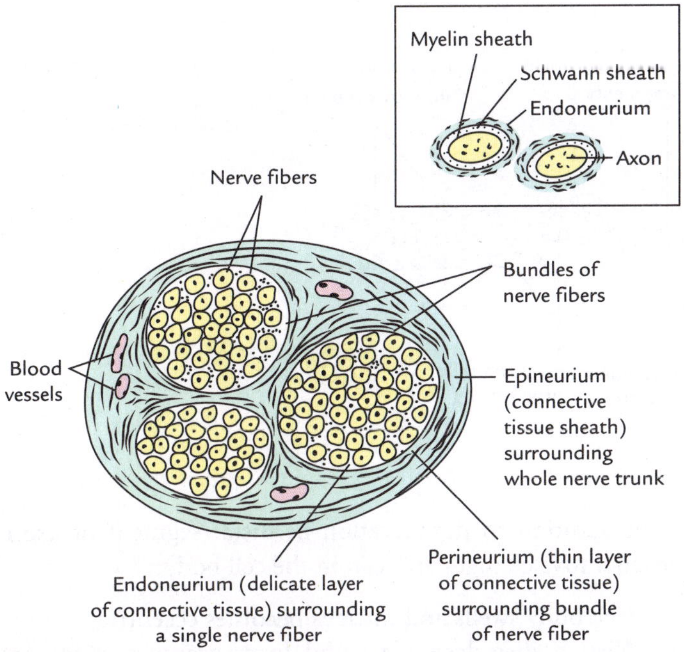

Fig. 12.11 Structure of a peripheral nerve. Inset shows covering of axon.

The **motor nerves** transmit motor impulse from CNS to the effector organ, *viz.* skeletal muscle. The loss of motor nerve supply leads to degeneration of skeletal muscle fibers.

The **mixed nerve** consists of both the motor and sensory fibers.

REFLEX ACTION

A reflex action is an automatic response to a stimulus without conscious thought. It is protective in nature. The structures involved to carry out this reflex are:

1. Sensory receptor
2. Afferent (sensory) neuron
3. Association (connector) neuron
4. Efferent (motor) neuron
5. Effector organ

The classic example of reflex action is a **withdrawal reflex** such as when a pin is pricked in the hand, the receptor is stimulated. The nerve impulse produced by a painful stimulus reaches the spinal cord through a sensory (afferent) neuron. The impulse is passed to the motor neuron via an association neuron (interneuron) which in turn stimulates the flexor muscles of hand (effector organ) and as a result hand moves (i.e. withdrawn) away from the pin (Fig. 12.12).

N.B.

Various other reflexes like ocular, cardiac, cough and intestinal operate in a similar fashion.

DEGENERATION AND REGENERATION OF NERVES AFTER INJURY

The injuries of peripheral nerves are quite common. They may occur due to compression, traction, trauma, intramuscular injection, cut, etc.

There are three types of nerve injuries as follows:

1. **Neurotmesis:** Interruption of axon and its myelin sheath.
2. **Axonotmesis:** Interruption of axon with preservation of myelin sheath.
3. **Neuropraxia:** Both axon and myelin sheath are preserved.

Recovery can occur in cases of neuropraxia and axonotmesis but some degree of function loss is inevitable with neurotmesis. When a nerve (axon) is cut, a series of degenerative and regenerative changes follows.

Degeneration (Fig. 12.13)

When the nerve fiber is cut, the distal segment of axon that is severed from the cell body degenerates. This is called

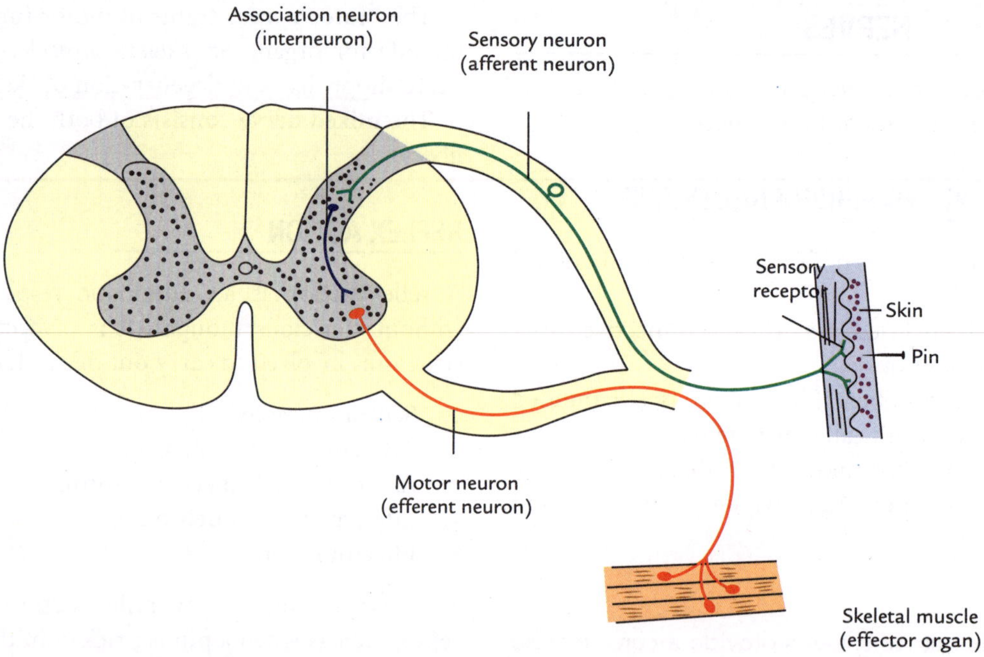

Fig. 12.12 Reflex arc (withdrawal reflex). The components of reflex are labeled in the order in which action potential passes through them. The five components are: sensory receptor, afferent neuron, association neuron, efferent neuron and an effector organ.

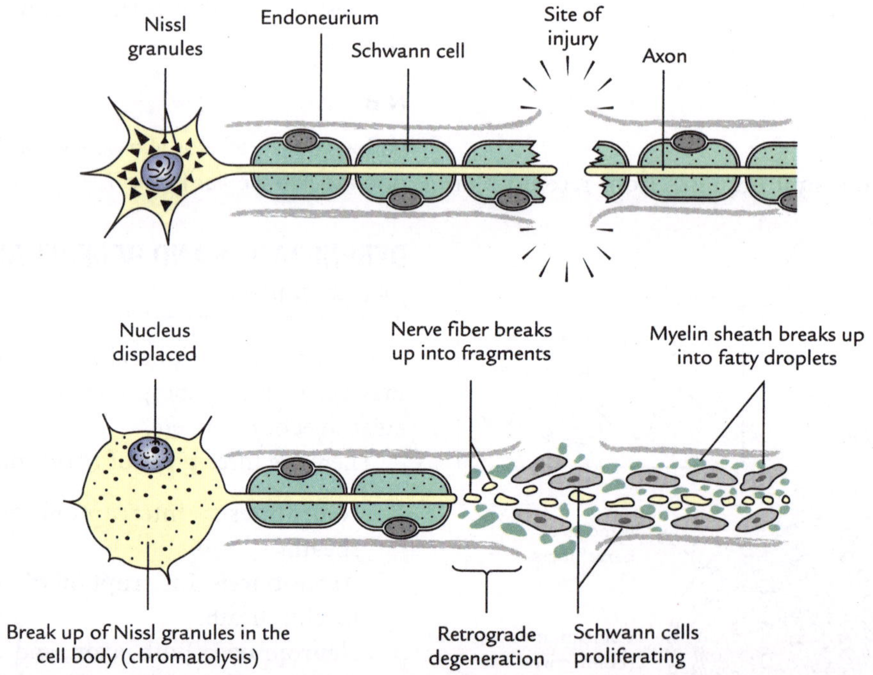

Fig. 12.13 Degeneration of nerve fiber (Wallerian degeneration).

Wallerian degeneration. The process is named after Waller, who first described (in 1850) the histological effects of nerve degeneration.

There is complete fragmentation of nerve fiber including its myelin sheath; however, myelin-producing sheath cells (Schwann cells) survive.

In addition to degeneration of distal segment of axon, degenerative changes are seen in the cell body:

1. Cell body swells and nucleus becomes eccentric.
2. Nissl bodies degenerate and form granules which are dispersed throughout within the cell body. This process is called **chromatolysis.**

The changes that occur in the cell body following an injury to its axon is called **'retrograde degeneration'**.

Regeneration (Fig. 12.14)

The macrophages migrate to the site of lesion and phagocytose the debris. The neurolemmocytes (Schwann cells) proliferate and form a cord of cells called **band fiber** within the endoneurium. The part of axon that is connected to the cell body begins to grow forming sprouts with bulbous tips and enters the cord of neurolemmocytes.

The neurolemmocytes of the cord secrete a chemical substance, the **nerve growth factor** that attracts the growing axon tip and guides it to its proper destination.

Factors Necessary for the Satisfactory Regeneration are:

1. Endoneurium and neurolemmal sheath should be present intact.
2. Distance between the cut ends should not be more than few millimeters.
3. Presence of nerve growth factor.
4. Infection should be absent at the site of lesion.

N.B.

The peripheral nerves, if damaged, may regenerate, but nerve fibers within the central nervous system cannot regenerate after damage due to absence of neurolemmal sheath and endoneurium.

> **Clinical correlation**
>
> **Nerve repair:** The severed major nerves may be surgically reconnected and the function of the nerve re-established, if the surgery is performed before the tissue death. The axon grows at a rate of 1 mm per day. The regeneration may take 3–6 months.

Types of Peripheral Nerves

The peripheral nerves are of following two types:

1. Cranial nerves
2. Spinal nerves

Cranial Nerves

There are 12 pairs of cranial nerves which arise from brain within the cranial cavity and come out of it through foramina in the skull. The cranial nerves are designated by Roman numerals in order of their attachment on the brain in craniocaudal direction. The 12 pairs of nerves are as follows:

I **Olfactory:** concerned with sense of smell (olfaction).
II **Optic:** concerned with sense of sight (vision).

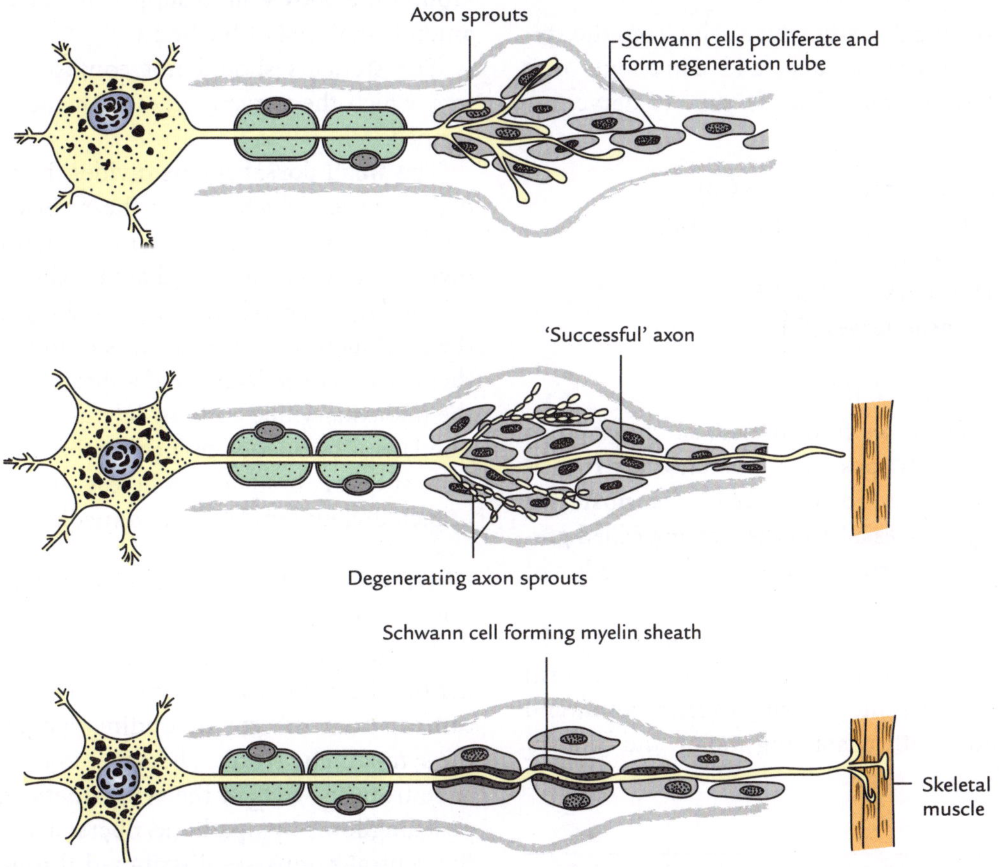

Fig. 12.14 Regeneration of a divided nerve.

III **Oculomotor:** supplies most of the extraocular muscles.
IV **Trochlear:** supplies one extraocular muscle.
V **Trigeminal:** provides sensory innervation to head and face, and motor supply to muscles of mastication.
VI **Abducent:** supplies an extraocular muscle.
VII **Facial:** supplies muscle of facial expression, and lacrimal, submandibular and sublingual salivary glands.
VIII **Vestibulocochlear:** concerned with the sense of hearing and balance.
IX **Glossopharyngeal:** provides sensory innervation to tongue and pharynx, and motor supply to a pharyngeal muscle.
X **Vagus:** provides motor supply to gut, heart and respiratory tract, and sensory innervation to tongue, thoracic and abdominal viscera.
XI **Accessory:** provides motor innervation to muscles of palate, pharynx, larynx and neck.
XII **Hypoglossal:** provides motor supply to muscles of tongue.

N.B.

A pair of small nerves called *nervi terminalis* is recently discovered. It is attached to the brain ahead of all other cranial nerves and is designated as *'O' pair*. It is thought to be concerned with smell-mediated sex behavior.

Spinal Nerves

There are 31 pairs of spinal nerves which arise from the spinal cord within the vertebral canal and come out of it through intervertebral foramina. The 31 pairs of nerves are as follows:

1. Eight pairs of **cervical nerves** (C1 to C8)
2. Twelve pairs of **thoracic nerves** (T1 to T12)
3. Five pairs of **lumbar nerves** (L1 to L5)
4. Five pairs of **sacral nerves** (S1 to S5)
5. One pair of **coccygeal nerves** (C1)

Typical Spinal Nerve (Fig. 12.15)

A typical spinal nerve* arises from the spinal cord by two roots: (a) anterior and (b) posterior. The **anterior root** is motor and arises from anterior horn cells. The **posterior root** is sensory and possesses a knot-like swelling called *posterior (dorsal) root ganglion* consisting of nerve cell bodies of sensory nerve fibers.

The two roots come out of the vertebral canal through the intervertebral foramen and then join each other to form **nerve trunk**, which divides into a small **posterior ramus** and large **anterior ramus**, both containing motor and sensory fibers.

* Thoracic spinal nerves from T3 to T11 are considered as typical spinal nerves.

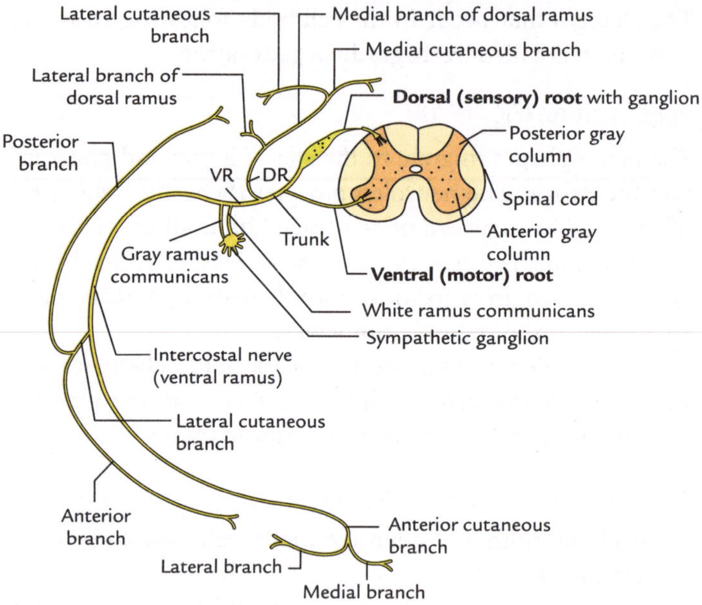

Fig. 12.15 A typical spinal nerve. (DR = dorsal ramus; VR = ventral ramus)

The posterior ramus curves backward around the vertebral column to supply the muscles of the back and skin covering these muscles. The anterior ramus runs anterolaterally around the body wall to supply the muscles and skin of the anterolateral wall of the body.

The students should not confuse the rami (branches) into which the nerve divides with the roots by which it is formed.

The **small dorsal ramus** divides the into lateral and medial branches which supply the muscles and one of them sends a branch called posterior cutaneous branch which divides into lateral and medial branches.

The **large ventral ramus** runs along the lower border of the corresponding rib and supplies intercostal muscles. Further it gives rise to lateral and anterior cutaneous branches in the midaxillary line and just lateral to sternum, respectively. The lateral cutaneous branch further divides into posterior and anterior branches, whereas the anterior cutaneous branch divides into lateral and medial branches.

Distribution of Sympathetic Fibers through Spinal Nerves (Fig. 12.16)

Soon after its formation, the ventral ramus receives a slender bundle of myelinated fibers, the **gray ramus communicantes,** from the corresponding sympathetic ganglion of the sympathetic trunk. The nerve fibers of each gray ramus arise from the cells in the sympathetic ganglion. These are postganglionic sympathetic fibers. The fibers which enter the ventral ramus are distributed through all its branches. They also enter every branch of each dorsal ramus by

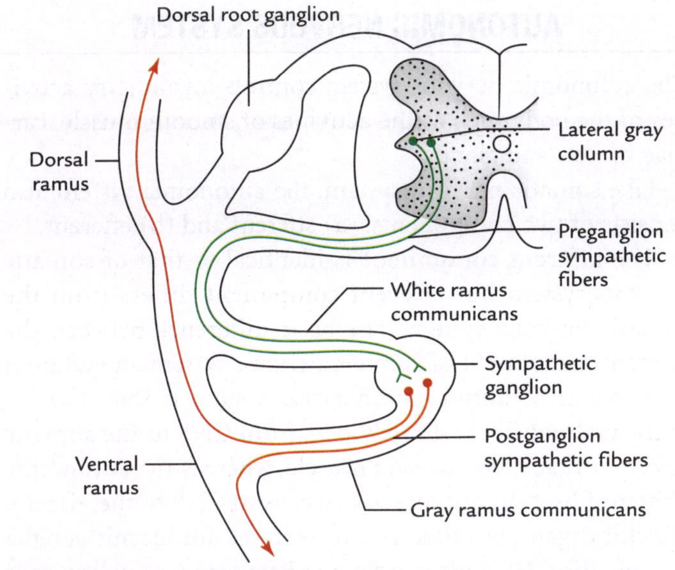

Fig. 12.16 Sympathetic contribution to the spinal nerve. Note that white ramus consists of preganglionic fibers while gray ramus communicans consists of postganglionic fibers.

coursing back in the corresponding ventral ramus to enter the dorsal ramus.

These sympathetic fibers supply the smooth muscle of blood vessels and muscles associated with hair (arrectores pilorum) and sweat glands.

The ventral rami of each thoracic and upper two lumbar spinal nerves are also connected with the corresponding sympathetic ganglion by another slender bundle of myelinated nerve fibers called **white ramus communicantes**. The fibers of this bundle are preganglionic sympathetic fibers which arise from lateral gray horn of spinal cord and relay in the sympathetic ganglion. The differences between the white and gray rami communicantes are given in Table 12.1.

Dermatome

The cutaneous area supplied by one spinal nerve, through both its rami is called **dermatome.** Figure 12.17 depicts the dermatomal map of the body for the sensory cutaneous distribution of the spinal nerves.

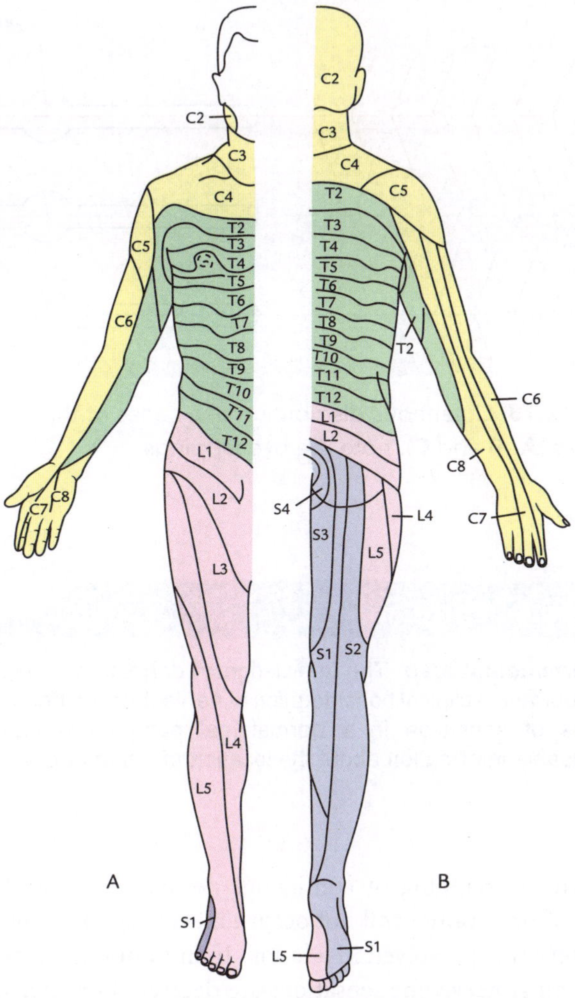

Fig. 12.17 Dermatomal map (i.e. pattern of peripheral distribution of spinal nerves): **A**, anterior view; **B**, posterior view.

N.B.

- With the exception of the first cervical nerve (C1), all the spinal nerves are associated with the specific dermatome.
- Typically, a dermatome extends around from anterior to posterior median line. The upper half of each zone is supplemented by the nerve above and lower half by the nerve below (Fig. 12.18).
- No area of skin is supplied by a single spinal nerve because adjacent dermatomes overlap.

Table 12.1 Differences between the white and gray rami communicantes

	White ramus communicantes	Gray ramus communicantes
Type of fibers	Myelinated	Nonmyelinated
Source of origin	Lateral horn cells of spinal cord	Cells of sympathetic ganglion
Destination	Relay in the sympathetic ganglion (preganglionic fibers)	Distributed to blood vessels, hair and sweat glands through branches of anterior and posterior rami of spinal nerves

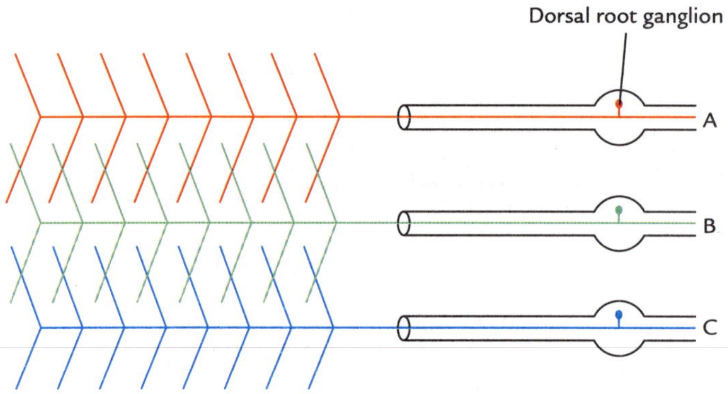

Fig. 12.18 Cutaneous distribution of a series of three spinal nerves (**A, B** and **C**); note the overlappings.

Clinical correlation

Dermatomal map: The knowledge of dermatomal map is important in clinical consideration of nerve damage because loss of sensation in a dermatomal pattern provides a valuable information about the location of nerve damage.

Due to overlapping of contiguous dermatomes, anesthesia (loss of sensations) will not occur unless more than two spinal nerves are involved in a lesion. If an injury involves only one spinal nerve, the sensations are decreased or altered but not completely lost.

In the trunk, the arrangement of dermatomes is simple as each dermatome extends around the body wall from posterior median line to the anterior median line. In the limbs, the arrangement of dermatomes is complicated, firstly because the spinal nerves supply the limbs form plexuses before innervating the skin, and secondly because the limbs rotate during the embryonic life.

Plexus Formation by Spinal Nerves

In general, except for thoracic nerves (T2–T12), the anterior primary rami of all the spinal nerves join and then split again to form a network of nerves called **nerve plexuses**. There are three major nerve plexuses:

1. **Cervical plexus:** It is formed by the anterior primary rami of C1, C2, C3 and C4 spinal nerves, and innervates the head and neck.
2. **Brachial plexus:** It is formed by the anterior primary rami of C6, C7, C8 and T1 and innervates the upper limb.
3. **Lumbosacral plexus:** It is formed by L1, L2, L3, L4 and S1, S2, S3 and innervates the lower limb.

AUTONOMIC NERVOUS SYSTEM

The autonomic nervous system controls involuntary activities of the body such as the activities of smooth muscle, cardiac muscle and glands.

Like somatic nervous system, the autonomic system also consists of two components: (a) afferent and (b) efferent.

The **afferent component** is identical to that of somatic nervous system but **efferent component** differs from the somatic nervous system. The basic difference between the efferent component of somatic nervous system and efferent component of autonomic nervous system is that: the somatic efferent fibers directly pass from CNS to the somatic effecter organs, *viz.* skeletal muscle, whereas the autonomic efferent fibers do not directly pass from CNS to the visceral effector organs, but first they relay in the autonomic ganglia outside the CNS and then fibers arising from ganglion cells supply the effector organs. Thus somatic efferent (motor) pathway consists of only first-order neurons arising from CNS while autonomic efferent (motor) pathway consists of first-order neurons arising from CNS and second-order neurons arising from autonomic ganglia. The first- and second-order neurons are autonomic efferent pathway and are called **preganglionic** and **postganglionic neurons,** respectively.

The nerve impulses passing through autonomic motor pathways cause stimulation or inhibition of glandular secretion and contraction or relaxation of smooth/cardiac muscles.

SUBDIVISIONS OF AUTONOMIC NERVOUS SYSTEM

The efferent (outflow) component of autonomic nervous system is divided into two divisions:

1. Sympathetic nervous system
2. Parasympathetic nervous system

Sympathetic nervous system: The preganglionic sympathetic fibers arise from spinal cord only, i.e. from lateral gray column of spinal cord from T1 to L2 segments; hence sympathetic outflow is termed as thoraco-lumbar outflow (Fig. 12.19).

Parasympathetic nervous system: The preganglionic fibers arise from brain as well as from spinal cord.

In the brain, they arise from visceral efferent nuclei and leave the cranium through 3rd, 7th, 9th and 10th cranial nerves—**cranial outflow.**

In the spinal cord, they arise from lateral gray column of 2nd, 3rd and 4th sacral segments—**sacral outflow.**

Therefore, in general, parasympathetic outflow is termed as **'cranio-sacral outflow'** (Fig. 12.19).

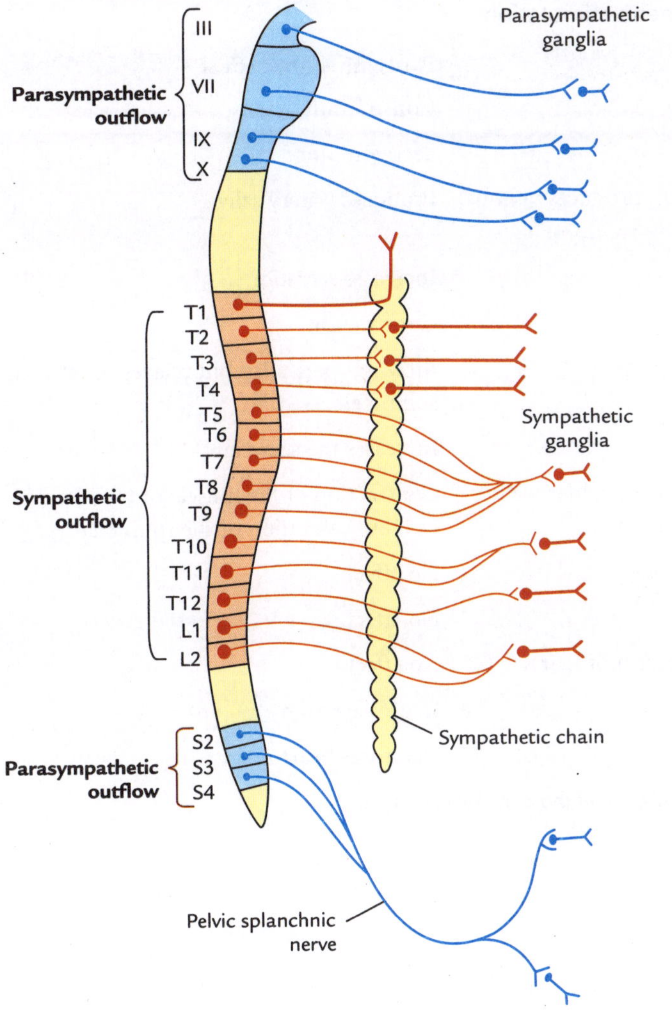

Fig. 12.19 Schematic diagram showing the efferent component of the autonomic nervous system. The parasympathetic (cranio-sacral) outflow is shown in blue, and sympathetic (thoraco-lumbar) outflow is shown in red.

Characteristic Features of Sympathetic and Parasympathetic Supply

All the parts of the body whether somatic or visceral receive sympathetic supply but parasympathetic supply has no somatic distribution, which supplies only viscera. Even some viscera like suprarenal glands and gonads have no parasympathetic supply.

Functions of Sympathetic and Parasympathetic Nervous System

In general, sympathetic stimulation mobilizes the body energy for **'flight and fright'**, e.g. fear (Fig. 12.20 A) whereas parasympathetic stimulation slows down the body processes to **conserve and restore energy**, e.g. sleep (Fig. 12.20 B).

The effects of sympathetic and parasympathetic stimulation of some organs are enumerated in Table 12.2.

From the interpretation of the effects presented in Table 12.3, it is clear that the effects of these two systems are:

1. *Antagonistic*, e.g. effects on heart, pupil, GIT and respiratory tract.
2. *Complementary*, e.g. effects on salivary glands.
3. *Cooperative*, e.g. effects on urinary and reproductive systems.

Clinical correlation

Effects of sympathetic and parasympathetic overactivity: The sympathetic system is stimulated at the time of stress and strain.

- *The sympathetic overactivity causes:*
  (a) Rise in blood pressure
  (b) Increased heart rate (tachycardia)
  (c) Increased respiratory rate
  (d) Sweating

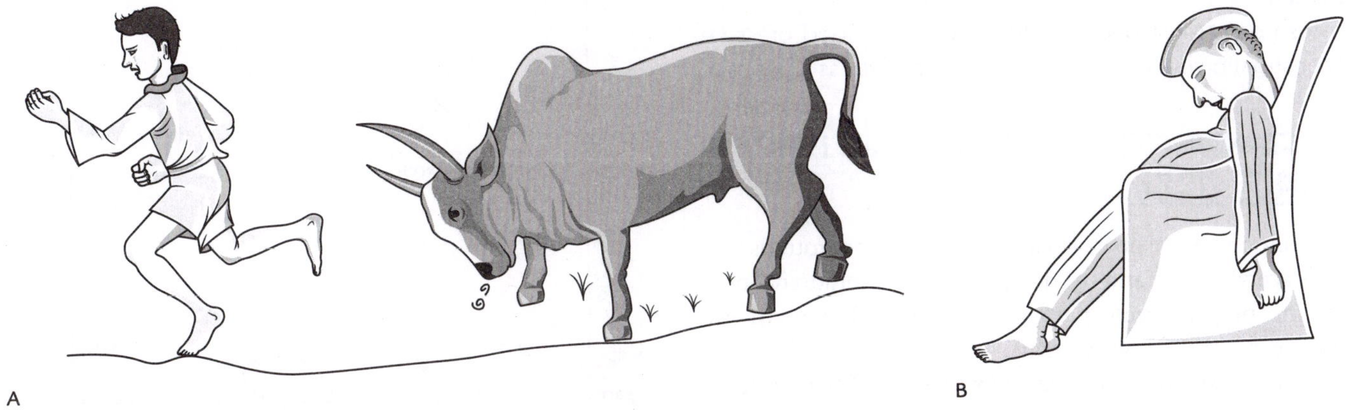

Fig. 12.20 Pictorial depiction of effects of sympathetic **(A)** and parasympathetic **(B)** activities.

Table 12.2 Organs and effects of sympathetic and parasympathetic stimulation

Organs	Sympathetic effect	Parasympathetic effect
Pupil of the eye	Dilatation	Constriction
Lacrimal gland	Vasomotor	Secretomotor
Salivary glands	Constriction of blood vessels, produces viscous saliva	Produces watery saliva
Bronchial gland	Inhibition of secretion	Increases secretion
Bronchioles	Dilatation	Constriction
Muscles of gastrointestinal tract	Inhibition of gastric motility but constricts sphincters	Increases peristalsis but relaxes (opens) the sphincters
Glands of gastrointestinal tract	Inhibition of secretions	Increases the secretion
Muscle of bladder	Relaxation of the muscle of the bladder wall but constriction of the sphincter	Contraction of the muscle of the bladder wall but relaxation of the sphincter
Blood vessels	Vasoconstriction* (vasomotor)	No effect
Sweat glands	Sudomotor (sweating)	No effect
Muscles of hairs follicles (arrector pili)	Pilomotor/Contraction (erection of hair)	No effect
Penis	Causes ejaculation	Causes erection
Heart	Increases heart rate	Decreases heart rate

*Sympathetic stimulation causes vasoconstriction of blood vessels all over the body, *except* those in skeletal muscles.

(e) Dilatation of pupil
(f) Dryness of mouth
(g) Loss of appetite
(h) Constipation

- The *parasympathetic overactivity* causes:
  (a) Constriction of the pupil
  (b) Decrease in heart rate (bradycardia)
  (c) Increase in motility of gut (to help evacuation)

N.B.

The sympathetic system is stimulated at the time of stress and strain

These days most people suffer from high blood pressure and constipation because they live in an era of stress and strain.

NEUROTRANSMITTERS OF THE AUTONOMIC NERVOUS SYSTEM (Fig. 12.21)

The autonomic nerve fibers release two types of neurotransmitters: (a) acetylcholine and (b) norepinephrine (noradrenaline)

All the preganglionic parasympathetic and sympathetic fibers release acetylcholine (Ach)

All the postganglionic parasympathetic fibers release acetylcholine (Ach)

All the postganglionic sympathetic fibers release norepinephrine *except* those supplying sweat glands and arrector pili muscles which release acetylcholine (Ach)

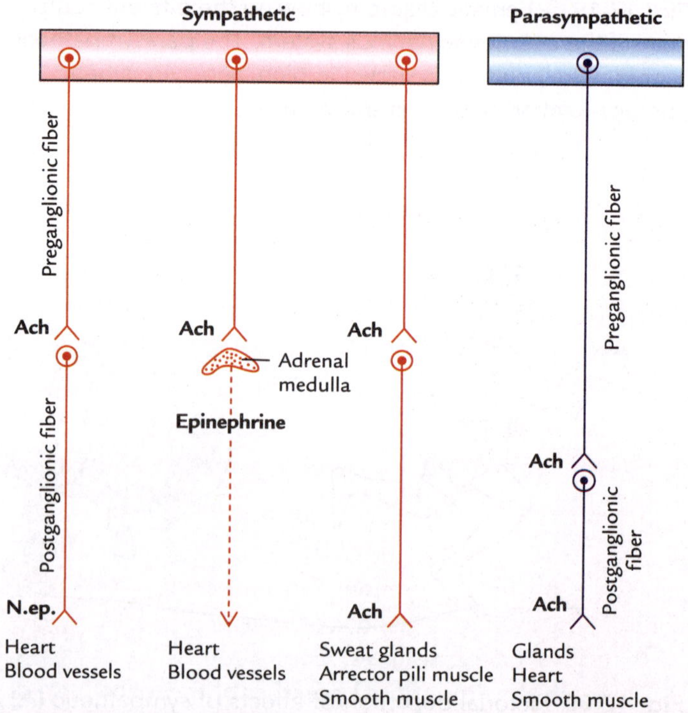

Fig. 12.21 Neurotransmitters released by sympathetic and parasympathetic nerve fibers.

Table 12.3 Segmental innervation of diseased viscera and areas of skin where the pain is referred

Diseased viscera	Site of referred pain	Segmental innervation
Appendix	Skin around umbilicus	T10
Gall bladder (causing irritation of right dome of diaphragm)	Skin over the tip of right shoulder	C3, C4, C5 (phrenic and supraclavicular nerves)
Spleen (causing irritation of left dome of diaphragm)	Skin over the tip of left shoulder (**Kehr's sign**)	C3, C4, C5 (phrenic and supraclavicular nerves)
Heart	Skin over precordium, medial side of arm and forearm	T1, T2, T3, T4
Ureter	Skin in loin, groin, scrotum, labium majus	T11, T12, L1, L2

N.B.

The fibers which release acetylcholine are termed as *cholinergic fibers* and the fibers which release norepinephrine (noradrenaline) are termed as *adrenergic fibers*.

Clinical correlation

The drug atropine, derived from deadly night shade plant (*Atropa belladona*), inhibits the parasympathetic stimulation of the constrictor pupillae muscle of the iris leading to dilatation of the pupil of the eye. Therefore, extracts of this plant were used by women during middle ages to dilate their pupils in order to enhance their beauty (*belladonna* = beautiful woman).

Nowadays in clinical practice, atropine is used to dilate the pupil during eye examination.

AFFERENT COMPONENT OF AUTONOMIC NERVOUS SYSTEM

As described earlier, afferent fibers of autonomic nervous system are identical to the afferent fibers of the somatic nervous system. The cell bodies of the afferent fibers (first-order sensory neurons) of ANS are located in dorsal root ganglia of spinal nerves and sensory ganglia of cranial nerves.

The impulses carried by afferent fibers of ANS are associated with:

(a) visceral reflexes usually at unconscious level,
(b) sensations of hunger, thirst, nausea, sex desire, distension of bladder and bowl and
(c) visceral pain.

The visceral pain is commonly encountered in day-to-day clinical practice. The sensations of visceral pain are conveyed by sympathetic afferent fibers.

The visceral pain is caused by either of the following:

(a) stretching of solid viscera,
(b) distension of hollow viscera,
(c) spasm of smooth muscles of viscera or
(d) ischemia of viscera.

Three types of pain may be encountered:

1. **True visceral pain:** It is dull and poorly localized over the viscera.
2. **Sharp pain:** It occurs due to inflammation and felt on the body surface close to the viscera.
3. **Referred pain:** It is localized acute pain felt on the body surface away from the affected viscera.The referred pain is of great clinical significance.

REFERRED PAIN

The pain arising from a diseased viscera is referred to an area of skin, which is supplied by the same segment/segments of spinal cord which supplies/supply that diseased viscera.

The segmental innervation of diseased viscera and areas of skin where the pain is referred are listed in Table 12.3. The important sites of referred pain are shown in Figure 12.22.

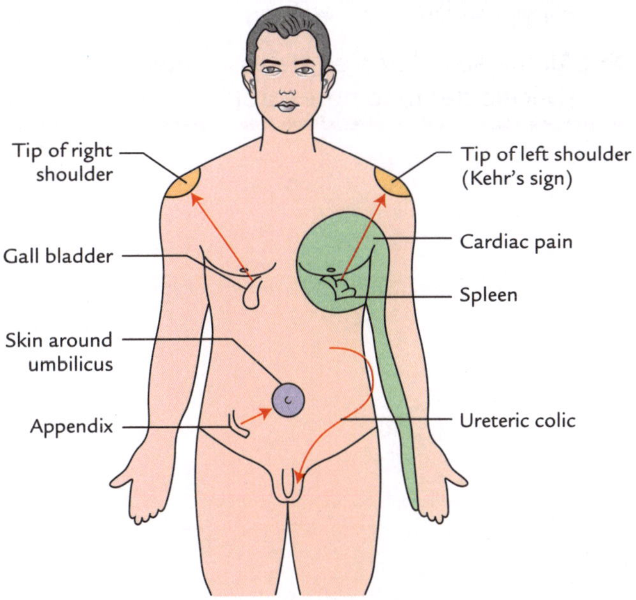

Fig. 12.22 Important sites of referred pain.

Golden Facts to Remember

➢ Number of neurons in the body	About 100 billion
➢ Number of neuroglia in the body	About 1000 billion
➢ Most important property of the neuron	Excitability and conductivity
➢ Most excitable part of the axon	Axon-hillock
➢ Longest neurons in the body	Sensory neurons of first sacral spinal nerve (S1)
➢ Largest neuroglia	Astrocytes
➢ Smallest neuroglia	Microglia
➢ All the neuroglia develop from neural crest except	Microglia which develops from mesoderm
➢ Commonest variety of synapse	Axodendritic
➢ Most common type of neurons in the body	Multipolar
➢ Largest sensory receptor	Pacinian corpuscles
➢ Cell bodies of all primary (first order) sensory neurons are located outside the CNS *except*	Cell bodies of primary sensory neurons forming mesencephalic nucleus of trigeminal nerve which are located within the CNS
➢ Cell bodies of all the motor neurons are located within CNS *except* those of	Postganglionic motor neurons of ANS which are located in the peripheral ganglia
➢ All the viscera are supplied by postganglionic autonomic fibers *except*	Adrenal medulla which is supplied by preganglionic autonomic fibers
➢ Largest cranial nerve	Trigeminal (5th cranial) nerve
➢ Longest cranial nerve	Vagus (10th cranial) nerve
➢ Smallest cranial nerve	Trochlear (4th cranial) nerve
➢ All the cranial nerves emerge from ventral aspect of brain *except*	Trochlear nerve which emerges from dorsal aspect of the brain
➢ All the spinal nerves are associated with a specific dermatome *except*	First cervical spinal nerve (C1) as it has no cutaneous distribution

Multiple Choice Questions

1. **Bipolar neurons are found at all of the following sites *except*:**
   (a) Retina
   (b) Olfactory epithelium
   (c) Cerebrospinal ganglia
   (d) Vestibulocochlear ganglia

2. **All the neuroglia are derived from neural crest *except:***
   (a) Astrocytes
   (b) Microglia
   (c) Oligodendrocytes
   (d) Neurolemmocytes

3. **Neuroglial cells that form myelin sheath around the peripheral nerve fibers are:**
   (a) Oligodendrocytes
   (b) Neurolemmocytes
   (c) Astrocytes
   (d) Microglia

4. **Which of the following neurons are pseudo-unipolar?**
   (a) Neurons of retina
   (b) Motor neurons forming tracts in CNS
   (c) Neurons of autonomic ganglia
   (d) Neurons of cerebrospinal ganglia

5. **A collection of nerve fibers outside the CNS is called a:**
   (a) Tract
   (b) Nerve
   (c) Ganglion
   (d) Nucleus

6. **The commonest type of synapse is:**
   (a) Axosomatic
   (b) Dendrosomatic
   (c) Axoaxonic
   (d) Axodendritic

7. **The commonest neurotransmitter is:**
   (a) Noradrenaline
   (b) Acetylcholine
   (c) Serotonin
   (d) Dopamine

8. **Select the incorrect statement:**
   (a) All preganglionic sympathetic fibers secrete acetylcholine
   (b) All preganglionic parasympathetic fibers secrete norepinephrine
   (c) All preganglionic sympathetic fibers secrete norepinephrine
   (d) All postganglionic parasympathetic fibers secrete acetylcholine.

9. **Nissl granules are absent in all *except***
   (a) Dendrites
   (b) Axon hillock
   (c) Axon terminal
   (d) Cell body/perikaryon

10. **Glial cell which acts as a phagocyte is**
    (a) Astrocyte
    (b) Oligodendrocyte
    (c) Microglia
    (d) Schwann cell

11. **The outer covering of the peripheral nerve is called:**
    (a) Epineurium
    (b) Perineurium
    (c) Endoneurium
    (d) Neurilemma

Answers

1. *c*, **2.** *b*, **3.** *b*, **4.** *d*, **5.** *b*, **6.** *d*, **7.** *b*, **8.** *b*, **9.** *d*, **10.** *c*, **11.** *a*

CHAPTER 13

Endocrine System

Learning Objectives

After studying this chapter, the student should be able to:

- define endocrine system and enumerate the important glands in the body
- describe the structure and functions of pituitary gland
- discuss the position of thyroid gland and its related structures
- describe the microscopic structure of thyroid gland and outline the action of the thyroid hormones
- elucidate the position and gross structure of parathyroid glands and outline the functions of parathyroid hormone
- demonstrate location and structure of suprarenal glands and discuss the action of hormones secreted by adrenal cortex
- state the position of pineal gland and outline its functions
- list the hormones secreted by the endocrine pancreas and describe the actions of insulin and glucagon
- correctly solve the review questions given at the end of the chapter

INTRODUCTION

The endocrine system is one of the two major control systems of the body (the other being the nervous system) and plays an important role in maintaining the homeostasis of the body. The disorders of the endocrine system lead to important clinical conditions such as diabetes mellitus, diabetes insipidus, Cushing's syndrome and varieties of reproductive malfunctions.

COMPONENTS OF ENDOCRINE SYSTEM

The endocrine system consists of:

1. **Endocrine glands**, which exist as separate distinct organs, *viz.* pituitary, thyroid and parathyroid glands.
2. **Scattered masses of endocrine cells within the exocrine glands,** *viz.* islet of Langerhans within pancreas, interstitial cells of testis, corpus luteum of ovary, etc.
3. **Diffuse neuroendocrine cells**, *viz.* neuroendocrine cells distributed in the lining epithelium of duodenum, etc.

ENDOCRINE GLANDS

The endocrine glands are ductless glands and pour their secretion directly into the bloodstream. The cells of endocrine glands abut directly against the vascular channels. Most of such groups of gland cells are arranged in cords or plates. These cords are separated by sinusoids or blood capillaries.

The secretion of endocrine glands is known as **hormone** or **chemical messenger** which cause activation or inhibition of even a distantly situated target tissues and/or organs.

The hormones/chemical messengers can be classified into the following four main types:

1. **Proteins** such as thyroid-stimulating hormone, growth hormone, parathormone, etc.
2. **Steroids** such as testosterone, progesterone, etc.
3. **Small peptides** such as vasopressin, thyroid-releasing hormone, etc.
4. **Amino acid derivatives** such as thyroxine, adrenaline, noradrenaline.

A clinician needs information on several aspects to understand the role of endocrine glands and their secretions in different tissues and organs of the body. This information pertains to:

1. Anatomy and location of each gland
2. Hormone/hormones secreted by each gland
3. Factors regulating the secretion of each hormone
4. Factors causing hypersecretion and hyposecretion of each hormone

The important endocrine glands of the body (Fig. 13.1) are as follows:

1. Pituitary gland or hypophysis cerebri
2. Thyroid gland
3. Parathyroid glands
4. Suprarenal (adrenal) glands
5. Pineal gland
6. Thymus gland

PITUITARY GLAND (HYPOPHYSIS CEREBRI)

The pituitary gland is the most complex endocrine gland. It weighs about 0.5 g and its normal dimensions are 10 mm × 13 mm × 6 mm. It is located in the bony fossa of the skull (pituitary fossa or hypophyseal fossa or sella turcica), below the hypothalamus and connected to it by a stalk of tissue called **infundibulum**. The optic chiasma is related to the roof of the hypophyseal fossa (Fig. 13.2 A).

Parts of Pituitary Gland

The pituitary gland consists of two distinct parts (Fig. 13.2 B):

1. Adenohypophysis (anterior pituitary)
2. Neurohypophysis (posterior pituitary)

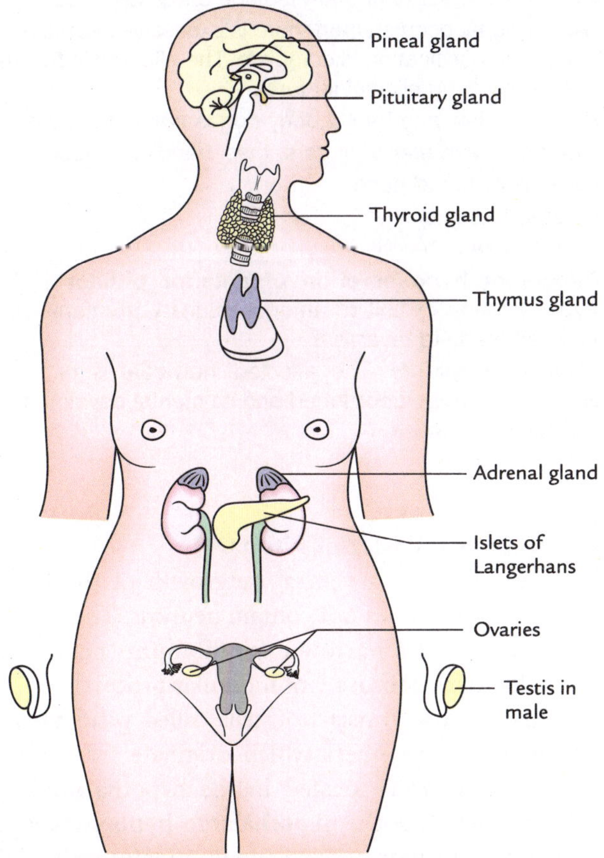

Fig. 13.1 Location of main endocrine glands.

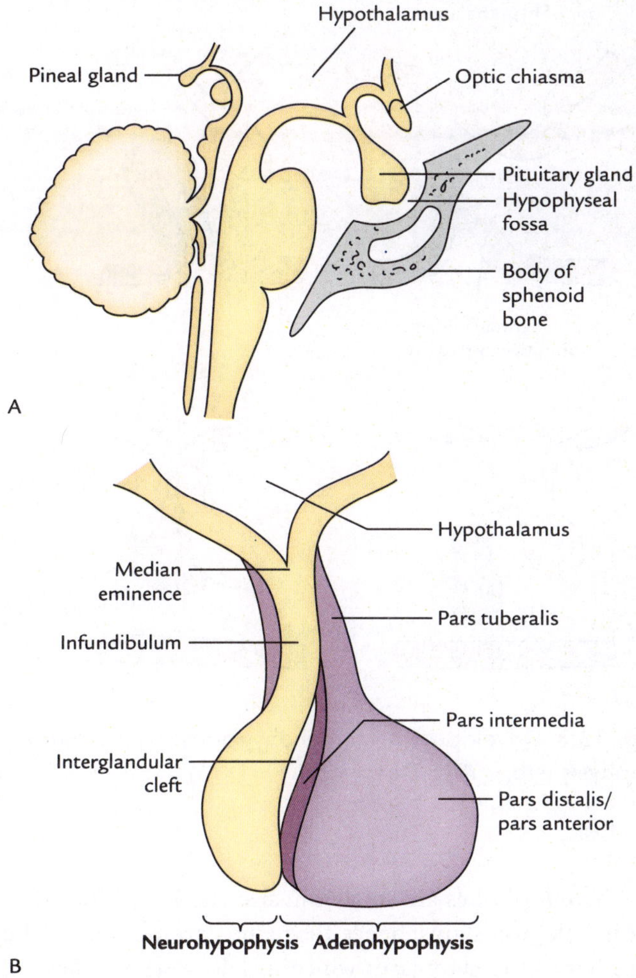

Fig. 13.2 Pituitary gland: **A**, location of the gland; **B**, subdivisions of the gland.

These two parts develop from two entirely different sources. Hence they have different structure and functions. The adenohypophysis develops from the ectodermal lining of the roof of the primitive oral cavity and neurohypophysis from the hypothalamus (Fig. 13.3).

Adenohypophysis (Anterior Pituitary)

It is divisible into three zones:

1. Pars anterior (pars distalis)
2. Pars intermedia
3. Pars tuberalis

Pars anterior (pars distalis): It forms the major part of adenohypophysis and consists of anastomosing cord of cells that are surrounded by sinusoids, the arrangement most suited for direct discharge of hormones into the blood stream. The cells forming the cords are of the following two types:

1. Chromophobes
2. Chromophils

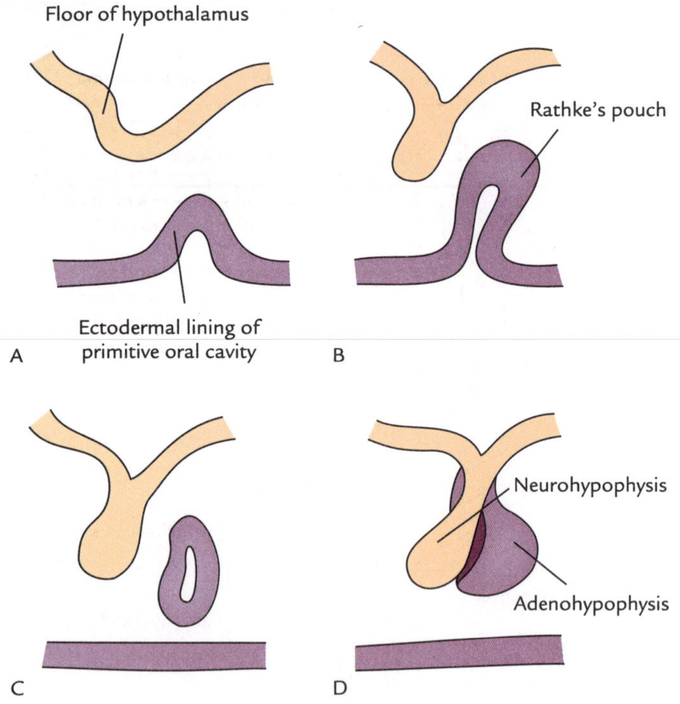

Fig. 13.3 Development of adenohypophysis and neurohypophysis (steps **A** to **D**).

Chromophobes are smaller in size and have little affinity for histological stains, hence the name chromophobe. These cells have little cytoplasm which usually does not have any granules. The chromophobes are considered as exhausted cells (or inactive phase of chromophils).

Chromophils are stainable and larger than chromophobes, and possess secretory granules. The chromophils are of two types: **acidophils** and **basophils**.

(a) *Acidophils*: According to the function, the acidophils are classified into the following three types:
   (i) **Somatotrophs**: They regulate body growth by secreting GH (growth hormone).
   (ii) **Corticotrophs**: They act on suprarenal glands by secreting ACTH (adrenocorticotrophic hormone).
   (iii) **Mammotrophs**: They act on mammary glands by secreting prolactin hormone.

(b) *Basophils*: According to their function, the basophils are classified into two types:
   (i) **Thyrotrophs**: They act on thyroid gland by secreting TSH (thyroid-stimulating hormone).
   (ii) **Gonadotrophs**: They act on gonads by secreting:
   - FSH (follicle-stimulating hormone)
   - LH (luteinizing hormone) in females
   - ICSH (interstitial cell-stimulating hormone) in males

Pars intermedia: It is a narrow zone consisting of small cells. The pars intermedia is separated from pars anterior by the interglandular cleft. The cells of pars intermedia secrete melanocyte-stimulating hormone (MSH).

N.B.

In amphibians, MSH controls the dispersal of melanin granules in melanocytes and are responsible for altering the color of their skin.

Pars tuberalis: It is an upward tubular extension of the pars anterior surrounding a part of the infundibulum. The cells within it are basophilic and contain some granules. The function of pars tuberalis is uncertain.

Clinical correlation

- **Effects of hypersecretion of anterior pituitary:** The hypersecretion of growth hormone (GH) of anterior pituitary leads to gigantism and acromegaly. The most common cause of hypersecretion of GH is pituitary tumor. The excessive secretion of GH leads to:
- excessive growth of bones
- enlargement of internal organs
- growth of excess connective tissue

Gigantism occurs when there is excess secretion of GH while epiphyseal cartilages of long bones are still growing. As a result, there is exaggerated and prolonged growth in long bones resulting in gigantism. The affected individual are abnormally tall, some of them may be 3 feet tall or so.

Acromegaly occurs when there is excessive secretion of GH after the ossification is complete. The affected individual presents following clinical features.

- Prominent jaw and heavy bony ridges above the eyes
- Increased diameter of fingers, toes, hands and feet
- Bulbous or broad nose
- Enlarged tongue
- No increase in height
- **Effects of hyposecretion of anterior pituitary:** The hyposecretion of GH of anterior pituitary in infants and children leads to *dwarfism*

Pituitary dwarfism: The affected individual is of small stature but is well proportioned and its mental development is not affected.

Neurohypophysis (Posterior Pituitary)

Developmentally, it is a ventral outgrowth of the floor of diencephalon but is does not contain neurons. The neurohypophysis consists of a narrow **infundibulum** (neural stalk) and a swollen **pars nervosa** (infundibular process).

The pars nervosa consists of cells called **pituicytes** and nonmyelinated nerve fibers which originate from the cell bodies of the neurons located in the hypothalamus. The nerve fibers constitute the **hypothalamo-hypophyseal tract** which passes to the pars nervosa and terminates with swollen endings close to the blood capillaries.

The *pars nervosa* itself does not secrete any hormone, rather it simply serves as a depot for the storage of the hormones (antidiuretic hormone and oxytocin) secreted in the hypothalamus.

The **oxytocin** stimulates the contraction of the uterine musculature during the later part of the pregnancy and also has a contractile action on the myoepithelial cells of the alveoli and ducts of the mammary gland, ejecting the milk.

The **antidiuretic hormone** (ADH) also known as vasopressin increases the permeability of the distal convoluted and collecting tubules of the kidney for the reabsorption of water, thus inhibiting diuresis.

N.B.

Besides secreting ADH and oxytocin, the neurosecretory cells of hypothalamus also secrete some hormone-releasing factors, which reach the pars anterior to cause the release of LH, FSH, TSH, etc.

Clinical correlation

Oxytocin injections

(a) The injections of oxytocin are given to women during labor if they are having difficulty in parturition. The increased amounts of oxytocin assist uterine contractions and generally speed up delivery.
(b) The injections of oxytocin are given after the parturition cause uterus to regress in size and the blood vessels to constrict and thus minimize the chance of *postpartum bleeding*.

The most important function of antidiuretic hormone (ADH) is to conserve water within the body. A failure of ADH secretion produces a clinical condition called diabetes insipidus which clinically presents as:

1. Passage of large amount of urine (5–10 L/day)
2. Excessive thirst

Blood Supply

The pituitary gland is supplied by superior and inferior hypophyseal arteries from the internal carotid artery.

The arterial supply of the pars anterior exhibits **hypothalamo-hypophyseal portal circulation.**

The superior hypophyseal arteries first break up into capillaries at the median eminence of hypothalamus to take up the hypothalamic-releasing hormones. Afterwards, these capillaries reunite to form vessels which again break up into capillaries in the pars anterior and discharge the releasing hormones into the sinusoids of the pars anterior.

THYROID GLAND

Thyroid gland is the largest endocrine gland of the body and weighs about 20 g. It lies in front of the lower part of the neck. It consists of two lateral lobes connected by an isthmus (Fig. 13.4). The lobes are conical in shape and are placed on either side of the upper part of trachea and lower part of larynx. The isthmus extends across the anterior aspect of the trachea opposite the 3rd and 4th tracheal rings.

The thyroid gland is invested by true and false capsules. The medial surface of lateral lobe is related to 2 tubes: respiratory and alimentary tracts, 2 nerves: recurrent laryngeal and external laryngeal nerves. The posterior surface of the lateral lobe is related to the carotid sheath containing common carotid artery, internal jugular vein and vagus nerve.

Structure

The unit structure of thyroid gland is called **follicle** which consists of a layer of cuboidal epithelial cells enclosing a cavity filled with colloid substance.

The **para follicular cells** are found in a delicate network of connective tissue between the follicles and amongst the cells that comprise the wall of follicles. Mostly they are found deep to the basement membrane of the wall of the follicles (Fig. 13.5).

The cells of thyroid gland develop from two different sources:

1. Follicular cells develop from endodermal cells of thyroglossal duct.
2. Parafollicular cells develop from neural crest.

Hormones Secreted by Thyroid Gland

The thyroid gland secretes three hormones:

1. **T3** (triiodothyronine or thyroxine) secreted by cuboidal cells of thyroid follicles.

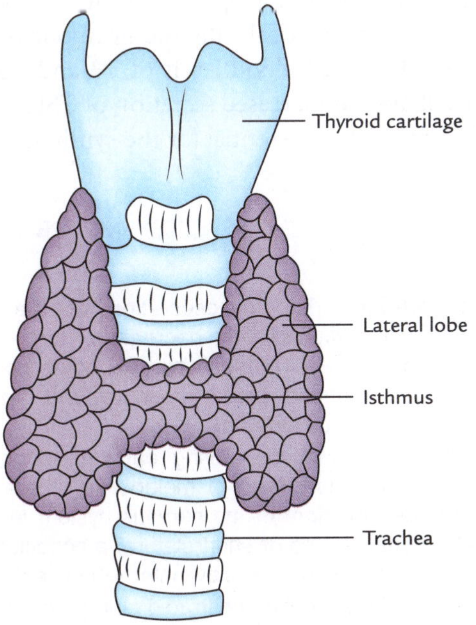

Fig. 13.4 Gross structure of thyroid gland.

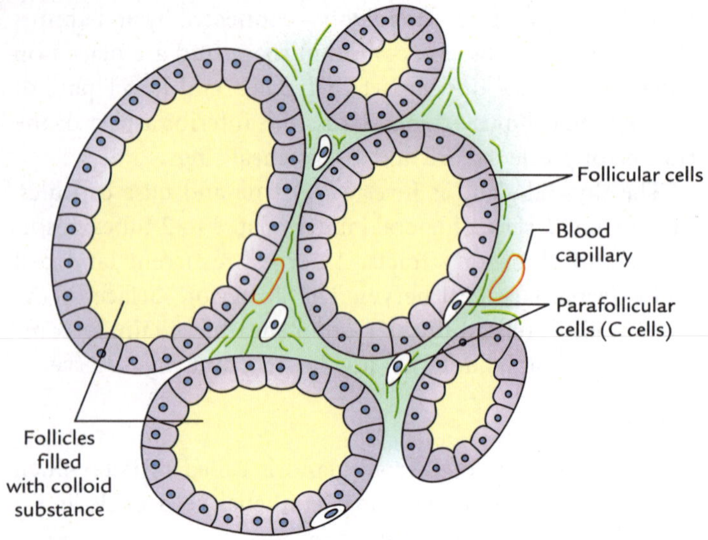

Fig. 13.5 Microscopic structure of thyroid gland.

2. **T4** (tetraiodothyronine or thyroxine) secreted by cuboidal cells of thyroid follicles.
3. **Calcitonin** (thyrocalcitonin) secreted by parafollicular cells.

***Thyroxine** forms the bulk of hormones secreted by the thyroid*. It includes mainly T3 and T4. The T3 and T4 are essential for psychosomatic growth of the body. They also maintain BMR (basal metabolic rate) of the body. In peripheral tissues, T4 is converted into more active T3. The normal growth and maturation of the organs is dependent on the thyroid hormone.

The **calcitonin** plays an important role in calcium homeostasis. It lowers the blood calcium level when calcium level is elevated. Its action is opposite to that of parathyroid hormone. The secretion of the thyroid hormone is regulated by TSH. The decreased blood levels of T3 and T4 lead (by negative feedback) to increased secretion of TSH.

The dietary iodine is essential for the synthesis of thyroid hormones, T3 and T4.

Clinical correlation

- **Hypothyroidism:** The hyposecretion of the thyroid hormone (*hypothyroidism*) decreases the rate of metabolism. Clinically it presents as: low body temperature, weight gain, reduced blood pressure and apathy, a condition called *myxoedema*.

  If hyposecretion occurs during early development, in addition to decreased rate of metabolism, there occurs abnormal development of the nervous system leading to mental retardation and/or short stature, a condition called *cretin*. The cretinism is caused by maternal iodine deficiency.
- **Goiter:** An enlargement of the thyroid gland is called *goiter*. An enlargement of thyroid gland without signs of hyperthyroidism is called *simple goiter*. It develops when there is iodine deficiency in the diet.

  The iodine deficiency leads to reduced secretion of T3 and T4. The low levels of T3 and T4 stimulate secretion of TSH from pituitary gland. The increased secretion of TSH causes hyperplasia of the thyroid gland.
- **Hyperthyroidism:** The hypersecretion of the thyroid hormone (*hyperthyroidism*) increases rate of metabolism. Clinically it presents as high body temperature, weights loss, high blood pressure, exophthalmos (protrusion of the eye balls) and an enlarged thyroid gland. This syndrome is also known as *thyrotoxicosis* or *Grave's disease*.

Blood Supply

The thyroid gland is profusely supplied by the blood. The arteries supplying the thyroid gland are:

1. **Superior thyroid artery**, a branch of external carotid artery.
2. **Inferior thyroid artery**, a branch of thyrocervical trunk of subclavian artery.

Venous drainage: The venous blood from the thyroid gland is drained by following veins:

1. **Superior and middle thyroid veins** into the internal jugular vein.
2. **Inferior thyroid veins** into the brachio-cephalic vein.

PARATHYROID GLANDS

There are four parathyroid glands. They are small, oval, yellowish brown bodies measuring about 2 × 3 × 5 mm, roughly equal to the size of a split pea. The two (superior and inferior) parathyroid glands are found embedded on the posterior surface of each lateral lobe of the thyroid gland (Fig. 13.6).

Structure

The cells of the parathyroid glands are densely packed in masses or cords rather than in follicles.

Hormones Secreted by Parathyroid Glands

The parathyroid glands secrete parathyroid hormone (PTH). The parathyroid hormone (also called **parathormone**) is important in maintaining blood calcium level. It mobilizes calcium from bones and raises blood calcium level. In addition, it inhibits osteoblastic activity and promotes osteoclastic activity of bone. Further, it converts vitamin D into an active principle 1,25-dihydroxycholecalciferol in the kidney and thus increases absorption of calcium into the kidney.

An increasing calcium level in blood, however, depresses the parathyroid activity. These balanced effects maintain blood calcium at a nearly constant level.

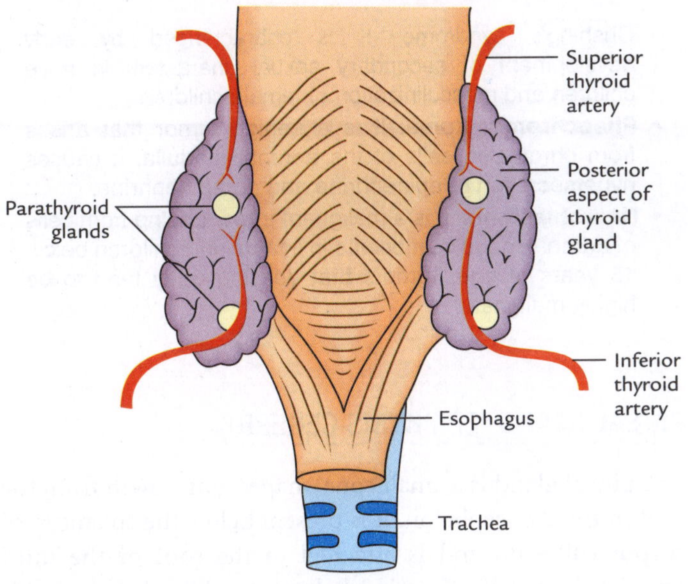

Fig. 13.6 Position of parathyroid glands.

Parathormone and calcitonin from the thyroid gland act in a complementary manner to maintain blood calcium levels within a normal range. This is needed for the following functions:

1. Muscle contraction
2. Blood clotting
3. Nerve impulse transmission

Blood Supply

The parathyroid glands are supplied by inferior thyroid artery.

> **Clinical correlation**
>
> - **Hypoparathyroidism:** It most commonly occurs due to *the atrophy or inadvertent surgical removal of the parathyroid glands*. It leads to by fall in blood calcium level (*hypocalcemia*) which causes hyperexcitability and painful skeletal muscle spasms, causing characteristic inward bending of hands, forearms and feet. This produces a clinical condition called *tetany*.
> - **Hyperparathyroidism:** It most commonly occurs due to parathyroid adenoma. It leads to osteoporosis and consequent pathological fractures, formation of renal calculi, muscle weakness and calcification of soft tissue.

SUPRARENAL GLANDS (ADRENAL GLANDS)

There are two suprarenal glands, the right and the left. One situated on the upper pole of each kidney. The right suprarenal gland is shaped like a hat and the left is semilunar in shape (Fig. 13.7). Like kidneys they are retroperitoneal and surrounded by abundant adipose tissue. They are about 4 cm long and 3 cm thick.

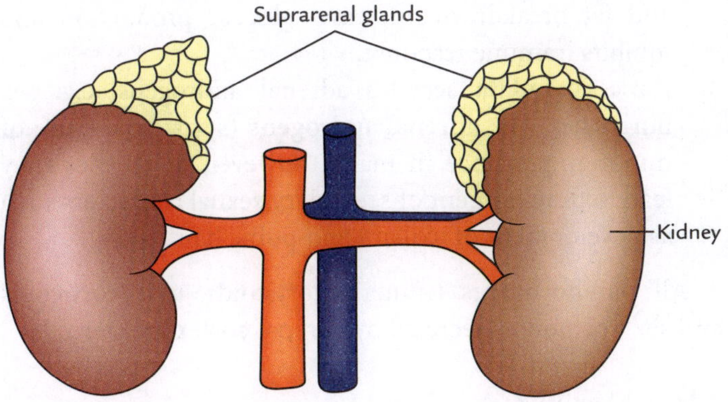

Fig. 13.7 Position of suprarenal glands.

Structure and Secretion of Hormones

Each suprarenal gland is a composite organ consisting of two distinct parts (Fig. 13.8) which are developmentally, structurally and functionally different. These parts are:

(a) an outer part, called **adrenal cortex**, and
(b) an inner part, called **adrenal medulla**.

The adrenal cortex develops from mesoderm whereas adrenal medulla develops from neural crest.

Adrenal Cortex

The adrenal cortex is the outer larger part of the adrenal gland.

It is divided into three distinct zones:

1. An outer zone, called **zona glomerulosa**.
2. A middle zone, called **zona fasciculata**.
3. An inner zone, called **zona reticulata**.

Each zone secretes its own hormones as follows:

1. **Zona glomerulosa** secretes mineralocorticoids, e.g. aldosterone. The **aldosterone** increases sodium ion reabsorption and potassium and hydrogen ion secretion.
2. **Zona fasciculata** secretes glucocorticoids, e.g. cortisol/cortisone. The **cortisol,** a glucocorticoid increases protein

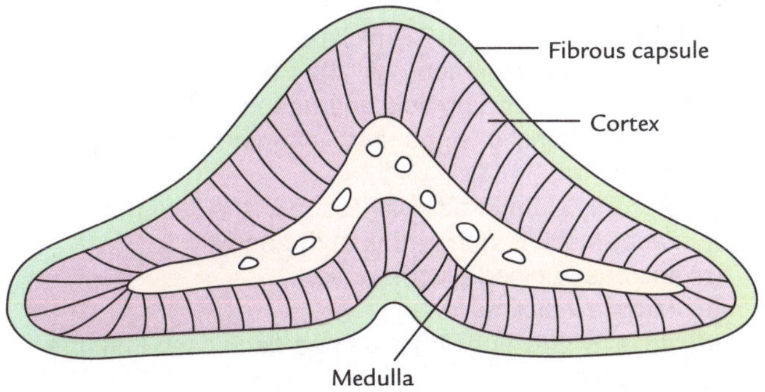

Fig. 13.8 Cross section through suprarenal gland showing adrenal cortex and adrenal medulla.

and fat breakdown, increases glucose production and inhibits immune response.

3. **Zona reticulata** secretes adrenal androgens, e.g. sex hormones. The **adrenal androgens** (sex steroids) are of minor importance in males; however, in females they lead to development of secondary sexual characters such as development of axillary and pubic hair.

All the hormones (mineralocorticoids, glucocorticoids and sex hormones) secreted by adrenal cortex are steroids.

Adrenal Medulla

The adrenal medulla is the inner soft part of the adrenal gland. It consists of cells which are arranged in anastomosing groups and are closely associated with sinusoids. The cells of adrenal medulla are called **chromaffin cells** because secretory granules within their cytoplasm specifically stain brown when treated with potassium dichromate solution. The chromaffin cells secrete **catecholamines** which are of two types, **epinephrine** and **norepinephrine**. Release of catecholamines from the medulla is controlled by sympathetic nerves.

Medullary secretions result from emotional reactions, sexual excitement or stress. In general, the hormones of adrenal medulla prepare the body for strong muscular activity and gear up the body for a fight-or-flight response.

Blood Supply

Arterial supply: Each suprarenal gland is supplied by three arteries:

1. **Superior suprarenal artery**, a branch of inferior phrenic artery
2. **Middle suprarenal artery**, a branch of abdominal aorta
3. **Inferior suprarenal artery**, a branch of renal artery

Venous drainage: The venous blood from each suprarenal gland is drained by one vein: right suprarenal vein drains into inferior vena cava and left suprarenal vein drains into the left renal vein.

Clinical correlation

- **Cushing's syndrome**: It is a clinical condition that results due to hypersecretion of the adrenal cortex, i.e. hypersecretion of cortisol, androgens and aldosterone. The characteristic signs and symptoms of Cushing's syndrome are:
  (a) Accumulation of adipose tissue in the face (moon face), neck and the trunk of the body
  (b) Increased blood glucose level
  (c) Muscle waisting
  (d) Atrophy of lymphoid tissue and decreased immune response
- **Adrenogenital syndrome**: It occurs due to hypersecretion of adrenal androgens and is usually associated with Cushing's syndrome. It is characterized by early development of secondary sexual characters in male children and masculinization of female children.
- **Pheochromocytoma**: It is a benign tumor that arises from chromaffin cells of the adrenal medulla. It causes hypersecretion of epinephrine and norepinephrine.
- **Neuroblastoma**: It is a malignant tumor arising from cells of adrenal medulla. It occurs in infants and children below 15 years of age. Tumors that develop early tend to be highly malignant.

PINEAL GLAND (EPIPHYSIS CEREBRI)

The pineal gland is a small cone-shaped outgrowth from the roof of the diencephalon. It is present below the splenium of corpus callosum and is attached to the roof of the third ventricle by a stalk. The pineal gland is reddish brown and is about 10 mm long. It is regarded as photosensitive neuroendocrine gland.

Structure

The pineal gland consists of epithelioid cells called **pinealocytes**, neuroglial cells and may contain calcareous granules called **'brain sand'**. It is richly supplied with capillaries and sympathetic fibers.

Hormones Secreted by Pineal Gland

The pineal gland secretes two hormones: **melatonin** and **serotonin**. The pineal secretion is influenced by light, i.e. secretion is more in darkness than in light.

The **melatonin** decreases gonadotrophin-releasing hormone (GnRH) secretion from the hypothalamus and thus inhibits the development of the reproductive organs. It probably holds the onset of puberty until the appropriate time. The **serotonin** is an effective vasodilator.

The **pineal concretions** composed of calcium, magnesium phosphates and carbonates begin to appear by middle age. They are not indicative of degenerative changes as it was thought earlier. The secretory status of the gland is not affected by the appearance of the pineal concretions.

Functions of Pineal Gland

The functions of pineal gland are contradictory and not yet fully known. However, following functions are being attributed to pineal gland:

1. Coordinates the circadian and diurnal rhythms of many tissues of the body
2. Inhibits the growth and development of the sex organs before puberty, i.e. pineal gland controls the onset of puberty
3. Modifies the activities of adenohypophysis, neurohypophysis, endocrine pancreas, parathyroids, adrenal glands,

and gonads (hence it is also called the master gland of the body).

Clinical correlation

Calcification of pineal gland: In middle age, calcareous deposits accumulate in pineal gland. The calcification of pineal gland is often detectable in skull radiographs, when it can provide a useful indicator of a space-occupying lesion as there is significant displacement of the gland from the midline in such lesions.

Blood Supply

The pineal gland is supplied by posterior choroidal artery, a branch of posterior cerebral artery.

THYMUS GLAND

The thymus gland is described in detail in Chapter 1.

Hormone Secreted by Thymus Gland

The thymus gland secretes a hormone called **thymosin** which is required for the development of T lymphocytes for cell-mediated immunity.

SCATTERED MASSES OF ENDOCRINE CELLS IN EXOCRINE GLANDS

In addition to the presence of endocrine tissues in distinct endocrine glands such as pituitary, thyroid, etc., some endocrine tissues such as **islets of Langerhans** of pancreas, **interstitial cells (Leydig cells)** of testis, corpus luteum of ovary occur as scattered mass within an exocrine gland.

ISLETS OF LANGERHANS OF PANCREAS

The pancreas is a gland with both exocrine and endocrine functions. The major exocrine function is performed by **pancreatic acini** which manufacture digestive enzymes. Its endocrine function is executed by **islets (islands) of Langerhans.** The islets are highly vascular epithelial masses scattered among the exocrine glandular tissue.

The well-defined cell types of islets include alpha (A) cells and beta (B) cells. The B cells are far more numerous than the A cells. The other types of cells are also now recognized, *viz.* delta cells, C cells, etc. (Fig. 13.9). The B cells produce **insulin** which plays an important role in carbohydrate metabolism. Without this hormone, the cells of the body cannot utilize glucose to form glycogen. As a result, there occurs a decrease in blood sugar level and increase in glycogen level in the liver. The A cells produce **glucagon**. Its effect is opposite to that of insulin. The glucagon increases the blood sugar level by promoting glycogenolysis in the liver.

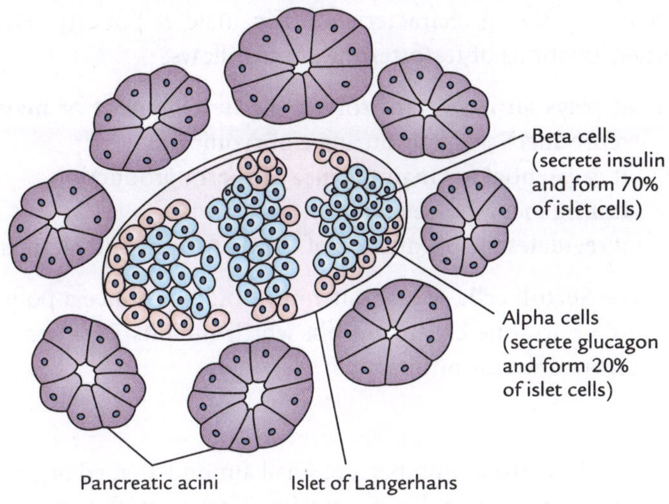

Fig. 13.9 Microscopic structure of pancreas. Note that alpha cells are towards the periphery and beta cells are towards the center.

N.B.

The blood sugar level is controlled by the opposing actions of insulin and glucagon:

- Insulin decreases blood sugar level.
- Glucagon increases blood sugar level.

Clinical correlation

Diabetes mellitus: It is a clinical condition that results from deficiency of insulin. It is characterized by hyperglycemia and glycosuria of variable severity. Clinically, it presents as polyphagia (excessive eating), polydipsia (excess drinking of water) and polyuria (excessive urine).

GONADS

Testes

The testes, two in number, are small ovoid organs, about 5 cm long and 2.5 cm wide located within the scrotum. The testis has both exocrine and endocrine functions. The exocrine function of testis is the production of spermatozoa, whereas endocrine function of testis is the production of steroid hormones (e.g. testosterone).

The testis is made up of large number of seminiferous tubules which produce spermatozoa. In between these tubules, there are loose interstitial cells also known as **Leydig cells.** These cells are endocrine cells. They produce male hormone **testosterone.** It is classified as an androgen (andro = male) because it stimulates the development of secondary sexual characteristics of a male at puberty. The other functions of testosterone are as follows:

1. It plays an important role in the development of male reproductive organs during embryonic life.
2. It is essential for maintenance of sperm production.
3. It influences the behavior.
4. It regulates the production of GnRH from hypothalamus.

The **Sertoli cells** of seminiferous tubules produce a polypeptide hormone called **inhibin** which inhibits FSH secretion from anterior pituitary.

Ovary

The ovaries, two in number, are small almond-shaped organs about 2.5 cm long and 1.25 cm wide. They lie in the ovarian fossa at the lateral pelvic wall one on each side. Each ovary is attached to the posterior surface of the broad ligament of uterus by a short peritoneal fold called **mesovarium**.

As an endocrine gland, the ovary secretes the **steroid hormones** which are required to prepare the endometrium suitable for the implantation of the fertilized ovum.

The hormones are produced by stromal cells which are arranged into two distinct zones around the ovarian follicles:

1. The inner zone known as **theca interna**.
2. The outer zone known as **theca externa**.

The *theca interna cells secrete estrogen hormone* which stimulates the proliferation of the endometrium. The *theca externa remains small and compact, and have no known secretory function.*

After ovulation, the granulosa cells of the follicle undergo changes. They divide rapidly and enlarge followed by progressive organization and fibrosis to form **corpus luteum**. *The corpus luteum acts as an endocrine gland.* The corpus luteum consists of central area of fibrosing blood clot and peripheral broad area made up of yellow lipid-rich granulosa lutein cells. The enlarged granulosa cells secrete **progesterone.** If fertilization takes place, the corpus luteum increases in size and continues secreting progesterone needed for maintaining the pregnancy till placenta is formed and takes over its function.

DIFFUSE NEUROENDOCRINE CELLS

There are certain scattered neuroendocrine cells such as (a) rennin-producing juxtaglomerular cells of the kidney and (b) gut-associated endocrine cells or enteroendocrine cells, found scattered in the epithelial layer of mainly stomach and small intestine.

The **enteroendocrine cells** of the stomach produce **gastrin** which acts on the fundic glands of the same organ, i.e. stomach to secrete hydrochloric acid (HCl) and cells of duodenum to produce four hormones:

1. **Secretin** causes secretion of pancreatic juice.
2. **Cholecystokinin** causes secretion of bile.
3. **Pancreozymin** causes secretion of pancreatic enzymes.
4. **Enterogastrone** inhibits peristalsis of stomach to reduce its acid secretion.

Golden Facts to Remember

➢ Most complex endocrine gland in the body	Pituitary gland
➢ Largest endocrine gland in the body	Thyroid gland
➢ Most vascular endocrine gland in the body	Thyroid gland
➢ Most variable endocrine gland in the body	Inferior parathyroid
➢ All the endocrine glands pour their secretion follicles directly into the bloodstream *except*	Thyroid gland which first stores its secretion within its and then release in bloodstream according to the need
➢ Third eye	Pineal gland
➢ Master endocrine gland	Pineal gland

Multiple Choice Questions

1. **Select the *incorrect statement* regarding the pituitary gland:**
   (a) Develops from two different sources
   (b) Is the largest endocrine gland
   (c) Secretes antidiuretic hormone
   (d) Is located on the inferior aspect of the brain

2. **Regarding the thyroid gland, all are true *except:***
   (a) It is the largest endocrine gland
   (b) Its unit structure is called thyroid acinus
   (c) It secretes three hormones
   (d) Dietary iodine is essential for the synthesis of T3 and T4

3. **Thyroid gland secretes all of the following hormones *except:***
   (a) Triiodothyronine
   (b) Tetraiodothyronine
   (c) Growth hormone
   (d) Calcitonin

4. **Regarding the parathyroid glands, which of the following statements is *not correct*?**
   (a) They are four in number
   (b) They are located on the posterior surfaces of thyroid lobes
   (c) Their removal leads to increase in blood calcium level
   (d) Their size is roughly equal to a split-pea

5. **Regarding the adrenal glands, which of the following statements is *not correct*?**
   (a) Right suprarenal gland is semilunar in shape
   (b) They are retroperitoneal in location
   (c) They secrete epinephrine and norepinephrine
   (d) Cortex of each gland is divided into three distinct zones

6. **All are correct regarding the pineal gland *except:***
   (a) It is a small outgrowth from the root of diencephalon
   (b) It is supplied by sympathetic fibers
   (c) It secretes calcitonin
   (d) It is photosensitive

7. **The hormone insulin:**
   (a) Is secreted by alpha cells of the islets of Langerhans
   (b) Is secreted by beta cells of the islets of Langerhans
   (c) Plays an important role in carbohydrate metabolism
   (d) Stimulates the production of glycogen

8. **The hormone testosterone is not responsible for:**
   (a) Development of male reproductive organs during embryonic life
   (b) Maintenance of sperm production
   (c) Production of GnRH from hypothalamus
   (d) Maintaining blood calcium level

9. **All are correct regarding pituitary gland *except:***
   (a) It weight about 25 g
   (b) Develops from two entirely different sources
   (c) It is located within cranial cavity
   (d) It secretes growth hormone

10. **A clinical condition called tetany occur due to:**
    (a) Hyperthyroidism
    (b) Hypothyroidism
    (c) Hyperparathyroidism
    (d) Hypoparathyroidism

Answers

1. *b*, 2. *b*, 3. *c*, 4. *c*, 5. *a*, 6. *c*, 7. *a*, 8. *d*, 9. *a*, 10. *d*

CHAPTER 14

Digestive and Respiratory Systems

Learning Objectives

After studying this chapter, the student should be able to:

- define the structures forming the digestive system and enumerate their functions
- describe salivary glands and discuss their functions
- elucidate the location and functions of pharynx, esophagus and stomach
- delineate the parts of small intestine and enumerate its functions
- describe the accessory glands of digestive system and discuss their role in digestion
- define the respiratory system and its two divisions
- enumerate the components of conducting and respiratory positions of the respiratory system
- name the air passage of the bronchial tree in descending order of the size
- describe the location of gross anatomy of the lungs
- correctly solve the review questions given at the end of the chapter

DIGESTIVE SYSTEM

INTRODUCTION

The digestive system consists of **digestive tract** and **associated organs of digestion:** teeth, tongue, salivary glands, liver, gallbladder and pancreas.

It provides water, electrolytes, vitamins and nutrients to the body with the help of the circulatory system.

The functions of digestive system are as follows:

1. **Ingestion:** taking in food through mouth.
2. **Mastication:** movements of the lower jaw during chewing to pulverize food and mix it with the saliva.
3. **Deglutition:** swallowing of food so that it passes from mouth to stomach.
4. **Digestion:** chemical breakdown of food material.
5. **Absorption:** nutrient molecules absorbed into circulatory system through mucous membrane of small intestine.
6. **Peristalsis:** rhythmic wave-like intestinal contractions that move food through digestive tract.
7. **Defecation:** elimination of solid/semisolid/liquid waste material of food (i.e. feces) through anus.

DIGESTIVE TRACT

The digestive tract extends from the mouth to the anus. Roughly, it is a tubular passage and measures about 10 m (30 ft) in length.

The digestive tract consists of the following parts from proximal to distal ends in succession (Fig. 14.1):

1. Mouth (oral cavity)
2. Pharynx
3. Esophagus
4. Stomach
5. Small intestine
6. Large intestine
7. Rectum
8. Anal canal

N.B.

The term *gastrointestinal tract* is not synonymous with digestive tract. It actually stands for stomach and intestine together.

MOUTH (ORAL CAVITY)

The mouth or oral cavity is the first part of the digestive tract. It is bounded anteriorly by **lips**, laterally by **cheeks**, superiorly by **palate** and inferiorly by a **muscular floor**.

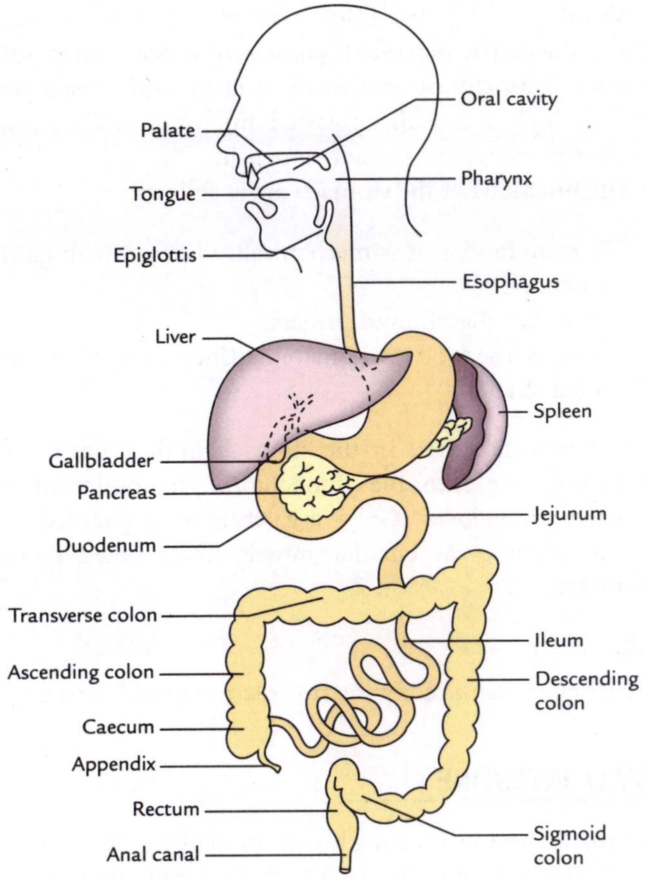

Fig. 14.1 Digestive system.

The oral cavity communicates externally through a cleft, between the upper and lower lips, called oral orifice and internally through fauces into the pharynx.

Oral cavity is divided into two parts: (a) vestibule and (b) oral cavity proper.

The **vestibule** is a horseshoe-shaped space outside the gums and teeth, and inside the lips and cheeks.

The **oral cavity proper** is a space surrounded by the teeth and gums. It contains a tongue which is attached to its floor.

The **teeth** form two dental arches—one set in the upper jaw and the other set in the lower jaw.

N.B.

- Oral cavity is lined by protective stratified squamous nonkeratinized epithelium.
- Mucous lining of palate, lips and cheeks contain minor salivary glands of the size of pinheads which keep the epithelial lining of oral cavity moist.

Lips and Cheeks

The lips are muscular folds guarding the oral orifice and cheeks form lateral walls of the oral cavity. The lips and cheeks are lined internally by mucosa and externally by skin.

The lips and cheeks play an important role in the process of mastication. They help manipulate the food within the oral cavity and hold the food in place for proper crushing and cutting by the teeth.

Teeth

The teeth are embedded in the sockets of alveolar process of mandible and maxilla. In an adult individual, there are 32 teeth, 16 in each jaw.

In humans, the teeth are replaced only once **(diphyodont)** in contrast to nonmammalian vertebrates where the teeth are constantly replaced throughout life **(polyphyodont)**.

The teeth in humans are **heterodont**, i.e. they vary structurally and are adapted to handle food in different ways. The teeth are of the following four types:

1. **Incisors** (4 pairs, upper and lower)—are chisel-shaped and adapted for cutting and shearing food.
2. **Canines** (2 pairs, upper and lower)—are cone-shaped and adapted for holding and tearing.
3. **Premolars**/bicuspids (4 pairs, upper and lower).
4. **Molars**/tricuspids (6 pairs, upper and lower).

The premolars and molars have irregular rounded surfaces called cusps and are adapted for crushing and grinding the food.

Tongue

The tongue is a large muscular organ that occupies the most of the oral cavity proper. It is made up of two types of muscles: **intrinsic muscles**, which are within the tongue itself, and **extrinsic muscles**, which are outside the tongue but attached to it.

The intrinsic muscles are responsible for changing the shape of the tongue, such as during drinking and swallowing, whereas the extrinsic muscles move the tongue.

The tongue is the major sensory organ for taste. The taste buds containing these receptors are located on the dorsal surface of the tongue. The ventral surface of the tongue is covered by the thin mucous membrane which is reflected onto the floor of oral cavity proper. There is a median fold of mucous membrane between tongue and floor of mouth called **frenulum linguae**. The oral cavity along with lips and cheeks holds the food in place during mastication. The tongue also plays a major role in swallowing the food and water, etc.

Clinical correlation

Sublingual route of drug administration: Certain drugs which are lipid soluble can diffuse through the mucous lining of the oral cavity and can be absorbed into the blood. An example is nitroglycerin, a vasodilator which is placed under the tongue in *angina pectoris.* In less than 1 minute, nitroglycerin dissolves and reaches the circulation.

PHARYNX

The pharynx is a funnel-shaped passageway, approximately 5 in. (12.5 cm) long, which connects oral and nasal cavities to the esophagus and larynx. It receives bolus of food from oral cavity and passes it to the esophagus. Pharyngo-esophageal junction is the narrowest site of the digestive tract.

For descriptive purposes, the pharynx is divided into three parts: **nasopharynx**, **oropharynx** and **laryngopharynx** according to location of part behind nasal cavity, oral cavity and laryngeal cavity, respectively. The nasopharynx is the part of respiratory system whereas oropharynx and laryngopharynx are passages common to both the respiratory and the digestive systems. (For details refer to volume IV.)

N.B.

- Musculature of pharynx is made up of voluntary muscles but it is not under voluntary control.
- Interior of pharynx is lined by protective stratified squamous epithelium.

ESOPHAGUS

The esophagus is a collapsible muscular tube about 25 cm (10 in.) long It has a diameter of 2 cm. It connects the pharynx to the stomach. Esophagus transports bolus of food from pharynx to stomach by peristaltic movements.

The esophagus is the most muscular part of the digestive tract. The musculature in the upper half of the esophagus is made up voluntary muscle but it is not under voluntary control. The musculature in lower half of esophagus is made of involuntary muscle. The lumen of the terminal portion of esophagus is narrowed due to thickening of circular muscle fibers in its wall, forming the **gastroesophageal/ lower esophageal sphincter**. The sphincter prevents the reflux regurgitation of food from stomach into the esophagus.

The presence of food in the esophagus causes gastroesophageal sphincter to relax and allows the food to enter the stomach. The swallowed food takes about 5–9 seconds to travel to the stomach.

The sphincter at the upper end of esophagus (upper esophageal sphincter) is formed by cricopharyngeus muscle of pharynx. It prevents the air from passing into esophagus during inspiration.

The lumen of esophagus is lined by protective nonkeratinized stratified squamous epithelium. Numerous mucous glands in the submucosa produce thick lubricating mucous.

STOMACH

The stomach (Gk. *gaster* = belly) is the most distensible part of the GI tract and lies in the epigastric region of abdominal cavity below the diaphragm. It is 'J-shaped' pouch that connects the esophagus with the duodenum.

About 2 L of gastric juice is secreted daily by secretary cells in the gastric mucosa. It consists of water, mineral salts, mucous, hydrochloric acid, intrinsic factor and pepsinogens. Hydrochloric acid kills ingested microbes and converts inactive pepsinogen into active pepsin.

The functions of the stomach are as follows:

1. To store food as it is mechanically churned with gastric secretions
2. To initiate digestion of proteins
3. To move the food into small intestine as a pasty material called **chyme**

The food is stored in the stomach until it passes at a controlled rate into the duodenum. The outlet of the stomach, the ***pylorus*** (Gr. = a gatekeeper) is guarded by a strong sphincter of circular muscle fibers called **pyloric sphincter**.

N.B.

The stomach can accommodate volumes from 0.5 to 5 L.

SMALL INTESTINE

The small intestine is a long hollow muscular tube about 6 m (20 ft) that connects stomach with the large intestine. It is located in the center of abdominal cavity surrounded by the large intestine.

The small intestine is divided into three parts:

1. Duodenum
2. Jejunum
3. Ileum

Duodenum: The duodenum is a fixed C-shaped tube about 25 cm (10 in.) long that connects the pylorus of stomach to the jejunum.

The concavity of the duodenum faces towards the left and is occupied by the head of pancreas.

The duodenum receives **bile** from the liver and gallbladder through **common bile duct** and **pancreatic secretions** through pancreatic duct. Both these ducts unite to form a common entry into the duodenum called **hepatopancreatic ampulla** which enters into the duodenum through its left concave aspect. In the duodenum, digestion continues and absorption of water and digestive products begins.

Jejunum and ileum: Clinically, jejunum and the ileum together form the small intestine.

The jejunum is about 2 m (6 ft) long and extends from the duodenum to the ileum. The ileum is about 3 m (9 ft) long and connects jejunum with cecum.

The small intestine is supported by mesentery proper. Since the root of mesentery is only 15 cm (6 in.) long, the small intestine is thrown into folds called **loops.** The loops of jejunum tend to be located in the left lateral region of the abdominal cavity while the ileal loops tend to be located in the pelvic cavity.

The main function of small intestine is absorption of nutrients from digested food. In order to suit this function, the surface area of mucosa of small intestine is extensively increased by: (a) circular folds of mucosa and submucosa called **plicae circularis** and (b) the presence of villi. The villi are finger-like projections of mucosa.

The intestine is exposed to toxins and microorganisms. To protect the intestine from toxins and microorganisms, there are aggregations of lymphoid tissue in the mucosa, called **Peyer's patches**, and are usually concentrated along the antimesenteric border. The concentration of Peyer's patches is maximum in the terminal portion of ileum. The Peyer's patches get ulcerated in typhoid fever if not treated timely and may cause intestinal perforation.

LARGE INTESTINE

The large intestine is 1.5 m (5 ft) long and extends from ileocecal junction to the anal orifice. It is called the large intestine not only it is longer than small intestine but also its diameter is larger than that of small intestine.

The large intestine is divided into the following parts:

1. Cecum and appendix
2. Ascending colon
3. Transverse colon
4. Descending colon
5. Sigmoid colon
6. Rectum
7. Anal canal

The large intestine has no digestive function, but it absorbs water and electrolytes from the chyme, which it receives from small intestine, a process that forms feces. The feces are stored in sigmoid colon and then evacuated through the rectum and anal canal.

The mucous membrane of large intestine does not have folds except in rectal portion. There are also no villi in the large intestine. The intestinal glands are long and characterized by great abundance of goblet and absorptive cells. In submucous layer, there is more lymphoid tissue than in any other part of the alimentary tract, providing nonspecific defense against resident and other microbes.

After meal, the motility of large intestine increases and as a result the fecal matter (feces) is pushed into the rectum. The distension of rectum acts as stimulus to initiate defecation reflex for the defecation to occur. But this local reflex is modified by higher centers so that defecation occurs at an appropriate time and place. For rectum and anal canal see *Textbook of Anatomy: Abdomen and Lower Limb,* Vol. III, 2E by Vishram Singh.

MAJOR DIGESTIVE GLANDS

SALIVARY GLANDS

These are accessory glands of digestion that produce saliva. The saliva acts as a solvent in cleaning the teeth and dissolving the food chemicals so that they can be tasted. It also contains enzymes (ptyalin, lysozymes, etc. and mucous). The ptyalin digests starch, lysozymes are bactericidal and mucous lubricates the food and the oral cavity.

The salivary glands can be classified into two types:

1. Minor salivary glands
2. Major salivary glands

Minor salivary glands: The minor salivary glands are numerous and are of the size of pinheads. They are located in the mucous membranes of palate, cheeks and lips. They produce small quantity of saliva.

Major salivary glands (Fig. 14.2): There are three pairs of major salivary glands—parotid, submandibular and sublingual which lie outside the oral cavity.

The **parotid gland** is largest and located below and in front of the external ear.

The **submandibular gland** is located inside and below the mandible.

The **sublingual gland** lies underneath the mucosa of the floor of mouth on the side of the tongue.

The **parotid duct** opens into the vestibule of mouth opposite the second upper molar tooth.

The **submandibular duct** opens in the floor of oral cavity proper onto a papilla on the side of root of frenulum of tongue behind the lower incisor teeth.

The **sublingual ducts**, several in number and small, open into the floor of mouth on a ridge posterior to the papilla of submandibular duct.

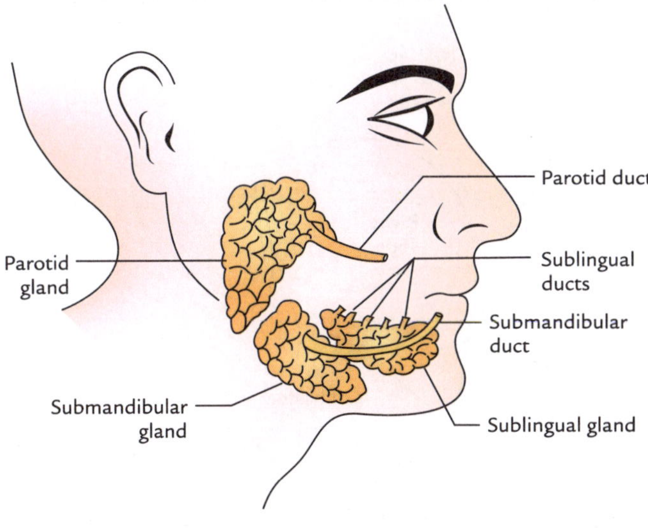

Fig. 14.2 Three major salivary glands: parotid, submandibular and sublingual.

N.B.

In humans, 1–1.5 L of saliva is secreted in a day.

> **Clinical correlation**
>
> **Diseases of salivary glands:** The commonest surgical diseases of the salivary glands are infection and calculus formation in the submandibular gland, and tumors of the parotid gland. *Mumps* (acute viral parotiditis) is the commonest medical disease of the salivary glands.

LIVER

The liver (Gk. *hepar* = liver) is the largest internal organ of the body weighing about 1500 g (1.5 kg) in an adult. It is reddish brown and is located in the upper right portion of the abdominal cavity, immediately below the diaphragm in right hypochondriac and epigastric regions of abdominal cavity.

The liver is roughly triangular (wedge-shaped). The base is directed towards the right while the apex is pointed and reaches the 5th intercostal space in the mid-clavicular line. Its diaphragmatic surface is related to the diaphragm and adjacent body walls and its visceral surface is related to the abdominal organs. It is divided into two major lobes—left and right, and two minor lobes—caudate and quadrate (Fig. 14.3). The vessels, ducts and nerves enter and exit the liver through a depressed area on its inferior surface called 'porta hepatis' (porta = gate).

The internal substance of liver is divided into segments (hepatic segments) on the basis of the ramification of the bile duct and hepatic vessels.

Structure

The liver has uniform structure consisting of anastomosing sheets of the hepatic cells called **hepatic plates**. These plates are only one or two cells thick and separated from each other by large capillary spaces called **sinusoids**. The sinusoids are lined with phagocytic **Kupffer's cells.**

The hepatic plates are arranged into functional units called **liver lobules**. Each lobule is hexagonal. In the center of each lobule is a central vein and at the periphery of each lobule are branches of portal vein and hepatic artery and interlobular bile duct which together form portal triad.

The liver has dual blood supply—from hepatic artery and portal vein. The blood of portal vein (nutrient rich and deoxygenated) and blood of hepatic artery circulates through sinusoids and supply the liver cells and then leaves the liver through hepatic veins into the inferior vena cava.

Recently and more correctly, it is found that **portal lobules** form the functional units of the liver. It consists of area of liver tissue supplied by one of the branches of portal vein. However, there are still smaller units in the liver called **portal acini**. Each portal acinus consists of an area of liver tissue supplied by one hepatic arteriole running along the line of junction of two hepatic lobules. At each end of acinus lies the central vein.

The hepatic cells secrete bile into thin channels called **bile canaliculi** located within each hepatic plate. These canaliculi are merely spaces present between plasma membranes of adjacent liver cells. Bile canaliculi join to form **interlobular ducts,** which in turn form larger interlobar ducts of portal triad. The larger interlobular ducts join to form hepatic ducts that carry bile away from the liver.

Functions of Liver

The liver is an extremely active organ. The important functions of liver are:

1. Metabolism of carbohydrates, fats, proteins and alcohol.
2. Detoxification of drugs and noxious substances.
3. Secretion of bile.
4. Production of heat.

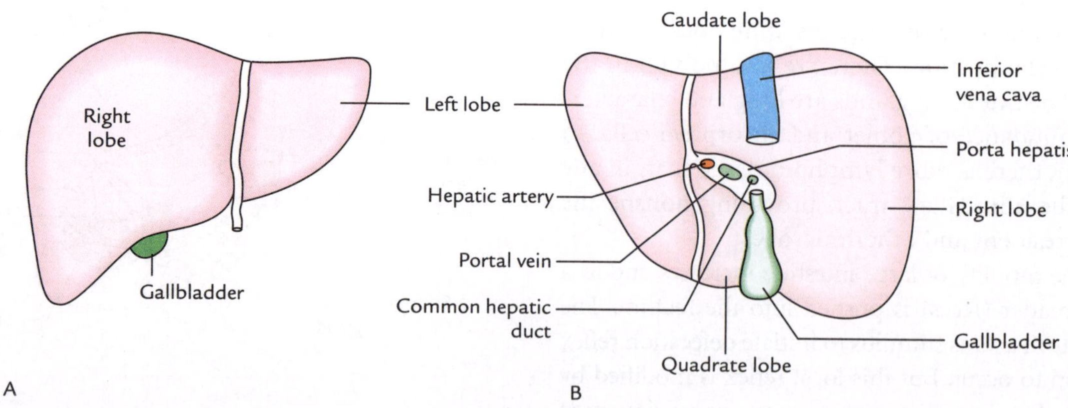

Fig. 14.3 Liver: **A**, anterior view; **B**, inferior view.

Bile Secretion

The liver secretes about 1L of bile every day into biliary tree. Among the constituents of bile are **bile salts** and **bile pigments.** The bile pigments produce distinctive color of feces. The bile salts help in the digestion of fat by emulsification.

> **Clinical correlation**
>
> **Common liver diseases:** They include hepatitis (viral, amoebic), cirrhosis of liver, amoebic liver abscess, tumors, etc.
>
> The liver diseases often present with jaundice. The jaundice is a yellow discoloration of skin caused by excess bile pigment in the blood plasma.

N.B.

Any obstruction of the biliary tree may produce *jaundice*, but the two most common causes are: (a) gallstones in the common bile duct and (b) carcinoma head of pancreas obstructing the common bile duct.

GALLBLADDER

The gallbladder is a pear-shaped sac attached to the inferior surface of the right lobe of the liver. The gallbladder stores and concentrates bile which it receives from liver through hepatic ducts and cystic ducts (Fig. 14.4).

The bile is a yellowish-green fluid containing bile salts and bile pigments. When the fatty chyme enters into duodenum from stomach, the intestinal glands in the duodenal mucosa release hormone called **cholecystokinin** which induces contraction of gallbladder musculature and bile is poured into the duodenum.

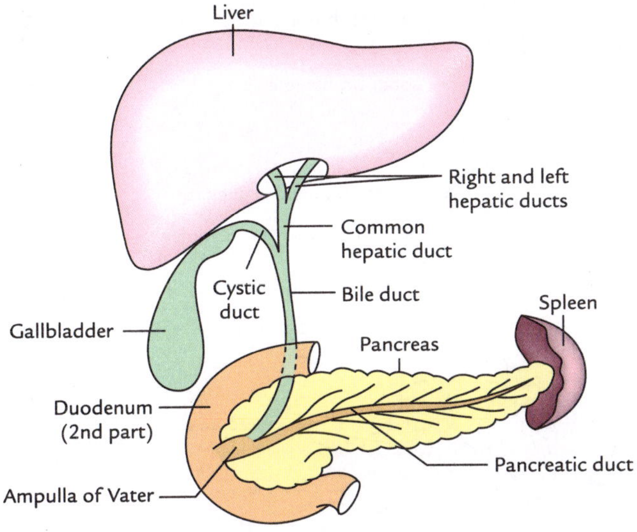

Fig. 14.4 Ducts of major digestive glands.

> **Clinical correlation**
>
> **Gallstones:** A common clinical problem of the gallbladder is the development of gallstones. The bile consists of various salts, pigments and cholesterol which become concentrated as water is removed. Normally cholesterol remain in solution, but under certain conditions they precipitate to form solid crystals called *gallstones*.

Extrahepatic biliary apparatus (Fig. 14.4): It consists of the following structures:

1. Right and left hepatic ducts
2. Common hepatic duct
3. Gallbladder and cystic duct
4. Bile duct

The right and left hepatic ducts after emerging from porta hepatitis join to form common hepatic duct, which in turn join the cystic duct to form the bile duct (commonly called common bile duct [CBD] by the clinicians).

PANCREAS

The pancreas is a long, soft and lobulated gland that extends across the posterior abdominal wall behind the stomach. It has expanded head near duodenum, a centrally located body, and a tapering tail near the spleen. It acts as both exocrine and endocrine glands. The pancreatic acini secrete **pancreatic juice** (**exocrine secretion**) that passes to the duodenum through pancreatic duct. The pancreatic duct joins the common bile duct (CBD) to form the **ampulla of Vater**, which opens into the second part of the duodenum. The pancreatic juice is highly alkaline (pH = 8) due to the presence of carbonates. This helps to neutralize the acidic chyme as it enters the duodenum. The enzymes in the pancreatic juice are: trypsin, amylase and lipase. The trypsin helps in the digestion of carbohydrates, amylase in the digestion of starch and lipase in the digestion of fat.

Pancreatic **islets of Langerhans** secrete hormones, namely insulin and glucagon (endocrine secretion). Insulin plays a major role in carbohydrate metabolism.

> **Clinical correlation**
>
> **Pancreatic cancer:** It is extremely fatal because of its vital exocrine and endocrine functions. Moreover, pancreatic surgery is a problem because pancreas is made of spongy vascular tissue, hence difficult to suture.

RESPIRATORY SYSTEM

INTRODUCTION

The respiratory system is concerned with breathing, which is the process of inhalation and exhalation of air during respiration. The respiration consists of the following four processes:

1. Movement of air into and out of lungs (i.e. ventilation).
2. Gaseous exchange between the air in the lungs and the blood.
3. Transport of oxygen (O_2) and carbon dioxide (CO_2) in blood.
4. Utilization of oxygen and production of carbon dioxide by the cells.

The respiratory tract allows oxygen from atmospheric air to enter the blood in the lungs and carbon dioxide to leave the blood and enter the atmospheric air.

COMPONENTS OF RESPIRATORY SYSTEM

Anatomically, respiratory system is broadly divided into the following two parts (Fig. 14.5):

1. **Upper respiratory tract (URT):** It comprises:
   (a) Nasal cavities
   (b) Pharynx and associated structures
2. **Lower respiratory tract (LRT):** It comprises:
   (a) Larynx
   (b) Trachea
   (c) Bronchi
   (d) Lungs

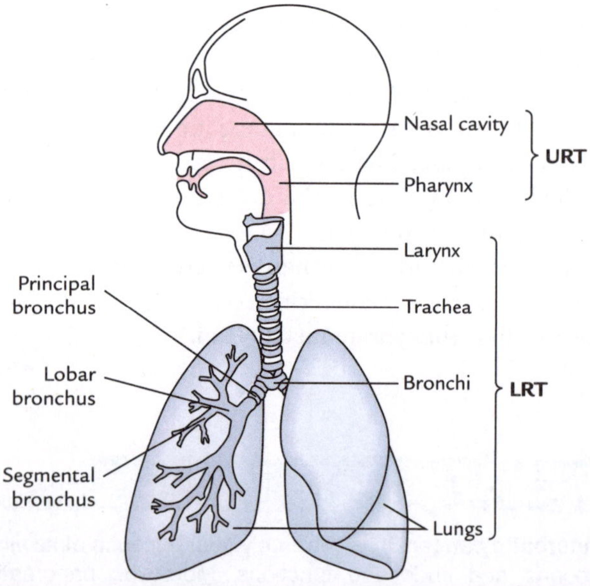

Fig. 14.5 Anatomical subdivisions of the respiratory system. Upper respiratory tract (URT) is shown in pink while lower respiratory tract (LRT) is shown in violet.

Functionally, however, the respiratory system is divided into the following two portions (Fig. 14.6):

1. Upper conducting portion
2. Lower respiratory portion

The **conducting portion of respiratory system** comprises:

1. Nasal cavities
2. Pharynx
3. Larynx
4. Trachea
5. Bronchi
6. Bronchioles
7. Terminal bronchioles

The **respiratory portion of respiratory system** comprises:

1. Respiratory bronchioles
2. Alveolar ducts
3. Alveolar sacs
4. Alveoli

The **main functions of the conducting portions** of the respiratory system are as follows:

1. Provide a conduit through which air can travel to and from the lungs.

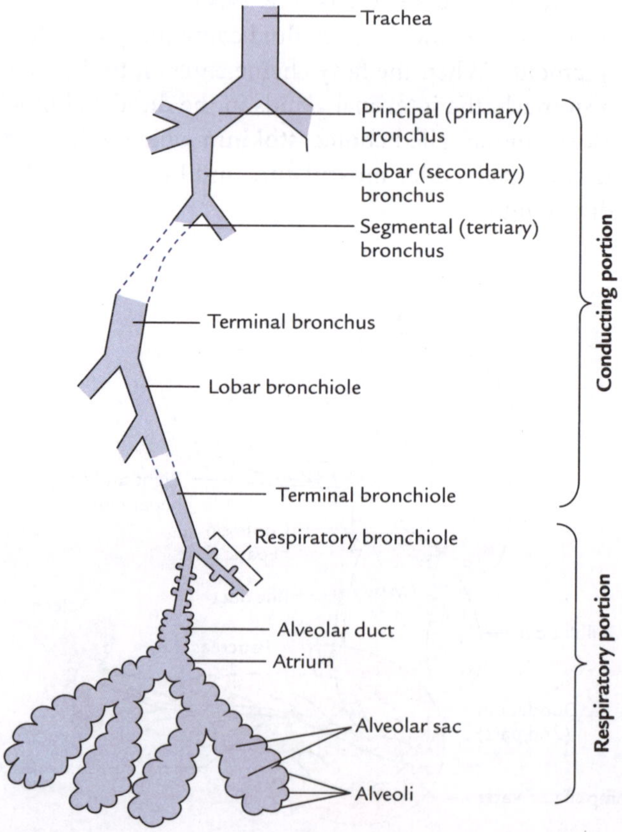

Fig. 14.6 Conducting and respiratory portions of trachea and lungs.

2. Condition the inspired air, i.e. filters, warms and moistens the air while it is passing through it.

The main function of respiratory portion of respiratory system is exchange of gases (oxygen and carbon dioxide) between air and blood, i.e. the air is absorbed and carbon dioxide is eliminated.

CONDUCTING AND RESPIRATORY PORTIONS OF THE RESPIRATORY SYSTEM

The following section describes the upper conducting portion and lower respiratory portion of the respiratory system.

NASAL CAVITY

The nasal cavity is located inside the external nose. It is divided into two nasal cavities, a right and a left by nasal septum. The external and internal openings of each nasal cavity are called nostril (external nare) and choana (internal nare), respectively. Each nasal cavity has floor, roof, medial wall and lateral wall. The lateral wall of nasal cavity presents three characteristic curved bony shelves called **conchae** which overhang three anteroposteriorly running passages called **meatuses**.

Lining of Nasal Cavity

The features of the lining of nasal cavity are as follows:

1. A small dilated area immediately above the nostril (**vestibule**) is lined by skin (*stratified squamous epithelium*) having coarse hair called **vibrissae**. The vibrissae filter large dust particles that might otherwise be inhaled.
2. The uppermost part (2 cm^2 in each nasal cavity) of medial and lateral walls where they meet to form a narrow roof (**olfactory region**) is lined by specialized **olfactory epithelium** concerned with the sense of smell.
3. The remaining large area of nasal cavity (**respiratory region**) is lined by pseudostratified ciliated columnar epithelium with goblet cells called **respiratory epithelium**.

Fine particles such as dust, pollen or smoke are trapped in moist mucous lining of the nasal cavity. The cilia are microscopic hair-like projections from cell surfaces that waft the mucous and entangle foreign particles in it, posteriorly into the nasopharynx.

The mucous membrane covering the inferior and middle conchae contains dilatable venous sinuses called **swell bodies**, which warm and humidify the inhaled air.

Thus, the respiratory functions of nose are: to warm, moisten and filter the air.

> **Clinical correlation**
>
> **Rhinorrhea:** The allergic reactions and inflammation of nasal mucosa lead to abnormal engorgement of *swell bodies* in nasal cavities causing difficulty in nasal breathing and excessive discharge of watery exudates from the nose (*rhinorrhea*).

PHARYNX

The pharynx is a funnel-shaped fibromuscular tube extending from base of skull to the lower border of the 6th cervical vertebra, where it becomes continuous with esophagus.

It acts as a passageway for both digestive and respiratory systems. It communicates anteriorly with nasal, oral and laryngeal cavities. Accordingly, it is divided into **nasopharynx** (upper part), **oropharynx** (middle part) and **laryngopharynx** (lower part):

1. The nasopharynx has only respiratory function, hence lined by respiratory epithelium. The paired auditory or eustachian tubes connect it with the middle ear cavities. The pharyngeal tonsils (or adenoids) are situated in the posterior wall.
2. The oropharynx has both respiratory and digestive functions. The paired palatine tonsils are located in its lateral walls near the oropharyngeal entrance.
3. The laryngopharynx directs the food into the esophagus, and air into the larynx.The air is further warmed and moistened as it passes through the pharynx.

LARYNX ('VOICE BOX')

It connects the laryngopharynx with the trachea. The lumen of larynx is kept patent by its rigid walls formed by hyaline and elastic cartilages that are united by membranes. The cartilages of the larynx are nine; out of which three are unpaired, *viz.* epiglottis, thyroid and cricoid, and three are paired, *viz.* arytenoid, corniculate and cuneiform. The thyroid cartilage is the largest and forms prominence on the front of neck (**Adam's apple**) in males. The cricoid cartilage completely encircles the lumen of larynx.

The larynx is lined internally by mucous membrane and covered externally with voluntary muscles. Two pairs of strong connective tissue bands are stretched anteroposteriorly across its lumen. The upper bands are called **false vocal cords** and lower bands the **true vocal cords**. The space between the false vocal cords is called **rima vestibuli**, whereas the space between the true vocal cords is called **rima glottidis**. The latter is the narrowest part of the laryngeal cavity.

The true vocal cords produce sounds whereas false vocal cords support the true vocal cords. Whole of the laryngeal cavity is lined with pseudostratified squamous epithelium *except* the vocal cords which are lined by stratified squamous epithelium.

The larynx serves three main functions:

1. It serves to prevent food or fluid from entering the trachea and lungs from pharynx during swallowing and thus it protects the lower respiratory tract.
2. It allows the passage of air into the lungs during breathing.
3. It serves to produce sounds hence the name **voice box**.

The humidifying, filtering and warming of air continue as the inspired air travels through the larynx.

TRACHEA

The trachea or **windpipe** is a flexible fibro-elastic cartilaginous tube about 10 cm (4 in.) long and 2.5 cm (1 in.) in diameter. It lies in front of esophagus partly in neck and partly in thoracic cavity. About 5 cm (2 in.) below the jugular notch, the trachea bifurcates into a right and left bronchi.

The lumen of trachea is kept patent by 16–20 incomplete C-shaped rings of hyaline cartilages. The gap between posterior free ends of C-shaped cartilage is bridged by a band of smooth muscle (trachealis) and a fibro-elastic ligament. It is lined by pseudostratified ciliated columnar epithelium containing many mucous-secreting goblet cells.

The arrangement of cartilages and elastic tissue in trachea prevents the kinking and obstruction of the airway during the movements of head and neck. The cartilages prevent collapse of tube when internal pressure is less than intrathoracic pressure, i.e. at the end of forced expiration.

Clinical correlation

Tracheostomy (creating an opening in the trachea and inserting a tube in it): It is a lifesaving measure for obstruction in the upper respiratory passages. It is done in the cervical part of trachea behind the isthmus of the thyroid gland through 2nd and 3rd tracheal rings.

BRONCHI, BRONCHIOLES AND TERMINAL BRONCHIOLES

After a short oblique course, each bronchus enters the respective lung and gives off branches to each lobe of lung called **lobar bronchi** which in turn branch and rebranch like a tree. When the bronchi are reduced to the diameter of 1.0 mm, they are called **bronchioles**. Bronchioles divide again and give rise to **terminal bronchioles** which are less than 0.5 mm in diameter. The terminal bronchioles are the last stage in the conducting portion of the respiratory system (Fig. 14.6).

RESPIRATORY BRONCHIOLES: ALVEOLAR DUCTS, ALVEOLAR SACS AND ALVEOLI

The terminal bronchioles branch to form respiratory bronchioles (Fig. 14.6), the level at which gaseous exchange begins. The respiratory bronchioles give rise to alveolar ducts which in turn lead to alveolar sacs. The wall of these sacs being sacculated, resembles a bunch of grapes called alveoli (L. *alveolus* = a bunch of grapes). The alveoli are the actual site of gaseous exchange and called functional units of the lungs. The alveoli form the parenchyma of the lung. The alveolar wall has characteristic elastic tissue made up of mainly elastin fibers. Because of these fibers, the alveoli can accommodate and expel air during inhalation and exhalation.

LUNGS

The lungs are the organs of oxygenation of blood in adults. They lie in the pleural cavity, one on either side of the mediastinum within the thorax. Lungs are largely made up of spongy tissue and feel like a rubber sponge. In this highly elastic framework, bronchus, pulmonary artery and pulmonary veins branch out.

Each lung is divided into lobes and lobules (segments):

1. The right lung is divided by two fissures (oblique and horizontal) into three lobes—superior, middle and inferior.
2. The left lung is divided by a single oblique fissure into two lobes—superior and inferior.

Each lobe is divided into segments called, broncho-pulmonary segments. Each lung has 10 broncho-pulmonary segments. The lobes are supplied by lobar bronchi, whereas broncho-pulmonary segments are supplied by tertiary bronchi.

The lungs are closely covered by a delicate and inseparable serous membrane called **visceral pleura**. Another layer of serous membrane lining the wall of thoracic cavity, diaphragm and mediastinum is called **parietal pleura**.

The two layers are continuous at the root of lungs formed by structures entering and leaving the lung.

The potential space between the visceral and parietal layers of pleura is called **pleural cavity**. Thus each lung is covered by a pleural cavity.

Clinical correlation

Asthma: It is an acute airway obstruction due to contraction of smooth muscle of bronchioles (bronchospasm), increased secretion of mucous and swelling of mucosa in response to allergy caused by variety of substances such as dust, pollen or a particular food, etc.

In patients suffering from asthma, the inspiration is normal but only partial expiration is possible. Consequently, the lungs become hyperinflated and there is severe difficulty in breathing (dyspnea) and wheezing. Asthma is treated with drugs which relax the smooth muscles of the bronchioles such as epinephrine.

Golden Facts to Remember

➢ Length of the digestive tract	10 m (30 ft)
➢ Most dilated part of the digestive tract	Stomach
➢ Most muscular part of the digestive tract	Esophagus
➢ Longest part of the digestive tract	Small intestine (6 m)
➢ Narrowest site of the digestive tract	Pharyngo-esophageal junction
➢ Largest internal organ of the body	Liver (1.5 kg)
➢ Largest salivary gland	Parotid gland
➢ Most important function of the small intestine	Absorption of nutrients from digested food
➢ Most important function of the large intestine	Formation of feces
➢ Ducts of all the major salivary glands open in the oral cavity proper *except*	Ducts of parotid glands which open in the vestibule of oral cavity
➢ Part of small intestine having maximum concentration of Peyer's patches	Terminal part of ileum
➢ Largest cartilage of larynx	Thyroid cartilage
➢ Narrowest part of laryngeal cavity	Rima glottidis
➢ Commonest site of tracheostomy	Cervical part of trachea through 2nd and 3rd tracheal rings

Multiple Choice Questions

1. Gastrointestinal tract includes all of the following structures *except*:
   (a) Esophagus
   (b) Stomach
   (c) Small intestine
   (d) Large intestine

2. Most of digestion of food occurs in:
   (a) Mouth
   (b) Stomach
   (c) Small intestine
   (d) Large intestine

3. All of the following are the accessory glands of the digestive system *except*:
   (a) Salivary glands
   (b) Liver
   (c) Spleen
   (d) Pancreas

4. Ducts of all of the following glands open in the oral cavity *except*:
   (a) Parotid gland
   (b) Submandibular gland
   (c) Sublingual gland
   (d) Liver

5. Mumps is related to which of the following glands?
   (a) Submandibular gland
   (b) Sublingual gland
   (c) Parotid gland
   (d) Lacrimal gland

6. The conducting portion of respiratory system consists of all *except*:
   (a) Bronchi
   (b) Bronchioles
   (c) Terminal bronchioles
   (d) Respiratory bronchioles

7. The term 'lower respiratory tract' includes all of the following structures *except*:
   (a) Pharynx
   (b) Larynx
   (c) Trachea
   (d) Bronchi

8. The term 'upper respiratory tract' consists of all of the following structures *except*:
   (a) Nasopharynx
   (b) Oropharynx
   (c) Laryngopharynx
   (d) Larynx

9. Regarding larynx, all of the following statements are correct *except*:
   (a) Connects laryngopharynx with trachea
   (b) Prevents food from entering the trachea
   (c) Is kept patent by its rigid walls formed by fibrocartilages
   (d) Serves to produce sound

10. The gaseous exchange takes place in all of the following structures *except*:
    (a) Terminal bronchiole
    (b) Respiratory bronchiole
    (c) Alveolar ducts
    (d) Alveolar sacs

Answers

1. ***a*****, 2.** ***c*****, 3.** ***c*****, 4.** ***d*****, 5.** ***c*****, 6.** ***d*****, 7.** ***a*****, 8.** ***d*****, 9.** ***c*****, 10.** ***a***

CHAPTER 15

Urogenital System

Learning Objectives

After studying this chapter, the student should be able to:

- identify the structures forming the urogenital system
- represent the gross structure of kidneys
- state the gross features and functions of ureters
- explain the structure and functions of urinary bladder
- characterize the structure and functions of urethra in males and females
- describe the main organs comprising the male reproductive system
- outline the structure and functions of accessory glands of the male reproductive system
- compare and contrast the male and the female reproductive systems
- elucidate the location, structure and functions of ovary, uterus, fallopian tubes and vagina
- describe the main structures comprising the female external genitalia
- correctly solve the review questions given at the end of the chapter

The urinary and genital organs develop together to constitute the urogenital system. The male urethra serves as a common outlet. Therefore, urinary and genital systems are discussed together in the same chapter.

URINARY SYSTEM

INTRODUCTION

The urinary system is the most important excretory system of the body. It plays a vital role in maintaining homeostasis of water and electrolyte concentrations within the body.

Components of the Urinary System

The urinary system includes following structures (Fig. 15.1):

1. Kidneys, paired
2. Ureters, paired
3. Urinary bladder, unpaired
4. Urethra, unpaired

The kidneys secrete urine, ureters convey urine from kidneys to the urinary bladder, the urinary bladder collects and stores urine and urethra discharges urine from urinary bladder to the exterior.

Functions of the Urinary System

The following are the functions of urinary system:

1. Formation and secretion of urine.
2. Maintenance of water and electrolyte balance to establish the internal environment of body cells.
3. Excretion of toxic metabolic products such as urea and creatinine.
4. Removal of various drugs that have been taken into the body.

N.B.

The end product of urinary system is urine which is discharged (voided) from the body during micturition.

KIDNEYS

Kidneys are the major excretory organs of the body and remove most waste products of the body, many of which are toxic.

They are reddish brown bean-shaped organs measuring 10 cm × 6 cm × 3 cm.

They lie retroperitoneally in the lumbar region, one on either side of vertebral column between T11 and L3 vertebral levels. The right kidney is slightly lower than the left due to the presence of liver above it. Each kidney is surrounded by a thin fibrous capsule—the **renal capsule** which in turn is

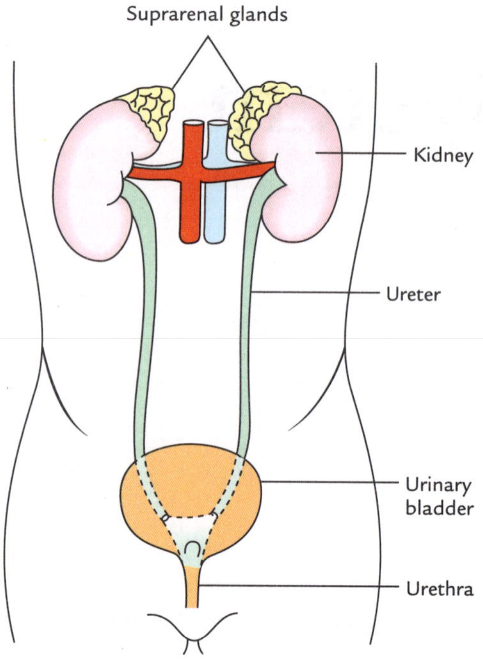

Fig. 15.1 Components of the urinary system.

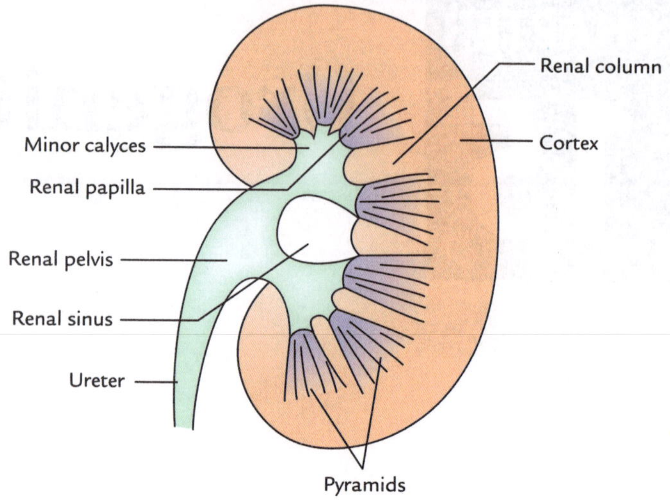

Fig. 15.2 Cross section of kidney showing the macroscopic structure.

surrounded by dense adipose tissue—the **perinephric fat.** The perinephric fat is enclosed in a thin fascial sheath—the **renal fascia**. The perinephric fat protects the kidney from mechanical shock.

The concave medial border of kidney presents hilum, through which renal artery and nerves enter the kidney and renal vein and ureter leave the kidney.

Macroscopic Structure of Kidney

The naked eye examination of coronal section of kidney (Fig. 15.2) presents following features:

1. The inner two-third of the cut surface of a kidney is occupied by darkly stained pyramidal-shaped areas called **pyramids** (8–15 in number). The tips of pyramids called *papillae* project into the minor calyces.
2. The outer one-third of the cut surface of a kidney, i.e. the part lying external to the bases of the pyramids is called **cortex.**
3. The *renal columns* similar to cortical tissue extend between the pyramids. The *renal columns* and *pyramids* constitute the **medulla.**

The minor calyces surround the renal papillae. These minor calyces from several pyramids joined together to form two or three major calyces. The major calyces converge to form a funnel-shaped channel called **renal pelvis.** The renal pelvis then narrows to form a narrow tube, the ureter, which leaves the kidney and connects it to the urinary bladder.

Microscopic Structure of Kidney

Each kidney is made of two components: (a) excretory and (b) collecting.

The **excretory component** consists of about 1,000,000 (one million) microscopic units called **nephrons**. The **collecting component** consists of collecting tubules, minor and major calyces.

Nephrons are the structural and functional units of a kidney. Each nephron (Fig. 15.3) consists of two parts: (a) a glomerulus and (b) a uriniferous tubule. A **glomerulus** (= a small ball) is **spherical bunch of looped capillaries** which invaginates the expanded blind end of uriniferous tubule called **glomerular capsule or Bowman's capsule.** This capsule is succeeded by the proximal convoluted tubule, Henle's loop, distal convoluted tubule and finally the junctional tubule which communicates with the collecting tubule.

The urine is formed as a filtrate from the blood by nephrons. **Collecting tubules** are the continuations of distal convoluted tubules. Several collecting tubules join to form a large duct called collecting duct/papillary duct/**duct of**

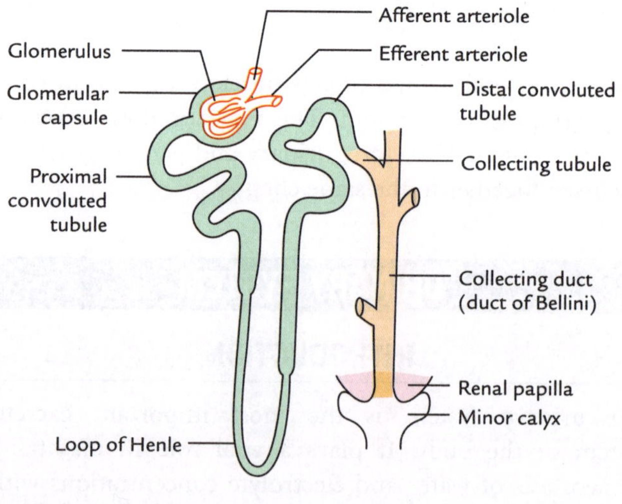

Fig. 15.3 A nephron.

Bellini. The collecting duct opens on the apices of pyramids (renal papillae) to pour urine in the minor calyces.

URETERS

Each ureter is a 25 cm (10 in.) long narrow muscular tube which connects the renal pelvis with the urinary bladder. The renal pelvis is the upper funnel-shaped portion of the ureter within kidney. The ureter conducts urine from renal pelvis to the urinary bladder by peristaltic contraction of smooth muscle in its wall.

Through a cystoscope, jets of urine are seen to squirt/spurt into the bladder from ureteral orifices, two or three times a minute. The peristaltic waves are initiated by the presence of urine in the renal pelvis.

The lumen of ureter is lined by transitional epithelium. The cells of this layer secrete a mucous that coats the walls of the ureter with a protective film, thus preventing absorption of toxic substances.

Clinical correlation

Even if kidneys are damaged extensively, they can still perform their important function of maintaining homoeostasis as long as one-third of one kidney remains functional and thus survival is possible.

The kidneys may be injured by a hard blow in the lumbar region leading to hemorrhage within the kidney. As a result such injury may produce blood in urine.

The urine from a healthy individual is virtually bacteria-free but easily becomes contaminated after voiding because its organic components serve as nutrients to the contaminating microbes. The breakdown of its organic components by bacterial action produces ammonia.

URINARY BLADDER

The urinary bladder is a muscular reservoir for urine. It is located in the true pelvis between the pubic symphysis and rectum in the male and between the pubic symphysis and uterus in the female. The bladder has widely varying capacity (average about 200–300 mL). In the male, the prostate gland is positioned below the urinary bladder. The shape of urinary bladder is determined by the volume of urine it contains. An empty bladder is pyramidal in shape with an apex, body, fundus and neck. The neck is the most fixed part of the urinary bladder. The apex is secured by median umbilical ligament. The body receives the ureters along the supralateral angles and the urethra exists at its neck.

The strong muscular coat in the wall of the urinary bladder is made up of smooth muscle fibers forming **detrusor muscle** in which muscle fibers are arranged in the form of whorls. The mucous membrane lining the cavity of bladder is composed of transitional epithelium that decreases in thickness as the urinary bladder distends and the cells are stretched. It is thrown into folds called **rugae** when the bladder is empty.

N.B.

The trigone of urinary bladder develops from the mesoderm whereas the rest of the bladder develops from the endoderm.

A triangular area between the two ureteric openings and a single urethral opening is called **trigone of the urinary bladder**. Over the trigone, the mucous membrane remains smooth even if the bladder is empty.

In males, a small grape-like bulging produced by median lobe of prostate gland (**uvula vesicae**) lies behind the internal urethral orifice. Uvula vesicae, if enlarged due to prostatic hypertrophy, obstruct the internal urethral orifice.

URETHRA

The urethra is a tubular continuation of the neck of the urinary bladder. It conveys urine from the urinary bladder to the outside of the body. The urethra has two muscular sphincters: (a) internal and (b) external.

The **internal urethral sphincter** at the junction of the bladder and urethra is formed by detrusor muscle of the urinary bladder. It is **involuntary in nature** and well-developed in females. The **external urethral sphincter** is formed by the sphincter urethrae muscle of the urogenital diaphragm. It is made up of skeletal muscle fibers, hence **voluntary in nature.**

The **female urethra** is short, about 4 cm (1.5 in.) long and empties urine into the vestibule of the vagina. In females, the urethra is exclusively a part of the urinary system. The male urethra is described later in this chapter.

Clinical correlation

- **Cystitis:** It is the inflammation of the urinary bladder that typically occurs due to infections. The urinary bladder infections often occur when bacteria from outside the body enter the bladder. Therefore, cystitis is more common in females because female urethra is short and opens on the surface of the body in the vestibule of vagina.

GENITAL/REPRODUCTIVE SYSTEM

INTRODUCTION

The reproductive system is concerned with the production of offspring, i.e. perpetuation of species. There are striking differences in the anatomy and physiology of male and female reproductive systems. The **male reproductive system** produces male gametes called *spermatozoa* and transfers them to the female through the process of coitus (sexual intercourse or copulation).

The **female reproductive system** not only produces female gametes called **oocytes** and receives the spermatozoa from male but also involved in the development of the embryo and fetus and nourishing the baby even after birth by breast milk.

N.B.

The reproductive organs become functional at puberty whereas the organs of other systems of the body become functional at birth or shortly thereafter.

In spite of these striking differences in the male and female reproductive systems, each sex has following similar features:

1. A symmetrical pair of sex glands
2. Two different pairs of passages for gametes
3. Accessory glands
4. External genitalia

N.B.

In early fetal life, the male and female organs of the reproduction are very similar.

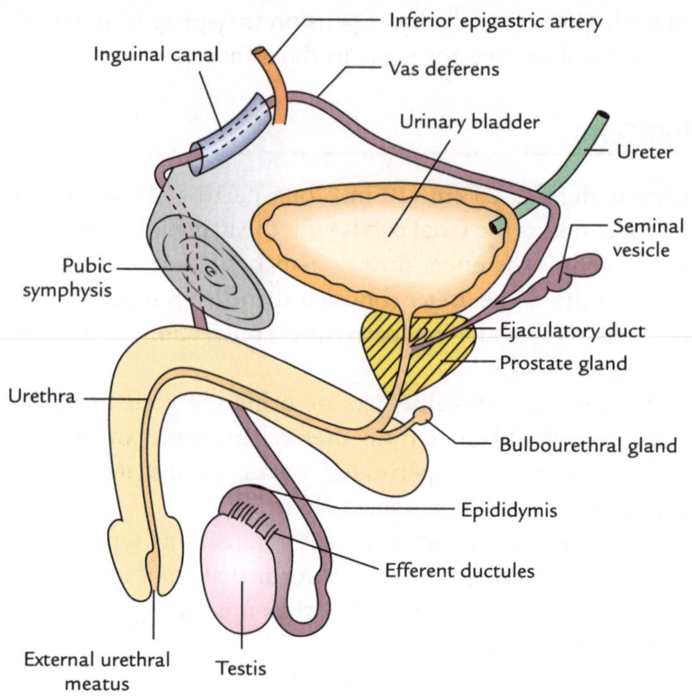

Fig. 15.4 Male reproductive system.

MALE REPRODUCTIVE SYSTEM

The *male reproductive organs* are:

1. Testes
2. Epididymis
3. Ductus deferens
4. Seminal vesicles (accessory glands)
5. Ejaculatory ducts
6. Prostate gland (accessory gland)
7. Bulbourethral glands (accessory glands)

The *male external genitalia* include:

1. Penis
2. Urethra
3. Scrotum

Figure 15.4 depicts the structures of the male reproductive system.

N.B.

All the male reproductive organs and male external genitalia are *secondary sex organs* except testes which are *primary sex organs*.

TESTES

The testes are male sex glands, one on each side located within the scrotum.

Each testis is a whitish ovoid organ, about 4 cm (1.5 in.) long and 2.5 cm in diameter. Each one consists of 200–300 lobules. Each lobule contains 1–4 seminiferous tubules. Between the tubules are the groups of interstitial cells (of Leydig) which secrete testosterone (hormone) at and after puberty. The seminiferous tubules contain only two types of cells: **germ cells** and **Sertoli cells**. The germ cells produce spermatozoa by progressive differentiation and Sertoli cells provide mechanical support and nourishment to the spermatozoa. The testosterone regulates the spermatogenesis and development of secondary sex organs. The testosterone also influences brain, and is responsible for the aggressive behavior and positive attitude of the males.

After production in the seminiferous tubules, the sperms leave the testis through 6–12 **efferent ductules** which emerge from the superior part of the testis and open into the duct of epididymis.

EPIDIDYMIS

The duct of epididymis, although 6 m long is so folded as to form a compact comma-shaped body called epididymis. The epididymis caps the superior pole of the testis and is applied to its posterior border. The spermatozoa are stored in the epididymis until release either by masturbation or coitus. During the storage period, the spermatozoa become mature and motile.

Clinical correlation

The final maturation of sperms occurs in the epididymis. The sperms taken directly from the testis in experimental animals are not capable of fertilizing but after spending one to several days in the epididymis, they develop the capacity to fertilize.

DUCTUS DEFERENS

The ductus deferens emerges from the tail of epididymis. It is a fibromuscular tube about 45 cm long that conveys spermatozoa from epididymis to the ejaculatory duct. The end of ductus deferens enlarges to form the ampulla.

The spermatozoa are transported along the vas deferens by muscular contractions of its walls.

SEMINAL VESICLES

These are sac-shaped glands adjacent to the ampullae of ductus differentia. In fact they are tubular outgrowths from the last part of the ductus deferens. Each gland is about 5 cm long and its short duct joins the ductus deferens to form the **ejaculatory duct**. From this point onward, the male urethra is a common passage for the urinary and genital systems. This is because the duct systems of both testes and kidney develop from a common embryonic structure called mesonephric duct.

EJACULATORY DUCT

It is formed near the prostate gland by the union of ductus deferens and duct of seminal vesicle. The ejaculatory duct, which is about 2.5 cm long, pierces the prostate gland and opens into the urethra close to its fellow of opposite side about 2.5 cm distal to the bladder.

Clinical correlation

Vasectomy: It is a surgical procedure to cut and tie the ductus deferens on each side so that the sperms do not pass from testis to the urethra. The vasectomy is a common method to render male permanently incapable of fertilization (i.e. they become sterile).

N.B.

Since sperms form only a small volume of the ejaculate, the vasectomy has little effect on the volume of the ejaculated semen. The sperms are reabsorbed in the epididymis.

PROSTATE GLAND

The prostrate is the largest accessory sex gland and weighs about 20 g in an adult male.

It is a cone-shaped gland about the size of chestnut, located below the neck of the urinary bladder with apex directed downward. It surrounds the first 3 cm of urethra just distal to the urinary bladder. It is partly glandular, partly muscular and partly fibrous. The glandular tissue of prostate gland consists of three types of glands, *viz.* mucosal, submucosal and main prostatic gland. Its glands secrete milky opalescent liquid, free from mucous which is nutritive to the sperms and forms the bulk of the semen. The prostate glands open into the prostatic part of the urethra. The prostatic secretion contains acid phosphatase, citric acid, amylase, fibrinolysin and prostatic-specific antigen (PSA). Fibrinolysin liquefies semen after ejaculation.

Clinical correlation

- **Benign hypertrophy of prostrate (BHP):** It occurs due to hypertrophy of mucosal and submucosal glands in almost 50% males after 50 years of age. The enlarged prostatic tissue compresses the prostatic urethra causing partial or total obstruction. This leads to difficulty in passing urine.
- **Carcinoma of prostate gland:** It occurs due to malignant hypertrophy of main prostatic glands. It is the second most common cancer in elderly men.

BULBOURETHRAL GLANDS (OF COWPER)

These are two small glands of the size of a pea which lie one on each side of the membranous urethra. Their ducts are 2–3 cm long and open into the penile urethra. They secrete mucous-like fluid that lubricates penile urethra before ejaculation.

Clinical correlation

The secretions of accessory glands of male reproductive system along with spermatozoa form the seminal fluid. The seminal fluid contains high concentration of fructose which provides nutrition to the spermatozoa.

PENIS

Penis (L. *penis* = a tail) is a male organ of copulation and transfers sperms from male to the female genital tract. In order to accomplish this, penis need to be rigid (erect) so that it can enter the vagina. Penis consists of three fibrous columns of erectile tissue, 2 paired and 1 unpaired (Fig. 15.5). Each column of erectile tissue is surrounded by a thick fibrous connective tissue sheath called **tunica albuginea**. These columns have enumerable cavernous spaces filled with blood. The three columns are enclosed in a single loosely fitting tube of skin. Note that there is no subcutaneous tissue around the penis. The paired columns are called

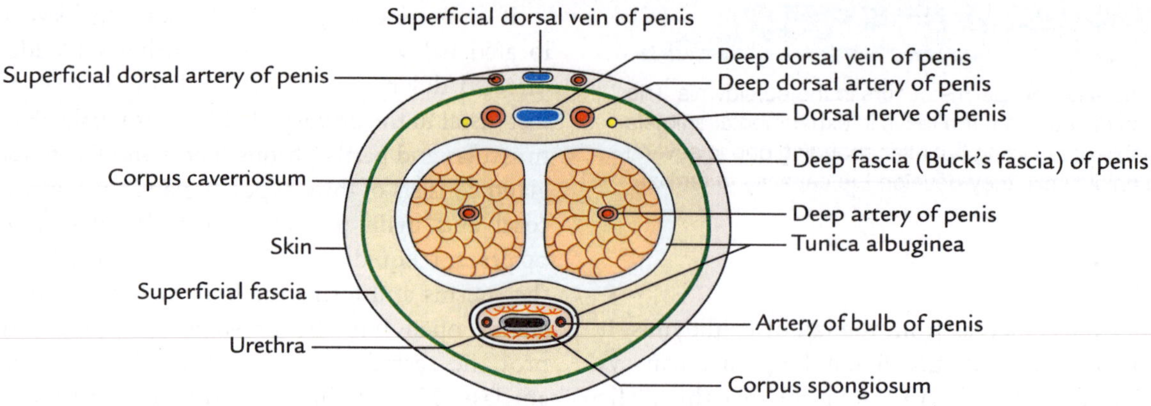

Fig. 15.5 Transverse section through the body of penis.

corpora cavernosa and unpaired column, the **corpus spongiosum**. The corpus spongiosum is traversed by urethra. The expanded proximal end (*bulb*) of corpus spongiosum is attached to the perineal membrane, which stretches between the sides of the pubic arch and its expanded distal end forms the **glans of penis.** A loose fold of skin covering the glans is called **foreskin or prepuce.** The corpora cavernosa are fused side by side. Distally they present a tapering ends whereas proximally they diverge into **right and left crura** which are firmly attached to the pubic arch on the respective sides.

During sexual arousal, the arteries feeding the cavernous spaces become dilated; consequently there is a great increase in blood volume flowing into the cavernous spaces and they expand. Meanwhile the veins draining the sinuses are compressed and prevent the blood leaving the penis. Thus the cavernous spaces become turgid and penis becomes stiff and erect.

URETHRA

The **male urethra** is long, about 20 cm (3 in.) in length and S-shaped. It traverses the prostate gland, urogenital diaphragm and penis to empty outside the body (Fig. 15.6). Accordingly, it is divided into three parts: prostatic part (3 cm long), membranous part (2 cm long) and penile/spongy part (15 cm long).

N.B.

The male urethra provides passage to both, urine and semen, i.e. it serves both the urinary and reproductive systems.

SCROTUM

It is a bag of skin and subcutaneous tissue. It is divided into two internal compartments by a connective tissue septum. Each compartment contains the testis and spermatic cord.

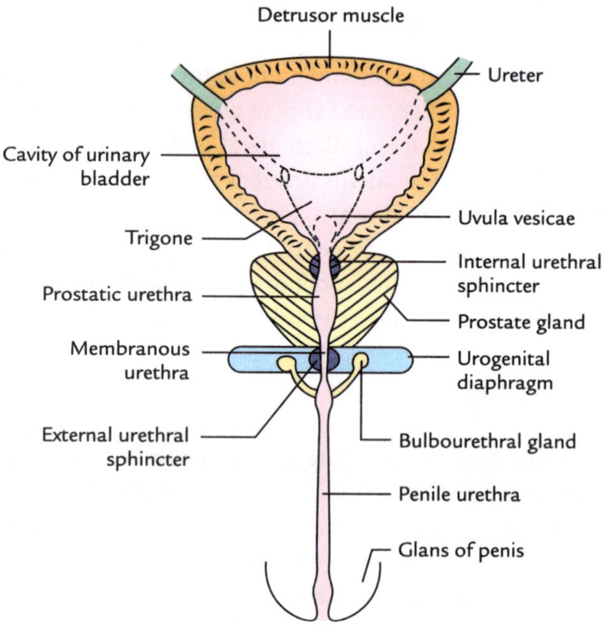

Fig. 15.6 Male urethra.

FEMALE REPRODUCTIVE SYSTEM

The *female reproductive organs* are:

1. Ovaries
2. Uterine tubes
3. Uterus
4. Vagina

The *female external genitalia* include:

1. Clitoris
2. Labia majora
3. Labia minora
4. Greater vestibular (Bartholin) glands

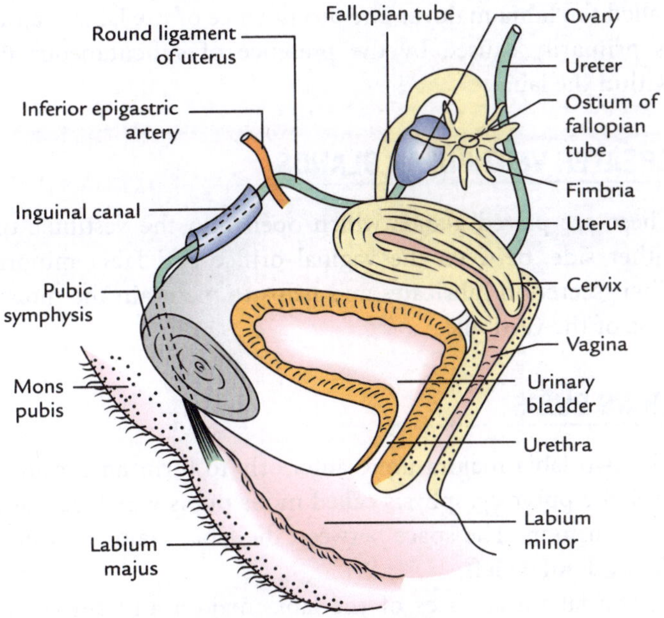

Fig. 15.7 Female reproductive system.

5. Mons pubis
6. Vaginal orifice

Structures of the female reproductive system are depicted in Figure 15.7.

OVARIES

The ovaries are female sex glands, one on each side, lying on the lateral wall of the pelvis. Each ovary is almond-shaped, solid body about half the size of the testis. It is attached to the posterior surface of broad ligament by a fold of peritoneum called **mesovarium** (i.e. mesentery of the ovary).

The ovary produces female gametes called **ova** and female sex hormones (estrogen and progesterone).

At birth each ovary contains about 2 million (200,000) immature ova. From puberty to the end of reproductive period (15–45 years of age), one ovum is shed into the peritoneal cavity once in a lunar month. In all, about 400 ova are shed in the whole reproductive life of a female and rest undergo degeneration and are absorbed in the ovary. The period between the successive ovulations is called **ovarian cycle**.

UTERINE TUBES

There are two uterine tubes, one on each side of the uterus. Each tube is about 10 cm long and lies in the free edge of a fold of peritoneum, the **broad ligament**.

Its narrow medial end opens in the uterus and the expanded distal (ovarian) end called **infundibulum** opens into the peritoneal cavity beside the ovary.

The opening of the infundibulum, the **ostium,** is surrounded by long thin finger-like processes called **fimbriae.** When an ovum is shed, the mouth of ostium lies ready to receive the ovum with the help of fimbriae and propelled in the tube with the peristaltic action of the wall of tube and movements of carpet of cilia in the mucous lining of the tube.

In the tube, the ovum may be met and fertilized by a sperm which is able to reach at this site through vagina and uterus. The ovum is fertilized in the widest and longest part of the tube near the infundibulum called **ampulla.** The part of the tube nearer the uterus is narrower and called **isthmus.**

> **Clinical correlation**
>
> **Tubectomy:** It is a surgical procedure in which uterine tubes are ligated and cut/clamped on both the sides so that the pathway between the sperms and oocyte is sealed. The tubectomy is a common method to render females permanently incapable of fertilization (i.e. they become sterile).

UTERUS

The uterus is a thick-walled hollow muscular organ located nearly in the center of true pelvis between the urinary bladder and the rectum. It is shaped like an inverted pear and flattened anteroposteriorly. Its rounded upper part is called **fundus** and narrower inferior part is called **cervix.** The main part of the uterus is between the fundus and the cervix. A slight constriction called **isthmus** marks the junction between the cervix and body. The fallopian tube opens into the uterus, one on either side at the junction of fundus and body of the uterus. The fertilized ovum is transported into the uterine cavity by the fallopian tube where it is implanted and develops into the fetus.

VAGINA

The vagina (L. *vagina* = a sheath) is thin-walled fibromuscular canal about 3–4 in. (7.5–10 cm) long which forms the organ of copulation in a female. The cervix of uterus projects into it superiorly; inferiorly the vagina opens into the vestibule of the external genitalia. Its functions are: to receive the penis during intercourse, and allow menstrual flow and child-birth.

The interior of vagina is lined by protective, moist stratified squamous epithelium. The smooth muscle in the vaginal wall can stretch to a great extent to accommodate the penis during intercourse and allow passage of baby during its birth. The lubricating fluid found in vagina comes from the glands of uterine cervix.

CLITORIS, LABIA MINORA AND LABIA MAJORA

The female external genitalia (also called vulva or pudendum) consists of vestibule and its surroundings structures

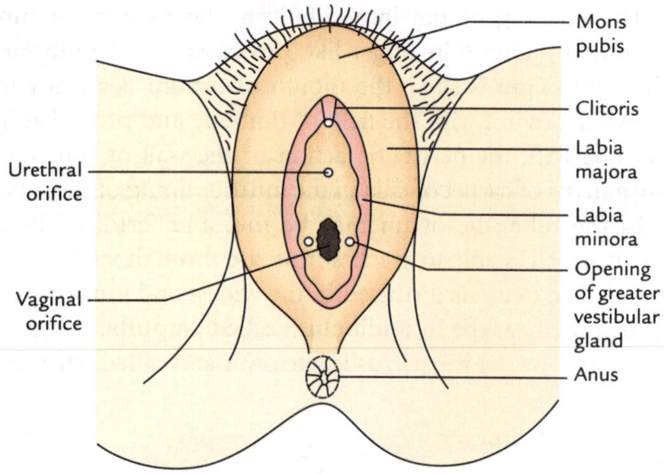

Fig. 15.8 Female external genitalia.

(Fig. 15.8). The **vestibule** is an elliptical space into which vagina opens posteriorly and urethra opens anteriorly.

The vestibule is guarded by a pair of thin longitudinal folds of skin called **labia minora.**

Clitoris

It is small erectile structure called the **clitoris**, which is located into the anterior margin of the vestibule. It is less than 2 cm in length and consists of a shaft and glans. It is made up of erectile tissue like penis (embryologically penis and clitoris are homologous structures). The clitoris is richly supplied with sensory receptors and functions to initiate and intensify sexual pleasure. Anteriorly, the labia minora unite over the clitoris to form a fold of skin called the **prepuce.** Lateral to the labia minora are two prominent rounded folds of skin called the **labia majora**. The prominence of the labia majora is primarily caused by the presence of subcutaneous fat within the labia.

GREATER VESTIBULAR GLANDS

These are paired glands which open into the vestibule on either side, between the vaginal orifice and labia minora. Their secretion lubricates and helps to maintain the moistness of the vestibule.

MONS PUBIS

The two labia majora unite anteriorly to form an elevation over the pubic symphysis called mons pubis which acts as a fatty cushion. The space between the labia majora is called the **pudendal cleft.**

The lateral surfaces of the labia majora and surface of mons pubis are covered with coarse hair.

VAGINAL ORIFICE

The vaginal orifice is located in the posterior part of the vestibule of external genitalia. The vaginal orifice is covered in virgin females by a thin mucous membrane called **hymen** (the word 'hymen' is named after a Greek mythological god of marriage and nuptial song, Hymen). Generally, hymen is perforated by one or several holes to allow menstrual flow. The hymen is completely perforated during first sexual intercourse. When ruptured, the remnants of hymen are seen as round tags called **carunculae hymenales** along the margin of vaginal orifice.

Golden Facts to Remember

➢ Most important function of the urinary system	Maintenance of water and electrolyte concentration within the body (homeostasis)
➢ Most important excretory organ of the body	Kidney
➢ Structural and functional units of kidney	Nephrons
➢ Number of nephrons in each kidney	One million
➢ All the organs in the body become functional at birth or shortly after birth *except*	Reproductive organs which become functional at puberty
➢ Primary sex organs in males	Testes
➢ Primary sex organs in females	Ovaries
➢ Longest duct of male reproductive system	Duct of epididymis (6 m long)
➢ Largest accessory gland of male reproductive system	Prostate gland
➢ Strongest smooth muscle in the body	Uterine muscle
➢ Largest accessory glands of female reproductive system	Mammary glands
➢ Most sensitive part of male external genitalia	Glans of penis
➢ Most sensitive part of female external genitalia	Glans of clitoris
➢ Most common cancer of male reproductive system	Carcinoma prostrate
➢ Most common cancer of female reproductive system	Carcinoma cervix
➢ Most of the bulk of semen is formed by	Secretions of seminal vesicles (60%)
➢ Commonest cause of sterility in modern Indian males	Oligospermia caused by wearing of tight jeans and the use of synthetic androgens (to increase muscle mass)
➢ Commonest cause of sterility in modern Indian females	Tubal-block caused by tubal infection due to decreasing tendency of females to take daily bath

Multiple Choice Questions

1. **Which of the following statements regarding the kidneys is *false*?**
   (a) They are retroperitoneal
   (b) Each kidney has distinct cortical and medullary regions
   (c) They are located between T11 and L3 vertebral levels
   (d) Each kidney contain 3 to 6 renal pyramids

2. **Which of the following statements about renal pyramids is *incorrect*?**
   (a) They are located in the renal medulla
   (b) They are separated from each other by renal columns
   (c) Their tips are called renal papillae
   (d) They do not contain nephrons

3. **Which of the following statements about ureter is *incorrect*?**
   (a) It is about 25 cm long
   (b) It is intraperitoneal
   (c) Its lumen is lined by transitional epithelium
   (d) It transports urine form kidney to the urinary bladder

4. **The detrusor muscle is located in the:**
   (a) Kidneys
   (b) Ureters
   (c) Urinary bladder
   (d) Urethra

5. **All of the following are accessory glands of male reproductive system *except:***
   (a) Prostate gland
   (b) Ejaculatory ducts
   (c) Bartholin glands
   (d) Seminal vesicles

6. **Which of the following statements about prostate gland is *false*?**
   (a) It surrounds the first 3 cm of the urethra
   (b) It is roughly of the size of walnut
   (c) Its secretion forms the bulk of ejaculated semen
   (d) It is shaped like an inverted cone

7. **Female external genitalia include all *except:***
   (a) Labia majora
   (b) Labia minora
   (c) Greater vestibular glands
   (d) Vagina

8. **The number of immature ova in ovary at birth is:**
   (a) 4 million
   (b) 3 million
   (c) 2 million
   (d) 1 million

9. **The fertilization most commonly occurs in:**
   (a) Ovary
   (b) Uterine tube
   (c) Uterus
   (d) Vagina

10. **The cervix is the portion of:**
    (a) Vulva
    (b) Vagina
    (c) Uterus
    (d) Uterine tube

Answers

1. *d*, **2.** *d*, **3.** *b*, **4.** *c*, **5.** *c*, **6.** *b*, **7.** *d*, **8.** *c*, **9.** *b*, **10.** *c*

CHAPTER

16 Radiological (Imaging) Anatomy

Learning Objectives

After studying this chapter, the student should be able to:

- define radiological anatomy and list the various methods used for its study
- describe x-rays and their properties
- outline the shadow cast by different objects on the radiographic film
- describe simple radiographic procedures and discuss their use in clinical medicine
- discuss contrast radiography and list the contrast media used in it
- outline the criteria for a good contrast medium and discuss the choice of different media
- describe CT scan, spiral CT and MRI, and discuss their properties
- present a brief account of positron emission tomography and discuss its main use
- briefly describe the ultrasound and discuss its properties
- correctly solve the review questions given at the end of the chapter

INTRODUCTION

The radiological anatomy or radiology is the science of medical imaging by means of x-rays. It has as its origin on one evening in November 1895 when Wilhelm Röentgen observed that a photographic plate was glowing when a high voltage was passed through an evacuated glass tube. Medical imaging provides a way of observing structures within the body without intervention. It is based on the principle that substances of different densities absorb different amount of x-rays, resulting in a differential exposure of the photographic film. Since the traditional radiograph had limitations as diagnostic tools, a large number of new techniques have been developed to produce the images of structures within the body. Some of them even do not use x-rays. Consequently, the term 'radiological anatomy' is replaced by **imaging anatomy.**

The imaging anatomy deals with different techniques/methods used to provide the images of internal organs of the human body to demonstrate the pathological lesions within them.

The imaging techniques used can be classified as follows:

1. Methods using ionizing radiation
   (a) Conventional imaging
      (i) Plain radiography
      (ii) Contrast radiography
   (b) Computed tomography (CT) scanning/computerized axial tomography (CAT) scanning
   (c) Radioisotope scanning (nuclear medicine imaging)
2. Methods not using ionizing radiation
   (a) Ultrasonography (USG)
   (b) Magnetic resonance imaging (MRI)

IMAGING TECHNIQUES: USING IONIZING RADIATION

CONVENTIONAL IMAGING

Plain Radiography

x-Rays were discovered in 1895 by Wilhelm Conrad Röentgen, a German physicist, who won the first Nobel Prize in physics in 1901. This was the starting point of modern medical radiology and radiotherapy.

x-Rays are produced by passing a high voltage electric current across a vacuum tube called x-ray tube. This induces a stream of electrons from an electrically heated metal element (*tungsten filament*) called **cathode.** When they strike a metal target (*tungsten plate*) called **anode** after passing across a vacuum tube, x-rays are produced (Fig. 16.1). At the time of discovery, nothing was known about x-rays. Thus they were named as x-rays. The term 'x-ray' stands for unknown rays.

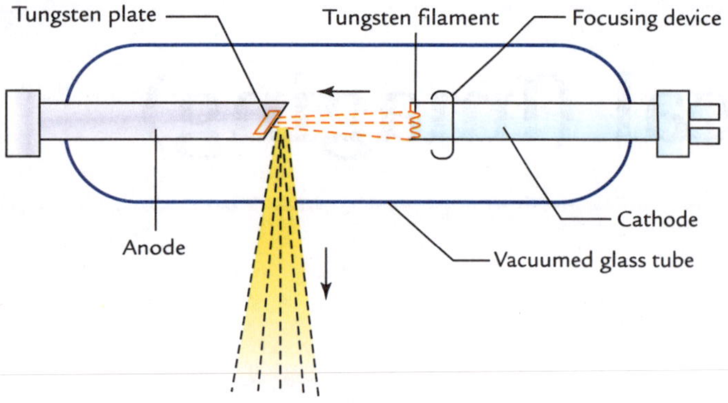

Fig. 16.1 X-ray tube (cathode ray tube) for the production of x-rays.

The x-rays are part of the spectrum of electromagnetic radiation (Fig. 16.2) where long electric waves are found at one end (long wavelength end) and cosmic rays at the other end (short wavelength end) of the spectrum. The radio waves, infrared waves, visible light rays, ultraviolet rays, x-rays and gamma rays are found in the middle of spectrum, in order of increasing frequency, between electric waves and cosmic rays. All these radiations travel at the same speed (300,000 km/sec) in straight lines.

The x-rays are electromagnetic waves similar to the visible light, but with much shorter wavelength (1/10,000). It is this characteristic that empowers the x-rays to penetrate materials which otherwise would absorb or reflect the light.

Properties of x-Rays

The x-rays have the following properties:

1. **Penetrating power:** The x-rays have the power to penetrate the different materials and tissues to variable extent, and the x-ray beam emerging from the other side of the body affects a photographic film, or a fluorescent screen, forming a shadow picture of the different parts of the body structures. The degree of penetration depends on the atomic weight and density of different substances. The higher the atomic weight and density and thickness of a substance, the greater the absorption, e.g. the less dense tissues such as soft tissues are readily penetrated than the more dense tissues such as bone, i.e. x-rays are absorbed more in dense tissues than in soft tissues. The scale of absorption of x-rays in an increasing order in various substances is as follows:
   (a) Air
   (b) Fat
   (c) Water/fluid
   (d) Soft tissues, *viz.* muscles, vessels, nerves, viscera, etc.
   (e) Bone
   (f) Enamel of teeth
   (g) Metals (ornaments, metallic fillings in teeth, etc.) and radiopaque contrast media

   From the above scale it is deduced that air absorbs x-rays a little, fat absorbs x-rays more than air but less than water.

   These differences in absorption (attenuation) of x-rays result in differences in the level of exposure of the film. Thus substances which absorb x-rays little appear more transparent (**radiolucent**) and those which absorb more appear opaque (**radiopaque**). For example, the bone appears white (radiopaque) in radiograph because this region of the film has been exposed to maximum number of x-rays, whereas air in the trachea, lungs, etc. appears dark (radiolucent) because these regions of the film have been exposed to the least number of x-rays.

   Radiology is, therefore, based on the principle of differential absorption of x-rays.

N.B.

Penetrating power/effect is the fundamental property of the x-rays.

2. **Photographic effect:** The x-rays affect the photographic emulsions of the film in much the same way as light waves.

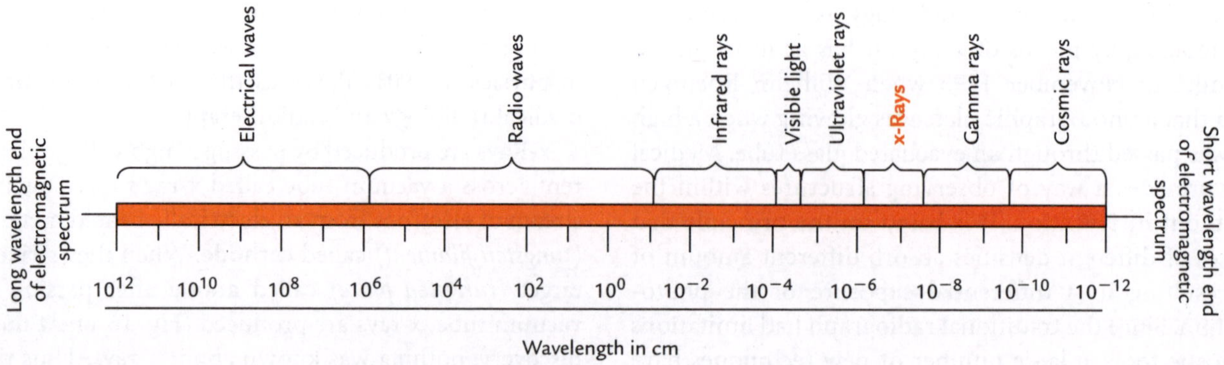

Fig. 16.2 The position of x-rays in electromagnetic spectrum.

After penetrating the tissue/substance, when the x-rays strike the photographic film, the film gets sensitized. The development of such film gives a radiographic image called **radiograph** (Fig. 16.2). The x-ray (radiographic) image is also called skiagram (*skia* = shadow) or Röentgenogram (named after the discoverer of x-rays, Röentgen).

The x-ray sensitive film emulsion consists of silver bromide in the form of a crystal or grains suspended in suitable emulsion. This sensitive emulsion is coated on both sides of the film.

N.B.

The skiagram is a negative picture and it is in this form that the skiagram is examined by radiologists and clinicians.

3. **Fluorescent effect:** When x-rays strike certain metallic salts such as phosphorous, zinc sulfide, cadmium sulfide, etc., they cause these substances to fluoresce, i.e. light rays are produced. This is called fluorescence. This property of x-rays is used in fluoroscopy.
4. **Biological effect (or radiobiological effects):** The x-rays can destroy abnormal cells (e.g. malignant cells) much more readily than the adjacent normal cells, because malignant cells are more radiosensitive than the normal surrounding tissue cells. This property of x-rays is utilized in the treatment of various cancers (*radiotherapy*).

Side Effects of Radiations (Radiation Hazards)

On repeated exposures, radiation can cause:

(a) burns,
(b) genetic mutations,
(c) carcinogenesis, etc.

The effects of radiations are always destructive. Therefore, the x-rays are potentially dangerous. The radiobiological effects depend on the magnitude of the radiation doses and the radiosensitivity of irradiated tissues.

The cells are most radiosensitive at the time of cell division. The rapidly growing cells, such as cancer cells, are usually more radiosensitive than normal or resting cells. This difference of radiosensitivity between normal and cancer cells is the basis of radiation therapy called **radiotherapy**.

Radiosensitivity of Normal Tissues and Cells

The most sensitive cells in the human body are lymphocytes, followed by leucocytes and reproductive cells of testis and ovary. Moderately radiosensitive is epithelial lining of gastrointestinal tract (GIT) and epithelial lining of skin. Least sensitive tissues are fibrous tissue, muscles, bones and nervous tissue.

Clinical correlation

Protective measures to avoid or minimize radiation hazards:

(a) Doctors and technical staff in radiological units should strictly follow the protection regulations. These include:
   - Use of protective materials, *viz.* lead screens, protective aprons, etc.
   - Personal monitoring of radiation doses.

(b) *The 10-day rule*: In women of reproductive age, there is always a possibility of pregnancy; therefore, in such women, x-ray examination of lower abdomen and pelvis should be carried out within 10 days following the first day of mensuration.

(c) *During pregnancy*, only essential x-ray examinations have to be carried out and every care should be taken to protect the fetus from exposure to radiations.

(d) Avoid unnecessary x-ray examinations.

N.B.

Keeping in view the radiosensitivity of cell and tissues, adequate protective measures must be taken against repeated exposures to x-rays. The basic principle of radiation protection is '*ALARA*', i.e. *A*s *L*ow *A*s *R*easonably *A*chievable. This means that only permissible doses of radiation should be given at permissible intervals (for details consult radiology books).

Radiographic Views

The radiographs are taken by passing x-ray beam through the patient on to the photographic film (Fig. 16.3).

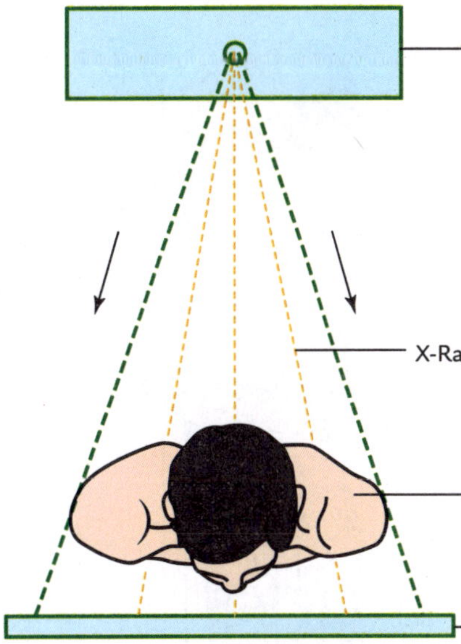

Fig. 16.3 Simple x-ray. Note that the x-rays are passed from posterior aspect of the body, and photographic film is in front of the body. The view of photograph thus taken will be posteroanterior (PA view).

The radiographs are taken at different positions of the subject in relation to the source of x-rays and photographic film, to have complete information about the entire structure by eliminating some particular overlapping shadow in a particular view. The view denotes the direction of the beam of x-ray.

Some of the common radiographic views are:

1. **Anteroposterior (AP) view:** In this view, x-rays pass from anterior aspect of the subject and x-ray (radiographic) plate is placed posteriorly. The posteriorly place structures are better visualized in this view.
2. **Posteroanterior (PA) view:** In this view, x-rays pass from behind (posterior aspect of) the subject and x-ray (radiographic) plate is placed anteriorly (Fig. 16.4). The anteriorly placed structures are better visualized in this view.

N.B.

The part of body closer to the x-ray plate casts sharper shadow than the part facing the x-ray tube.

For this reason, the chest x-ray for visualizing the lesion in the lungs and heart are taken in PA view, whereas for visualizing the thoracic spine, AP view is preferred.

The more commonly taken x-ray chest is a PA view.

Simple Radiological Procedures

The simple radiological procedures include:

1. Fluoroscopy
2. Plain radiography (plain x-ray)
3. Xeroradiography
4. Tomography

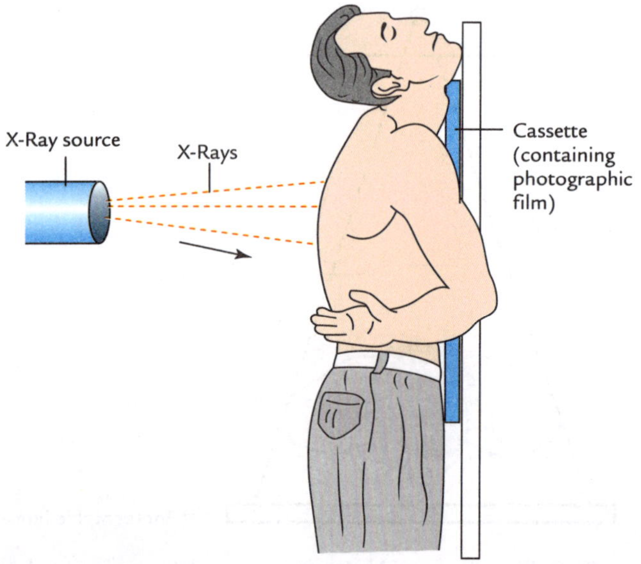

Fig. 16.4 Method of taking chest x-ray; posterior–anterior view. Note the position of x-ray source and cassette containing photographic film.

Fluoroscopy

The human eyes cannot see x-rays. But when x-rays strike certain substances, they cause them to fluoresce (i.e. production of light rays) and can be perceived by the human eye. Hence one can see the fluorescence of the x-ray beam. This forms the underlying principle of fluoroscopy.

The fluoroscopy is done in the dark room and fluoroscopic image is directly visualized on the fluorescent screen. The sharpness of fluoroscopic image is inferior to that of a radiograph.

The fluoroscopy is of special advantage in observing the movements of organs such as lungs, stomach, intestine, diaphragm, etc.

The fluoroscopic image can be photographed by a camera in a miniature form. These films are very cheap; hence masses can be surveyed for detection of widespread diseases such as tuberculosis. This is called **mass miniature radiography** (MMR).

Plain Radiography (Plain x-Ray)

In this procedure, x-ray beam is passed through the patient on to the photographic plate and a natural x-ray image is directly obtained without using any contrast medium.

The plain radiography is useful in the study of normal and abnormal bones, lungs, paranasal air sinuses and gaseous shadows in the abdomen.

Silver bromide is used as the photosensitive material in x-ray.

The characteristic features of plain radiography are as follows:

1. Plain radiograph cannot show the pathological differences among various organs.
2. It can show gross differences between gas, fat, soft tissue and calcification, metal and fluid by different grades of shadows (Table 16.1).

Interpretation of common plain radiographs

Although comprehensive interpretation of plain radiographs is beyond the scope of this book, a brief outline of interpretation of common radiographs is given here.

Table 16.1 Shadows cast by different substances in plain radiograph

Substance	Shadow
Gas/air	Black
Fat	Dark gray
Soft tissue	Light gray
Fluid	Hazy (haziness)
Bone/calcification	White
Metal	Brilliant white

Chest radiograph: It is one of the most commonly requested plain radiograph. The chest radiograph is obtained in erect posture on inspiration and includes the upper abdomen to demonstrate the normal air bubble in the fundus of stomach and right subphrenic area. A good quality chest radiograph will demonstrate the lungs, cardiomediastinal contour, diaphragm, rib cage and peripheral soft tissue (Fig. 16.5). One should check the following features:

1. The heart is of normal size (less than the width of the chest) or enlarged (greater than the width of the chest).
2. There is the normal outline of aortic arch called aortic knuckle.
3. The lung fields are lucent (dark areas) on either side of cardiomediastinal shadow, or there are focal mass/masses seen as areas of increased density.
4. The trachea (lucent track in midline) is in normal position or shifted to the side.
5. The ribs are normal or showing fracture or malignant destruction.
6. There is free gas under the diaphragm.
7. The costodiaphragmatic recess is clear or contains fluid.

Abdominal radiograph: It is obtained in supine position (AP view). The plain radiographs of abdomen demonstrate intestinal gas pattern and size and contour of the liver and spleen. The position of the kidney is outlined due to lucency of the perinephretic fat surrounding them. The presence of calcified opacities such as biliary and renal tract calculi may be seen. Areas of abnormal calcification may be seen in pancreas due to chronic pancreatitis. Then the obstruction of lumen of the bowel is seen as abnormal air-filled levels on erect film and distended bowel loops proximal to obstruction in supine position.

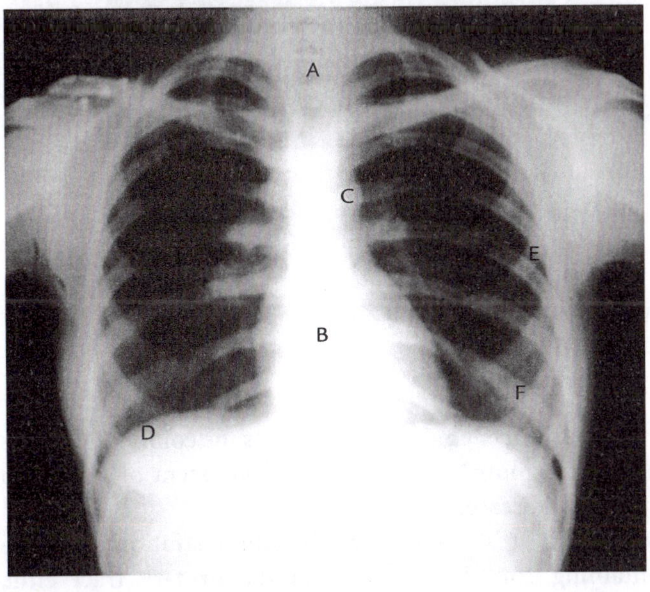

Fig. 16.5 Chest x-ray; posteroanterior view: **A,** tracheal shadow; **B,** cardiac shadow; **C,** aortic knuckle; **D,** dome of diaphragm; **E,** lung shadow; **F,** rib.

Peripheral radiographs of limbs: They are obtained in AP, PA and lateral views. The plain radiographs of films are widely used to detect fractures. The osteomyelitis and bone tumors are often well seen on plain films.

Xeroradiography

It is a variation of the plain radiography. In this procedure, an x-ray beam is passed through a patient onto the aluminum plate which is coated with a thin layer of selenium and electrically charged. This causes an alteration of the electrostatic charge corresponding with the image. The image can be obtained/seen by blowing a thin powder which adheres in proportion to the local charge onto the plate. This is then transferred to a special paper and permanent record is obtained. This procedure provides better soft tissue contrast than seen in simple plain radiography.

Tomography

It is also a variation of the simple radiography performed to take radiographs of body sections. In this procedure during x-ray exposure, the x-ray tube and x-ray film are moved in opposite direction so as to produce the equivalent of a body section. The x-ray tube and x-ray film are connected by a rod, which can be made to pivot a variable point.

Special Radiological Procedures

Contrast Radiography

In this procedure, different contrast media (either radiopaque or translucent) which have permeability to x-rays different than that of body tissues are inserted into various cavities and organs or even into blood vessels to achieve greater contrast in a radiograph.

Since the contrast media have different permeability to x-rays than that of the body tissues, x-ray pictures of the interiors of hollow organs and vessels can be obtained.

With the advent of new imaging modalities, the contrast media is also used to improve the visibility between a focal mass and surrounding parenchyma of an organ. This is commonly known as **lesion enhancement**.

Thus, the functions of contrast media include:

1. **Delineation of normal structures**, e.g. gastrointestinal tract, biliary tree, thecal sac, joint space and blood vessels.
2. **Lesion enhancement**, e.g. mass in liver, renal calculus, etc.

Contrast Media

The contrast media generally used are:

1. **Radiopaque:** The contrast media are ingested or injected into the body. These include:
   (a) *Salts of heavy metals*, e.g. barium sulfate
   (b) *Organic iodide preparations*.
2. **Radiolucent:** It includes gas, e.g. air and other gases.

N.B.

- The barium sulfate and iodine compounds produce radiopaque shadows, whereas air and oxygen produce radiolucent shadows.
- Barium is most widely used contrast media in radiography.

Criteria for a good contrast medium

The contrast medium should be:

1. nontoxic,
2. reasonably radiopaque or radiolucent,
3. easily administrable and
4. easily available.

Choices of different media

1. *Barium sulfate suspension* (emulsion) in water is used for visualizing gastrointestinal tract.
2. The *aqueous solution of iodine compounds* is used to visualize the biliary passage, urinary passage and blood vessels.
3. The *iodized oil* is used for visualizing bronchial tree and genital passage.
4. The *air and gases* are used for visualizing the body cavities like ventricles of the brain and serous cavities of the body.

N.B.

Air can be used along with barium for *double contrast studies* of the GIT. The barium coats the mucosa is studied in detail following air distension of the organ.

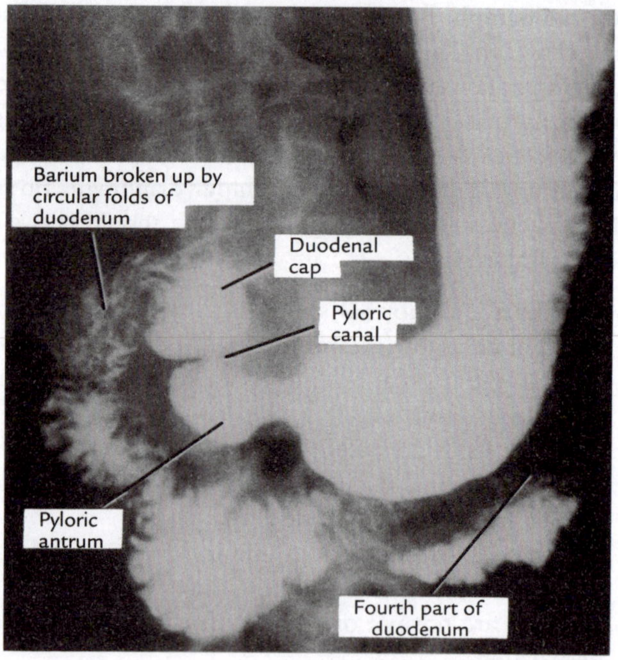

Fig. 16.6 Barium meal x-ray. (*Source*: Fig. 5.25, Page 250, *Last's Anatomy: Regional and Applied*, 12th ed, Chummy S Sinnatamby. Copyright Elsevier Ltd. 2011, All rights reserved.)

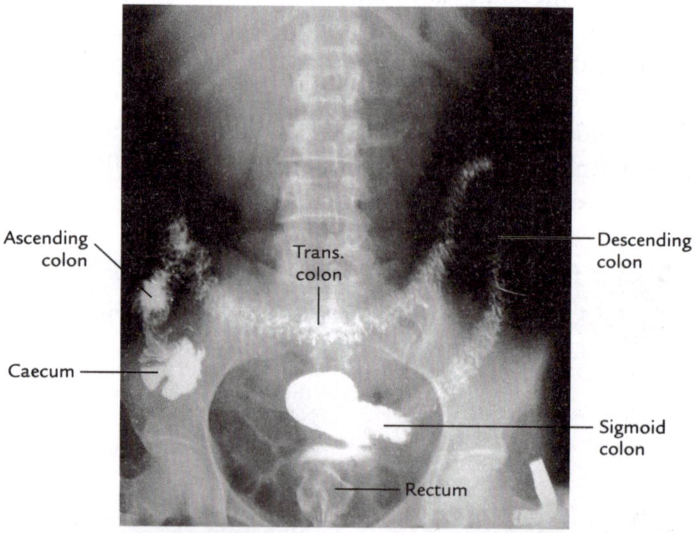

Fig. 16.7 Barium enema x-ray.

Interpretation of Common Contrast Radiographs

Barium meal x-ray (Fig. 16.6): It is obtained by oral administration of barium meal in erect posture. The barium meal contrast radiograph demonstrates J-shaped shadow of stomach, with lucent shadow of air bubble in its fundus, angular notch (incision angularis) at the junction of pylorus and lesser curvature of stomach, and narrow pyloric canal at the junction of pylorus and duodenum. The first part of duodenum typically presents a triangular shadow called **duodenal cap**. The remaining part of the duodenum presents a floccular appearance; alteration in the mucosa of esophagus, stomach and duodenum is seen filling the defects. Peptic ulcers cause craters, called **ulcer craters**, in the wall of the stomach and duodenum.

Barium enema x-ray (Fig. 16.7): It is obtained by the administration of 2–3 pints (1 L) of barium sulfate emulsion through the anal canal. The barium enema x-ray demonstrates the characteristic sacculations in the wall of large intestine. The rectum is seen to have a wider caliber than the colon. Appendix may sometimes be seen as arising from the base of cecum.

The barium enema is used to assess the colon for the presence of carcinomas, diverticulosis and extent of inflammatory bowel disease.

Pyelogram: It is obtained by the administration of iodine-containing contrast medium in the urinary tract either intravenously or through catheter, and pyelography thus performed is termed as descending (intravenous) and ascending pyelography, respectively. Intravenous pyelography is the standard method to visualize the urinary tract. The pyelogram demonstrates calyces, ureter and bladder. Haematuria, dysuria and loin pain are important indications for intravenous pyelography. The stones in the pelvicaliceal system, ureter and urinary bladder are readily visualized as radiopaque shadows.

Hysterosalpingogram: It is obtained by injecting contrast medium (lipiodol) into cervix and uterus through a suitable canula. The hysterosalpingogram outlines the uterine cavity, fallopian tubes and spilling of contrast medium in the peritoneal cavity through ostia of fallopian tubes. The hysterosalpingography is useful in cases of sterility to prove or disprove the patency of the uterine tubes.

COMPUTED TOMOGRAPHY (CT) SCANNING/ COMPUTERIZED AXIAL TOMOGRAPHY (CAT) SCANNING

It is a new method of forming images from the x-ray. In this method, a movable x-ray tube and computer scanner are used. The computed tomography permits the study of tissue slices so that minor differences in tissue density can be recognized. The x-ray source/tube rotates in an arc around the body part being studied and send out a beam of x-rays. The x-ray having passed through the part of the body are collected by a special x-ray detector, the scanner. The scanner receives intensity information of the body part from many positions. These data are entered as a matrix and the radiodensity at each point in three-dimensional space of the part is calculated. With a sufficiently narrow x-ray beam, sensitive detectors and digital signal processing techniques, small difference in radiodensity can be converted into an image. Since the information is gathered for the full volume of the part, the computed matrix contains information about the entire part, it is therefore possible to generate 'slices' or tomograms (Greek word *tomo* means '*cut*' or '*slice*') of various planes through the part, visualizing internal structures at any desired level. Thus CT scan obtains a series of images of the body (slices) in the axial plane and displays a cross-sectional image (Fig. 16.8).

N.B.

CT scanning is based on same principle as conventional x-rays but combines it with computer technology. This procedure is more safe as it is quick and lasts only a few seconds to generate each slice.

Features

The characteristics of computed tomographic imaging are as follows:

1. Computerized tomography uses x-rays.
2. It gives excellent cross-sectional image of internal structures.

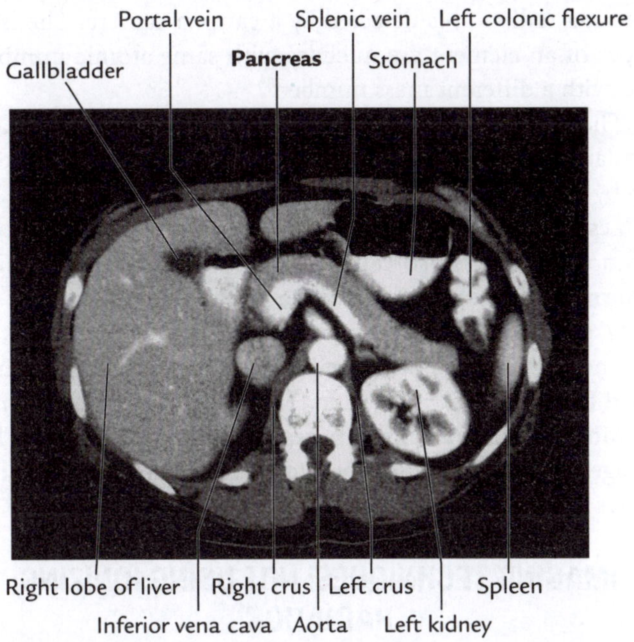

Fig. 16.8 CT scan of abdomen with contrast in axial plane. (*Source*: Fig. 4.88A, Page 289, *Gray's Anatomy for Students*, Richard L Drake, Wayne Vogl, Adam WM Mitchell. Copyright Elsevier Inc. 2005, All rights reserved.)

3. It is very useful in detecting deep seated lesions.
4. It is less harmful than conventional x-ray due to shorter exposure time.
5. It is generally called computed axial tomographic scanning (CAT scan).
6. It was invented and introduced for clinical use by Godfrey N. Hounsfield in 1970.

Spiral CT (SCT)

In this procedure, the patient moves longitudinally and the x-ray tube moves in a circular motion. As a result, the x-ray beam takes a spiral path through the organ being studied. The vast information thus achieved is manipulated by using modern computer system to get an image that can be viewed from any angle.

The unwanted tissues, obstructing the details, can also be removed by computer manipulation.

The presentation can be further improved by color coding.

RADIOISOTOPE SCANNING (NUCLEAR MEDICINE IMAGING)

During the last two decades, the radioisotopes are being used for organ imaging. The radioisotope imaging (or nuclear medicine imaging) is based on the principle that certain isotopes emit gamma radiation. By introducing isotopes in the body, it is possible to visualize specific regions of interest.

Gamma radiation is detected by a gamma camera. The isotopes of an element are nuclides with same atomic number but with a different mass number.

The technique of scanning depends on the fact that particular isotope can be so designed as to be selectively taken up by a particular organ.

Lesions of organ such as tumors may take up more of isotope resulting in so-called '*hot*' areas on scan as in brain. Alternatively, they may fail to take up the isotope resulting in '*cold*' areas as in liver and thyroid.

The common isotopes used in nuclear medicine imaging are those of iodine (^{123}I, ^{125}I and ^{131}I) and technetium (99Tcm).

Most nuclear medicine images are functional studies. The images are generally directly interpreted on a computer and series of representative films are obtained for clinical use.

IMAGING TECHNIQUES: NOT USING IONIZING RADIATION

ULTRASONOGRAPHY (USG)

In ultrasonography, the high frequency sound waves are used. The frequency of waves is so high that they cannot be heard by the human ear, hence the name **ultrasonic waves**.

The principle of medical ultrasound imaging lies in the passing of a beam of high frequency sound into the patient and detecting the returning echoes.

The ultrasonic waves are produced from a **transducer** and travel through the human tissues at a velocity of some 1500 m/sec. When the wave reaches an object or surface with a different texture, it is reflected back to the source, the transducer, as echoes. These echoes received by the transducer are amplified and electronically converted into real-time anatomical images, which are shown on a monitor (Fig. 16.9).

The sound waves that are passed through gas, solid and fluid-filled structures travel at different rates and are reflected back with differing degrees of echoes. The gas and bone are not suitable for ultrasonography; hence gas-filled structures such as the lungs and bowel are very difficult to be visualized.

The ultrasound is very useful in assessing the nature of masses in abdomen and soft tissues, because one can differentiate between solid and fluid-filled masses. For example, if mass in kidney is first observed by intravenous pyelography, one can more accurately assess it with ultrasound. During ultrasonography, if it is solid, it is likely to represent a tumor and if cystic, it represents a simple cyst.

Nowadays, ultrasound is widely used to visualize fluid-filled structures such as gallbladder, urinary bladder, etc.

N.B.

The ultrasound is now the primary means of investigation to assess the gallbladder disease since the ultrasonologist can also look at the liver, kidneys and pancreas at the same time. Pathology in these closely related organs, which may mimic biliary pathology, can be detected.

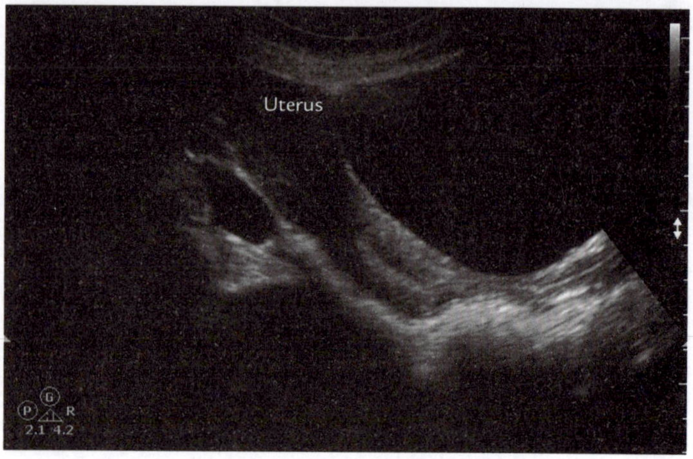

Fig. 16.9 Ultrasound image of lower abdomen.

Features

The characteristics of ultrasound imaging are as follows:

1. Ultrasound imaging of internal organs is noninvasive.
2. Is safe as it does not involve electromagnetic radiation.
3. Can be safely used to evaluate the condition of fetus such as gestational age, congenital defects (anencephaly, spina bifida), etc.
4. Can detect tumors that differ in density from surrounding tissues.
5. Can provide valuable information regarding the size, location, displacement, etc.
6. Is very useful in diagnosing defects in various internal organs like heart, kidneys, gallbladder, etc.

Ultrasound is very useful in assessing the nature of masses either in the abdomen or soft tissues. It is widely used in visualizing fluid-filled structures such as gallbladder, urinary bladder or abdominal aorta.

It is now the primary mode of investigating suspected gallbladder disease since ultrasonologists can look at the liver, kidneys and the pancreas at the same time.

Doppler images are currently being used to assess blood flow in major blood vessels.

MAGNETIC RESONANCE IMAGING (MRI)

This new imaging modality is a method of visualizing physiological distribution of protons of hydrogen ions within the body, enabling high quality of anatomical images to be obtained by using high powered magnets. The magnetic resonance imaging is the most exciting advancement in imaging technology since the beginning of medical radiology in 1895. It is based on the generalized phenomenon called nuclear magnetic resonance (NMR). The magnetic resonance is the study of interaction of molecules (specifically atomic nuclei such as hydrogen) with the radiofrequency field in the presence of strong external magnetic field. Since the human body contains nearly 70–80% of water (H_2O), as it is present in almost all the tissues of the body and water contains hydrogen (H); hence hydrogen proton is ideal. These protons behave like tiny magnets; hence it is possible to get the distribution of these protons present in the body, which is shown in the form of an MRI image.

To take an MRI image, the patient is placed in a strong magnetic field, i.e. he/she positioned in the center of the machine which has powerful magnets. When a pulse of radio waves is passed through the patient, the magnets are deflected and as they return to their aligned position they emit small radiopulses. The strength and frequency of emitted pulses and time taken by protons to return to their pre-excited state produce a signal. These signals are analyzed by a powerful computer, and an image is obtained (Fig. 16.10).

To summarize, the MRI images obtained are from abundant and strong signals of mobile protons (of atomic nuclei of hydrogen ions) of the water and fat present in the body. These images are nothing but the pictorial representation of the spatial distribution of the mobile protons of hydrogen ions. The NMR signals can be altered by introducing new contrast agents (*viz.* paramagnetic substances). Nowadays, by using these new contrast agents, enhanced images of very small lesions can also be demonstrated within the brain.

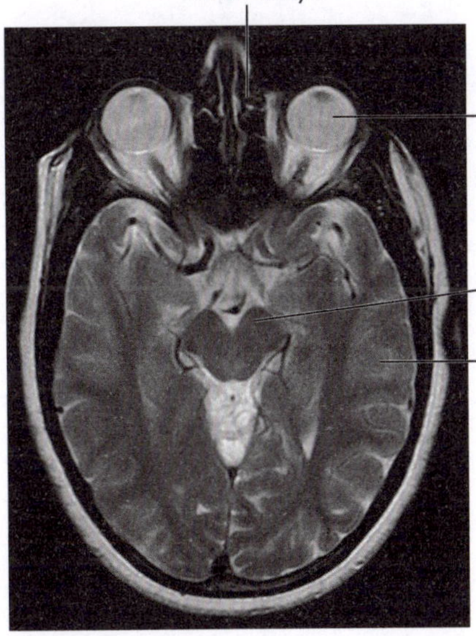

Fig. 16.10 MRI of the head.

WEIGHTING OF IMAGING

The different properties of protons can be assessed by altering the sequence of pulses subjected to protons. These properties are called *weighting*.

Two types of images are obtained by altering the pulse sequence and scanning parameters, which provide differences in image contrast as under:

1. **T1-weighted images:** They show dark on fluid and bright on fat, e.g. cerebrospinal fluid (CSF) in the brain appears dark.
2. **T2-weighted images:** They show a bright signal on fluid and an intermediate signal on fat, e.g. CSF in the brain appears white.

N.B.

The technique of MRI uses the magnetic properties of the hydrogen nucleus excited by the *radiofrequency radiation* transmitted by a coil around the body part. It provides better differentiation between different soft tissues, because some tissues contain more hydrogen in the form of water than the other tissues.

Features

The characteristics of an MRI are as follows:

1. An MRI is completely noninvasive and x-rays are not used.
2. Provides two- and three-dimensional pictures of any organ of the human body.
3. Is superior to CT and provides good soft tissue contrast.
4. Produces not only axial images resembling those of CT but also images of any direction and plane including sagittal and coronal.
5. Absence of ionizing radiation or any other apparent biological hazard.
6. Is the first investigation of choice to detect tumor in brain and spinal cord.
7. Can be used to assess the blood flow within the vessels and produce angiograms.

POSITRON EMISSION TOMOGRAPHY (PET)

The PET scan is a radiological technique used to determine the metabolic activity in the organs such as in brain, heart or other organs, after injecting a radioactive substance into the blood.

The metabolic activity is determined by tracking the movements and concentration of a radioactive tracer which is injected into the blood. A camera records the tracer's signals as it travels. A computer converts these signals into three-dimensional images of the organ under examination.

Table 16.2 Summary of radiological terms

Imaging modality	Brightness (white shade)	Darkness (dark shade)
Plain radiograph	Radiopaque	Radiolucent
Ultrasound	Hyperechoic	Hypoechoic
Computed tomographic (CT) scan	High attenuation	Low attenuation
Magnetic resonance imaging (MRI)	High signal	Low signal
Nuclear magnetic resonance (NMR)	'Hot' areas	'Cold' areas

Features

The characteristics of PET are as follows:

1. PET scan combines computed tomography and nuclear scanning.
2. This reveals the metabolic and functional changes at the cellular level in an organ.
3. PET scan detects these changes very early, whereas CT scan or MRI detects these changes late when the disease has caused structured changes in the organ.

RADIOLOGICAL TERMS IN PRESENT PERSPECTIVE

The images on screen or photographic films are composed of shades of gray ranging from white to black. In plain radiographs, only four densities or shades can be distinguished, *viz.* bone = white, soft tissues = gray fat = a darker gray, and air = black. But with the development of new imaging modalities, the radiologists use different terminologies to describe the shades of brightness and darkness. The accepted terminologies are listed in Table 16.2.

ORIENTATION OF IMAGES

The radiological images are viewed in standard orientations. In recent years, the advent of CT and magnetic resonance has greatly increased the possible orientations that the final image can be constructed by a process called **multiplanar reformatting (MPR)**. However, conventional orientations are still based on anatomical planes as under:

1. *Sagittal images* shows a slice through the long axis from anterior to posterior.
2. *Coronal images* shows a slice through the long axis from right side to left side.
3. *Axial (transverse or horizontal) images* shows a horizontal slice at right angle to the long axis of the body. These images are created as if standing at a patient's feet and looking towards his head.

Golden Facts to Remember

➢ X-rays were invented by	Wilhelm Conrad Röentgen in 1895
➢ Most important property of x-rays	Penetrating power
➢ CT scan was invented by	Hounsfield in 1970
➢ Most exciting advancement in imaging technology since the discovery of x-rays in 1895	Magnetic resonance imaging (MRI)
➢ Most sensitive cells in the body to ionizing radiation	Lymphocytes (followed by leucocytes and reproductive cells)
➢ Least sensitive tissue in the body to ionizing radiation	Fibrous tissue (followed by muscle, bone marrow and nervous tissue)
➢ Commonest view of x-ray chest desired by clinicians	Posteroanterior (PA) view
➢ Most commonly used contrast medium in radiography	Barium sulfate
➢ Most commonly used isotopes in imaging	Technetium, radio-iodine
➢ Most commonly used imaging technique to visualize the condition of fetus	Ultrasound
➢ Most efficient imaging technique used to detect gall-bladder disease	Ultrasound
➢ Most efficient imaging technique used to detect disc prolapse	MRI
➢ First choice of imaging technique used to detect tumor in brain and spinal cord	MRI
➢ Imaging technique used to detect metabolic activity in the organs	Positron emission tomography (PET)

Multiple Choice Questions

1. Regarding Wilhelm Conrad Röentgen, all of the following facts are true *except*:
   (a) He was a German physicist
   (b) He discovered x-rays
   (c) He won the Nobel Prize in 1895
   (d) He won the Nobel Prize in 1901

2. Which of the following structures absorb maximum x-rays?
   (a) Air
   (b) Bone
   (c) Soft tissue
   (d) Fat

3. Radiation exposure occurs in all *except*:
   (a) CT scan
   (b) Fluoroscopy
   (c) MRI
   (d) Plain x-ray

4. Calcification is best detected by:
   (a) CT scan
   (b) MRI
   (c) Ultrasound
   (d) Plain x-ray

5. x-Rays are produced when electrons hit:
   (a) Cathode
   (b) Anode
   (c) Water
   (d) Radium source

6. x-Rays are produced by:
   (a) Positrons
   (b) Protons
   (c) Electrons
   (d) Neutrons

7. Imaging technique commonly used to see the condition of fetus is:
   (a) Plain x-ray
   (b) Ultrasound
   (c) CT scan
   (d) MRI

8. x-Rays were discovered by Röentgen in:
   (a) 1885
   (b) 1895
   (c) 1901
   (d) 1907

9. x-Rays are:
   (a) Electrons
   (b) Protons
   (c) Neutrons
   (d) Electromagnetic waves

10. CT scan was invented by:
    (a) Röentgen
    (b) John Snow
    (c) Godfrey Hounsfield
    (d) Takashita Koba

11. Xeroradiography is generally used for detection of tumor in:
    (a) Breast
    (b) Stomach
    (c) Colon
    (d) Pancreas

12. First investigation of choice to detect tumor in spinal cord is:
    (a) Plain x-ray
    (b) Ultrasound
    (c) CT scan
    (d) MRI

13. The photosensitive material used in x-ray films consists of:
    (a) Cellulose
    (b) Silver bromide
    (c) Zinc sulfide
    (d) Cadmium

14. Most radiolucent substance is:
    (a) Fat
    (b) Soft tissue
    (c) Brain
    (d) Bone

Answers

1. *c*, **2.** *b*, **3.** *c*, **4.** *d*, **5.** *b*, **6.** *c*, **7.** *b*, **8.** *b*, **9.** *d*, **10.** *c*, **11.** *a*, **12.** *d*, **13.** *b*, **14.** *a*

CHAPTER 17

Medical Genetics

Learning Objectives

After studying this chapter, the student should be able to:

- describe the structure of DNA and RNA, and discuss the differences between them
- discuss the morphological types of chromosomes
- state what karyotyping is and discuss its significance in clinical medicine
- provide a brief account of sex chromatin
- outline the various types of chromosomal abnormalities
- present a brief account of genes and discuss autosomal and sex-linked inheritance
- describe in brief the clinical conditions that occur due to chromosomal abnormalities
- discuss briefly the single gene inherited diseases
- describe Down's syndrome, Klinefelter's syndrome, Turner's syndrome and Cat's cry syndrome
- correctly solve the review questions given at the end of the chapter

INTRODUCTION

Genetics is the branch of bioscience which deals with the underlying principles of heredity. The heredity/inheritance is a process by which children inherit certain characteristics (traits) from their parents.

The expression of inherited character is however modified by the environment around the individual in which he grows. These characteristics (traits) pass from parents to children through the inheritable material (**genetic code**) present in the nucleus of the cell. The genetic code is carried by the deoxyribonucleic acid (DNA) molecules. The functional unit of DNA is called ***gene***.

The DNA molecules are arranged in linear sequences in chromosomes inside the nucleus of the cell. The total genetic information present in a cell is called **genome.** The human genome comprises about 50,000–100,000 genes.

The gene expression occurs by formation of different types of proteins. The protein is synthesized by transcription of genetic code into ribonucleic acid (RNA), perpetuated by DNA replication. The RNA forms protein by translation using the genetic code. Thus RNA is an intermediary molecule to execute gene expression.

DEOXYRIBONUCLEIC ACID

The DNA is a double-stranded molecule, made up of two chains of nucleotides, coiled around each other, forming what is commonly described as a **double helix.** The double helical model of DNA was first introduced by James Watson and Francis Crick in 1953 (Fig. 17.1).

The nucleotides are the basic structural units of the DNA. Each nucleotide consists of three subunits:

1. A sugar
2. A phosphate group
3. A nitrogenous base

Each strand of the double helix consists of alternate units of sugar and phosphate. The sugar is **deoxyribose**. The two strands are held together by **hydrogen bonds** between the nitrogenous bases which are attached to the sugars as side groups and point towards the center of the helix. Thus the structure of a DNA molecule is likened to a twisted ladder. The nitrogenous bases are adenine (A), guanine (G), thymine (T) and cytosine (C). The nitrogenous base of two strands in normal conditions pair by hydrogen bonds in a specific manner. For example:

1. Adenine binds with thymine by two hydrogen bonds (A = T).
2. Guanine binds with cytosine by three hydrogen bonds (G ≡ C).

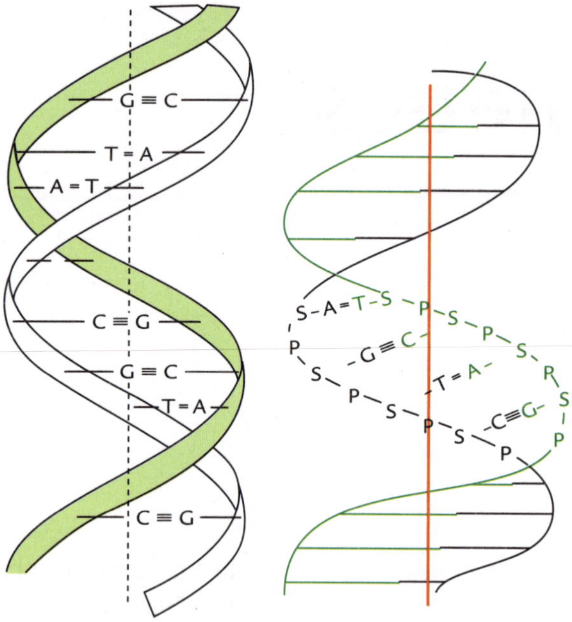

Fig. 17.1 Double helical model of DNA.

However, under abnormal conditions when the bases are in **enol form**, adenine may pair with cytosine and guanine with thymine. This is the basis of **mutation of genes**.

The two strands of a DNA molecule are complementary to each other, i.e. if the base sequence of one strand is known, then the base sequence of other strand can be formulated.

The functions of a DNA molecule are as follows:

1. **Self replication:** During nuclear division, the two strands of DNA separate and each strand acts as a template to form a new complementary strand (Fig. 17.2).

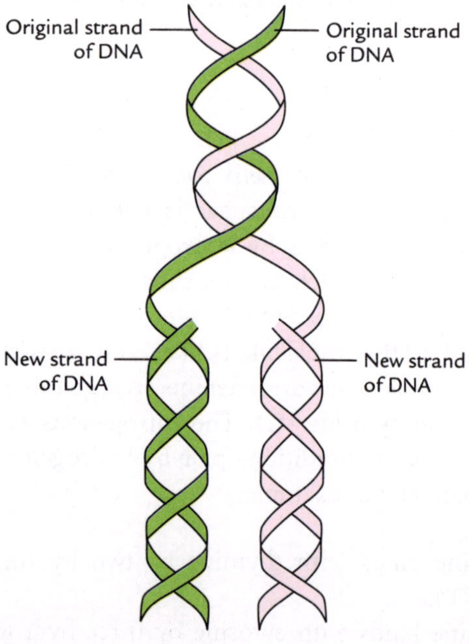

Fig. 17.2 DNA replication.

2. **Synthesis of RNA and proteins:** The certain regions of DNA serve as template for the synthesis of RNA which in turn synthesizes proteins.
3. **Recombination:** During crossing over in meiosis, there is an exchange of genetic material between homologous chromosomes, which leads to shuffling of genes, and the process is called recombination.
4. **Mutation:** It is the major source of genetic variation. The change of base sequence in a gene or gene sequence in the DNA molecule is called **gene mutation**. The mutation may be spontaneous or induced. The inducing agents include chemicals, radiation, etc.

N.B.

The DNA molecules are associated with globular histone proteins to form chromatin. The histone proteins are involved in regulating the function of DNA. Normally, the chromatin is organized as string with beads within cell nucleus but during cell division, the chromatin condenses into structures called *chromosomes*.

RIBONUCLEIC ACID

The ribonucleic acid (RNA) is synthesized in the nucleus by transcription of one strand of DNA. RNA is structurally related to DNA. Its structure is similar to a single strand of DNA with the difference that the sugar molecule in RNA is **ribose sugar** and **uracil** substitutes for thymine. The uracil can bind only to adenine.

Biosynthesis of RNA and Proteins

The DNA molecule acts as a template for the synthesis of RNA (Fig. 17.3) and the latter conveys the genetic message

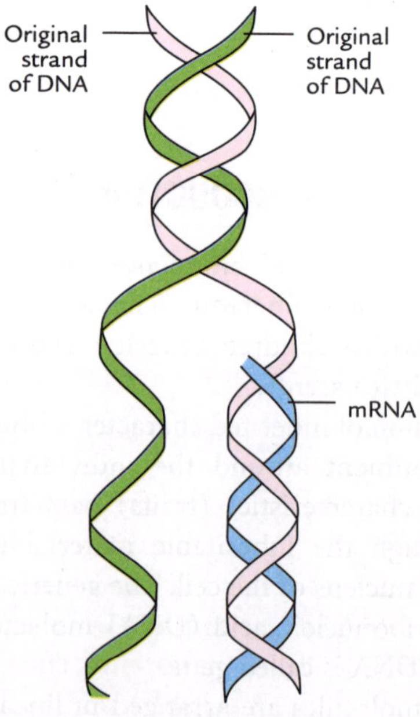

Fig. 17.3 Transcription of mRNA.

and deciphers genetic codes for synthesis of specific polypeptide chain of proteins by linear linkage of amino acids. Therefore, the central dogma of molecular genetics is that genetic information flows from DNA to proteins during gene expression. The flow of information from DNA to protein occurs in the following two steps:

1. DNA → RNA (by transcription)
2. RNA → protein (by translation)

N.B.

The RNA plays a key role in gene expression.

Types of RNA

There are three types of RNA which play important roles in protein synthesis:

1. **mRNA (messenger RNA):** It is synthesized in nucleus from DNA and copies the nucleotide sequence from DNA. It moves into cytoplasm through the nuclear pores and then dictates the sequence of amino acid in polypeptide chains.

   The mRNA contains the information required to determine the sequence of amino acids in protein. The information called **genetic code**—is carried in groups of three nucleotides known as **codons**.
2. **tRNA (transfer RNA):** It is also formed in the nucleus from DNA. The function of tRNA is to match a specific amino acid to a specific codon of mRNA. Each tRNA can pick up a particular amino acid. In other words, before formation of a peptide linkage, the amino acid are activated and attached to one end of specific transfer RNA (tRNA) molecule.
3. **rRNA (ribosomal RNA):** Like mRNA and tRNA, the rRNA is also produced in the nucleus from DNA. It is rich in guanine and cytosine in comparison to mRNA and tRNA. rRNA plays an important role in the formation of protein at the ribosome.

N.B.

The synthesis of a protein in ribosome is also produced in the nucleus from DNA

The differences between the DNA and RNA are given in Table 17.1.

Table 17.1 Differences between the DNA and RNA

DNA	RNA
Present within nucleus	Present within cytoplasm
Consists of two stands of polynucleotides	Consists of single strand of polynucleotides
Contains deoxyribose sugar	Contains ribose sugar
Nitrogenous bases are: adenine, thymine, cytosine and guanine	Nitrogenous bases are: adenine, uracil, cytosine and guanine
Replicates and transcribes	Does not replicate and transcribe
Stores genetic information	Helps in the expression of genetic information

CHROMOSOMES

The chromosomes (German: *chromosome* = a readily staining body) are deeply stained minute rod-like structures in nucleus of the cell formed by condensation of chromatin during cell division. They contain DNA encoding genetic information inherited from the parents. The individual chromosomes are best defined (visible) under microscope only during metaphase stage of cell division.

Each chromosome presents a primary constriction called **centromere** or **kinetochore**. During cell division (prophase), each chromosome splits longitudinally into two **chromatids** except at centromere. The centromere divides each chromatid into two arms and is associated with the movement of chromosomes during cell division. The free ends of chromatids are known as **telomeres**. The chromatids of some chromosomes present a secondary constriction near one end. The segment of chromatid distal to secondary constriction is called a **satellite body** (Fig. 17.4). Such chromosomes are sometimes called **SAT-chromosomes.**

CHEMICAL STRUCTURE

The chromosome consists of DNA, small amount of RNA, proteins (histone and nonhistone) and metallic ions. The DNA is the key constituent of the chromosome. It is the most essential and stable molecule. It exists as a highly coiled structure. In active state, it is lightly stained and most extended and is called **euchromatic**, whereas in inactive state, it is dark-staining and remains highly coiled and is called **heterochromatic.**

The **histones** are basic proteins which are aggregated as spheroidal particles. The DNA strand is coiled around each particle to form **a nucleosome.**

The nonhistone proteins are acidic and form many enzymes.

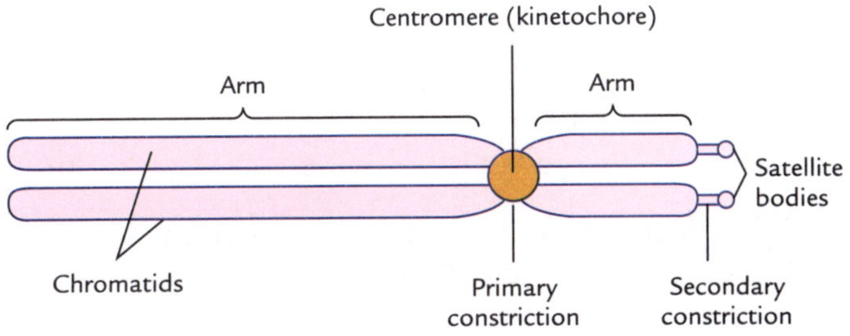

Fig. 17.4 Morphological structure of a chromosome.

MORPHOLOGICAL TYPES

Depending upon the location of centromere, the chromosomes are classified into four types (Fig. 17.5):

1. **Metacentric:** Centromere is located in the middle of the chromosome.
2. **Submetacentric:** Centromere is located close to the middle of the chromosome.
3. **Acrocentric:** Centromere is located close to the end of chromosome.
4. **Telocentric:** Centromere is located at the end of the chromosome.

NUMBER OF CHROMOSOMES

The number of chromosomes is constant in a species. In humans, this number is 46 in somatic cells* and 23 in germ cells. In somatic cells, they are arranged into 23 pairs, whereas in germ cells, they are not arranged in pairs. A cell with 23 pairs of chromosomes is called **diploid** cell and a cell with 23 chromosomes is called **haploid cell**.

In each pair of chromosomes, one is inherited from the mother and one from the father. The chromosomes belonging to the same pair are called **homologous chromosomes**. The complete set of chromosomes from a cell is called its **karyotype**.

Two of the 46 chromosomes are called **sex chromosomes** and the remaining 44 chromosomes are called **autosomes**.

A normal female has two **X** chromosomes (XX) in each somatic cell, whereas a normal male has one **X** and one **Y** chromosome (XY) in each somatic cell. For convenience, the autosomes are numbered in pairs from 1 through 22.

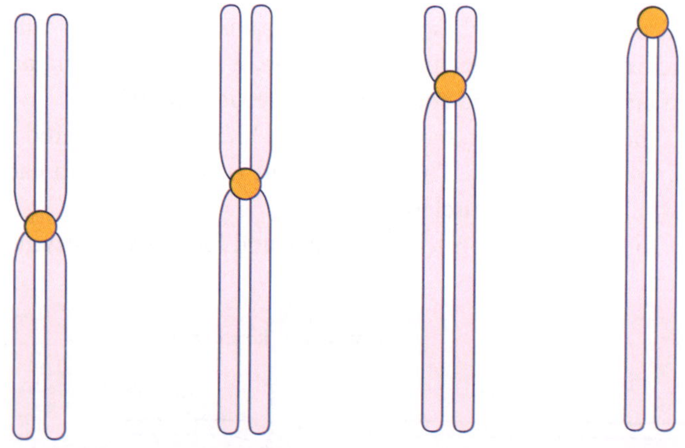

Fig. 17.5 Morphological types of chromosomes: **A,** metacentric; **B,** submetacentric; **C,** acrocentric; **D,** telocentric.

*All the cells of body are somatic cells *except* the germ cells.

Clinical correlation

Abnormalities in sex chromosome number are most easily transmitted chromosomal abnormalities.

The presence of a Y chromosome makes a person male, and the absence of a Y chromosome makes a person female, regardless of the number of X chromosomes. Therefore, persons with chromosomal complement XO, XX, XXX or XXXX are females, and persons with chromosomal complement XY, XXY, XXXY or XYY are males.

A YO condition is lethal, because genes on X chromosome are necessary for survival.

KARYOTYPING

It is a process of arranging the chromosomes of a cell in order to study the complete chromosomal complement of an individual. According to Denver system of classification (1960), the chromosomes, including sex chromosomes, are arranged into seven groups depending upon their (a) size, (b) position of centromere, (c) length-ratio between their arms and (d) presence of satellite bodies on their arms. These groups are referred to by the capital letters A to G.

Method

First, an enlarged photomicrograph of a **chromosome spread** is taken from a stained slide (Fig. 17.6). Then individual

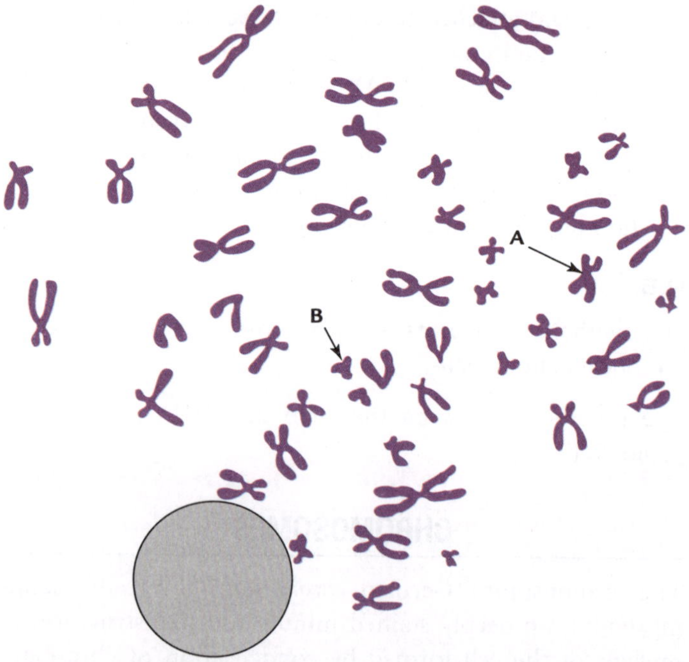

Fig. 17.6 Schematic photomicrograph of chromosome spread (at metaphase stage of cell division of male human leucocytes). The two sex chromosomes are marked by arrows: **A,** X chromosome; **B,** Y chromosome.

chromosomes are cut out from the photograph, the homologous chromosomes are paired and are arranged in a sequence. The longest chromosomes are placed at the beginning and the shortest at the end. This arrangement of chromosomes is called **karyotype** (Fig. 17.7). The karyotype provides the chromosomal constitution of a cell or an individual.

The features of chromosomes in different groups are presented in Table 17.2.

The precise identification of individual chromosome is now made possible by noting the patterns of bands on chromosomes by special staining techniques such as Q-banding, G-banding, R-banding and C-banding (Fig. 17.8).

Clinical correlation

The karyotyping is of clinical significance for, one can identify the structural and numerical variations in chromosomes, and with chromosomal banding pattern, one can note certain abnormalities of chromosome structure such as *deletion* and *translocation* of specific regions of chromosomes.

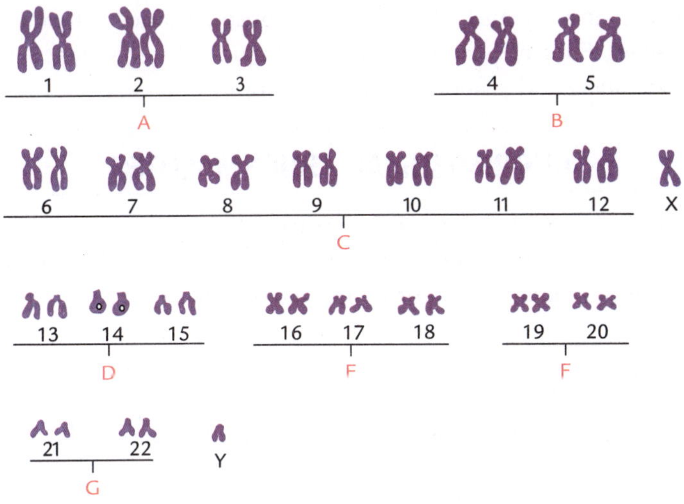

Fig. 17.7 Karyotype of a normal male.

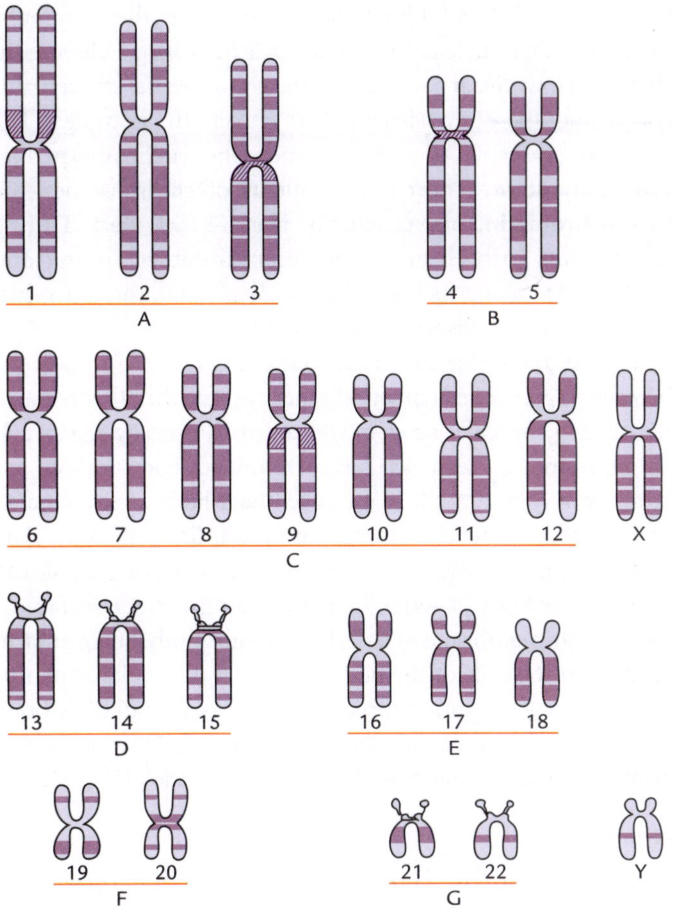

Fig. 17.8 G-banding pattern of chromosomes.

SEX CHROMATIN (BARR BODY)

It is a darkly stained condensed clump of chromatin located subjacent to the nuclear membrane of somatic cells of normal (XX) females. It represents inactivated X chromosome.** During interphase (resting phase) of cell cycle, the chromosomes

**In female embryo at a particular stage of embryogenesis (usually at the blastocyst stage), one of the two X chromosomes is inactivated on a random basis.

Table 17.2 The characteristic features of pairs of chromosomes in karyotype

Group	Pairs of chromosomes	Features
A	1, 2 and 3	Long and metacentric
B	4 and 5	Fairly long and submetacentric
C	6 to 12 +X chromosome	Medium sized and submetacentric
D	13 to 15	Medium sized and acrocentric with a *satellite body* attached to the free end of short arm of each chromosome
E	16 to 18	Fairly short and submetacentric
F	19 and 20	Short and metacentric
G	21 and 22 + Y chromosome	Very short and acrocentric with *satellite bodies* on their short arms

become uncoiled and thinned out; consequently, they cannot be identified. The nucleus thus contains a network of **chromatin threads**. However, at some places, the chromosome still remains coiled and these are visualized as **chromatin granules**. The uncoiled segments of chromosomes, the **euchromatin**, are genetically active. The coiled segments of chromosomes, the **heterochromatin**, are genetically inactive, i.e. inert. During cell division, each chromosome becomes thicker, shorter and tightly coiled along its entire length. As a result, the individual chromosomes are visualized and identified.

During interphase, in females, one out of two X chromosome becomes highly coiled (genetically inactive) and the other remains uncoiled (genetically active). The coiled, genetically inactive X chromosome is seen as heterochromatic body called **sex chromatin** (Fig. 17.9). It is also called **Barr body** after the name of a Canadian geneticist Murray Barr. It was first noticed by Barr and Bertram (in 1949) in the nucleus of nerve cell of a female cat.

The Barr body is generally located on the inner surface of the nuclear membrane as a dark basophilic body of chromatin in most of the cells of the body. It is generally ovoid or planoconvex. However, in neurons, it appears as a small dark body opposite to the nucleolus and in neutrophils, it appears as a knob of 1.5 μm in diameter known as drumstick (Fig. 17.10).

N.B.

Structurally, the sex chromatin is an extra X chromosome which is heterochromatic and genetically inactive.

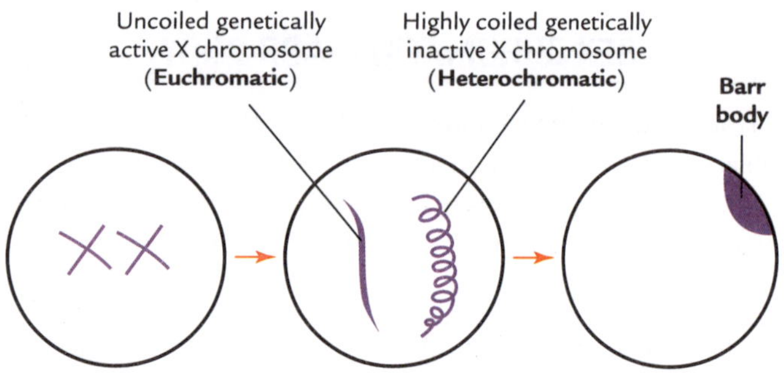

Fig. 17.9 Formation of sex chromatin in a female.

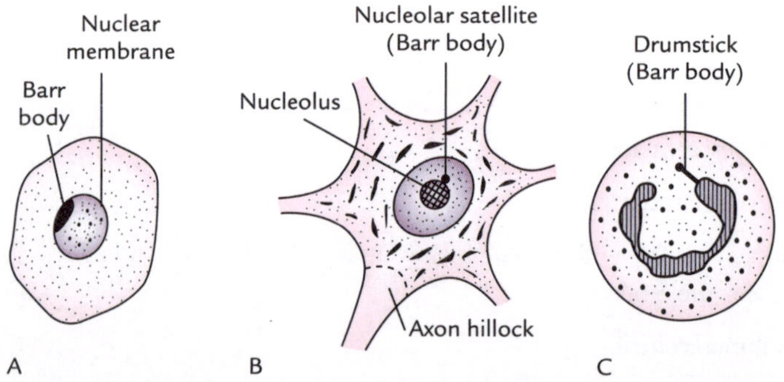

Fig. 17.10 Location of Barr body in: **A,** buccal smear; **B,** neuron; **C,** neutrophil.

Table 17.3 Individual's sex chromosome constitution and number of Barr bodies per cell

Individual	Sex chromosome constitution	Number of Barr bodies
Normal male	XY	Nil
Turner's syndrome	XO	Nil
Normal female	XX	One
Klinefelter's syndrome	XXY	One
Triple X syndrome (super female)	XXX	Two

Lyon's hypothesis: According to this hypothesis (formulated by Lyon), the number of Barr bodies in a cell is equal to the total number of X chromosomes minus one. It is also known as '**n−1 rule**', where **n** represents the number of X chromosomes in the cell. The number of Barr bodies per cell in different conditions in given in Table 17.3.

N.B.

During interphase, the Y chromosome in male exhibits within the nucleus of a cell an intensely fluorescent mass called **'F-body'** when stained with fluorochrome dye and examined under fluorescent microscope.

CHROMOSOMAL ABNORMALITIES

The study of chromosomal abnormalities is of great clinical importance because they produce number of genetic disorders causing various clinical conditions.

CLASSIFICATION

The chromosomal abnormalities may be classified in a number of ways:

1. **On the basis of type of abnormality:**
   (a) *Numerical,* involving changes in the number of chromosomes, e.g. polyploidy, aneuploidy
   (b) *Structural,* involving change in the structure of chromosomes, e.g. deletion, translocation
2. **On the basis of types of chromosomes involved:**
   (a) *Involving autosomes,* e.g. Down's syndrome
   (b) *Involving sex chromosomes,* e.g. Turner's syndrome, Klinefelter's syndrome

NUMERICAL ABNORMALITIES

The numerical abnormalities of chromosomes occur due to failure of meiotic division to occur or due to abnormal meiotic division during the formation of gametes. In normal meiotic division during gametogenesis, both primary spermatocytes and primary oocytes produce four daughter cells, each with 23 chromosomes, and when haploid sperm fertilizes haploid ovum, the diploid zygote is produced (Fig. 17.11).

Sometimes separation of two chromosomes does not occur (nondisjunction) either during first meiotic division (Fig. 17.12A) or during second meiotic division (Fig. 17.12B), and then both the members of a pair move into one cell.

As a result of the nondisjunction of the chromosome (Fig. 17.13), one gamete receives 24 chromosomes and the other 22. Consequently, at fertilization, when a gamete (e.g. sperm) having 23 chromosomes fuses with gamete (e.g. ovum) having 24 or 22 chromosomes, the result will be an individual with either 47 chromosomes (**trisomy**) or 45 chromosomes (**monosomy**).

The numerical abnormalities include the following conditions:

1. **Polyploidy:** It is a condition in which chromosome number is increased in multiple of haploid (23) set of chromosomes, of course, in addition to the diploid number. In other words, polyploidy is the condition of extra haploid set/sets of chromosomes (i.e. 23) to normal diploid set of chromosomes (i.e. 46); examples are:
   (a) *Triploidy*: A condition in which the cells contain 69 chromosomes (23 × 3). It occurs either due to failure of meiosis in germ cell, e.g. fertilization of diploid ovum by a haploid sperm or fertilization of haploid ovum by two haploid sperms (dispermy).

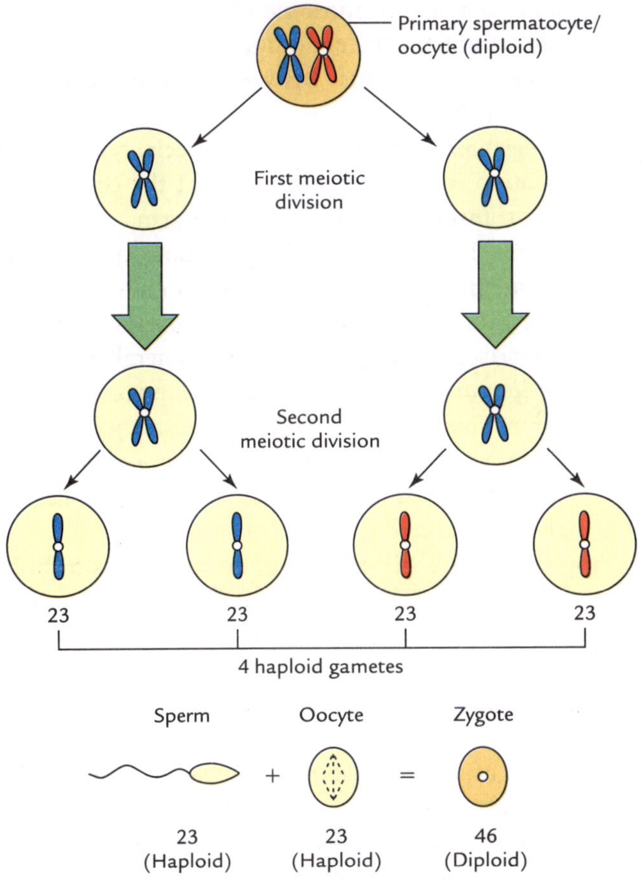

Fig. 17.11 Normal meiotic division producing gametes with 23 chromosomes.

N.B.

Triploidy results in spontaneous abortion of the conceptus or brief survival of liveborn infants after birth.

   (b) *Tetraploidy*: A condition in which the cells contain 92 chromosomes (23 ×4). It occurs due to failure of the first cleavage division.

N.B.

Tetraploidy results in spontaneous abortion of the conceptus.

2. **Aneuploidy:** It is a condition in which chromosome number is altered by one, i.e. there is addition of one chromosome (**trisomy**) or loss of one chromosome (**monosomy**). It occurs due to nondisjunction during meiosis (Figs 17.10–17.12).

N.B.

Trisomy usually results in spontaneous abortion of the conceptus; however, trisomy 13 (Patau's syndrome), *trisomy 18* (Edward's syndrome), *trisomy 21* (Down's syndrome) and Klinefelter's syndrome are found in liveborn population.

Monosomy also usually results in spontaneous abortion of the conceptus; however, monosomy of X chromosome (45 : XO), i.e. Turner's syndrome is found is live born population.

STRUCTURAL ABNORMALITIES

These abnormalities involve change in the structure of chromosome. The types of structural abnormalities include deletions, microdeletions, translocation, fragile sites, isochromosomes, inversions and breakage.

The abnormalities in structure cause following conditions:

1. **Deletions:** In this condition, there is a loss of segment of a chromosome. The clinical conditions caused due to deletions include: Wolf–Hirschhorn syndrome (due to deletion in the short arm of chromosome 4), Cri-du-chat or Cat's cry syndrome (due to deletion in the short arm of chromosome 5).

N.B.

Sometimes chromosome is deleted at both ends, and then the two broken ends adhere/unite to form a ring called *ring chromosome*, commonly seen due to break points of chromosome 14.

2. **Microdeletions:** In this condition, there is a loss of segment of a chromosome which can be detected only by

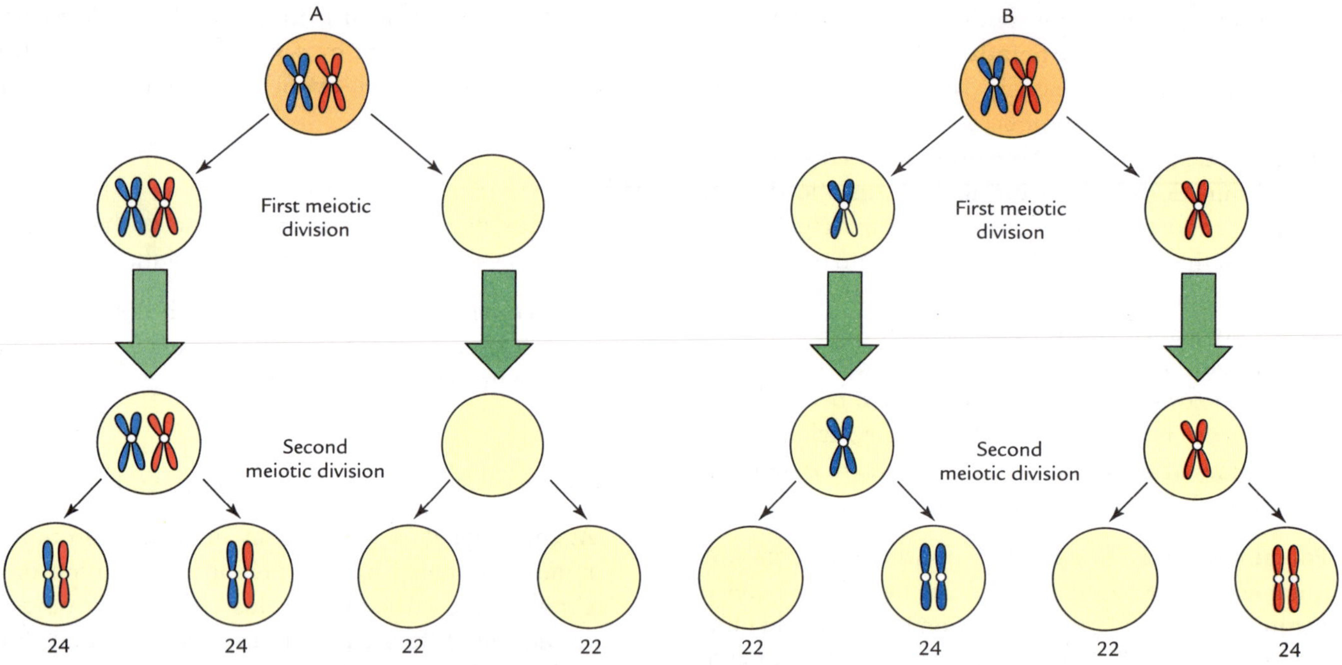

Fig. 17.12 Nondisjunction occurring during meiosis: **A,** Nondisjunction in meiosis I producing gametes with 24 and 22 chromosomes; **B,** nondisjunction occurring during meiosis II producing gametes with 24 and 22 chromosomes.

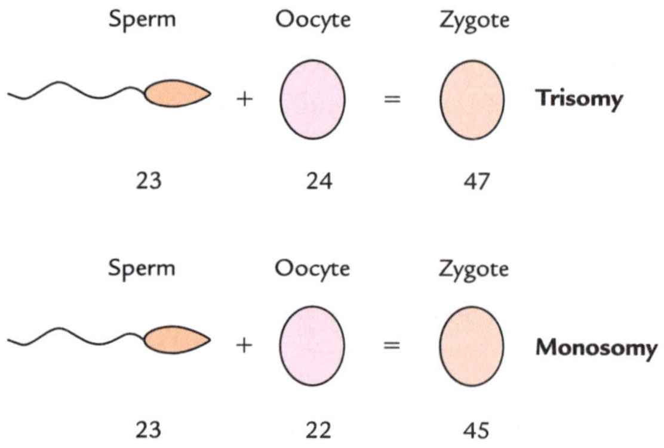

Fig. 17.13 Nondisjunction during oogenesis. Note that if abnormal oocyte with 24 chromosomes is fertilized by a normal sperm with 23 chromosomes, a zygote with 47 chromosomes is produced (i.e., trisomy). If abnormal oocyte with 22 chromosomes is fertilized by a normal sperm with 23 chromosomes, a zygote with 45 chromosomes is produced (i.e., monosomy).

a high resolution banding. The clinical conditions caused by microdeletions include:

(a) *Prader–Willi syndrome*: Due to microdeletion in long arm of chromosome 15 derived from the father.
(b) *Angelman's syndrome or Happy puppet syndrome*: Due to microdeletion in the long arm of chromosome 15 derived from the mother.
(c) *DiGeorge syndrome*: Due to microdeletion in the long arm of chromosome 2.
(d) *Miller–Dieker syndrome*: Due to microdeletion in the short arm of chromosome 17.

3. **Translocation:** In this condition, there is breakage and exchange of segments between chromosomes. The examples include:
   (a) *Robertsonian translocation*: Is a special type of translocation in which breaks occur at the centromeres, e.g. translocation between long arms of chromosomes 13 and 14 (**most common translocation found in humans**) and chromosomes 21 and 22. The short arms of these chromosomes involved in Robertsonian translocations are generally lost.
   (b) *Reciprocal translocation between chromosome 15 and chromosome 17*: Leads to *acute promyelocytic leukemia.*
   (c) *Reciprocal translocation between chromosome 9 and chromosome 22 (Philadelphia chromosome)*: Leads to *chronic myeloid leukemia.*
4. **Fragile sites:** In this condition, there are gaps or breaks in chromosome. The clinical conditions caused due to this condition include **Fragile X syndrome** (*Martin–Bell syndrome*).
5. **Isochromosomes:** In this condition, the centromere divides transversely instead of longitudinally. As a result, two arms of a chromosome are separated forming two isochromosomes.
6. **Inversions:** In this condition, a part of the chromosome is detached and later unites with same chromosome in inverted position. As a result, there is reversal of order of DNA between two breaks in the chromosome.

It can be **pericentric** if inversions occur on sides of the centromere or **paracentric**, if inversions occur on the same side of the centromere.

7. **Breakage:** In this condition, there occurs a break in chromosome due to ultraviolet radiation, ionizing radiation.

   The clinical conditions caused by breaks in chromosomes include:
   (a) *Xeroderma pigmentosum*: Affected individuals are hypersensitive to sunlight (ultraviolet radiation).
   (b) *Ataxia-telangiectasia*: Affected individuals are hypersensitive to ionizing radiation.
   (c) *Fanconi's anemia*: Affected individuals are hypersensitive to DNA cross-linking agents.
   (d) *Bloom's syndrome*: Affected individuals hypersensitive to a wide variety of DNA-damaging agents.
   (e) *Hereditary non-polyposis colorectal cancer*: Accounts for 15% of all cases of colorectal cancer.

Symbols Used in Genetics

These are as under:

p = short arm of chromosome
q = long arm of chromosome
t = Translocation
i = Isochromosome
inv = Inversion
r = Ring chromosome

Further when + or – signs are placed before a symbol, it stands for addition or missing of complete chromosome. On the other hand when + or – sign is placed after a symbol, it indicates increase or decrease of the length of the chromosome.

GENES

The term *gene* refers to a combination of DNA subunits which together constitute a unit of inheritance. The term 'gene' was first coined by the Danish botanist Wilhelm Johannsen (1909). It contains the information needed to synthesize a particular protein/enzyme. There are about 50,000 to 100,000 genes in the human cell.

Structure (Fig. 17.14)

The gene consists of a transcription unit flanked by regulatory sequences.

The transcription unit is made up alternating pattern of *exons* (functional parts) and *introns* (nonfunctional parts). The exon is a segment of gene that codes for mRNA (code for a particular protein). An intron is a segment of gene which when transcribed into RNA is spliced out during maturation process and does not code for a particular protein. The introns and exons may vary in length. Every gene requires a promoter to begin transcription. A promoter consists of DNA sequences that allow RNA polymerase to bind and initiate the polymerization of ribonucleotides.

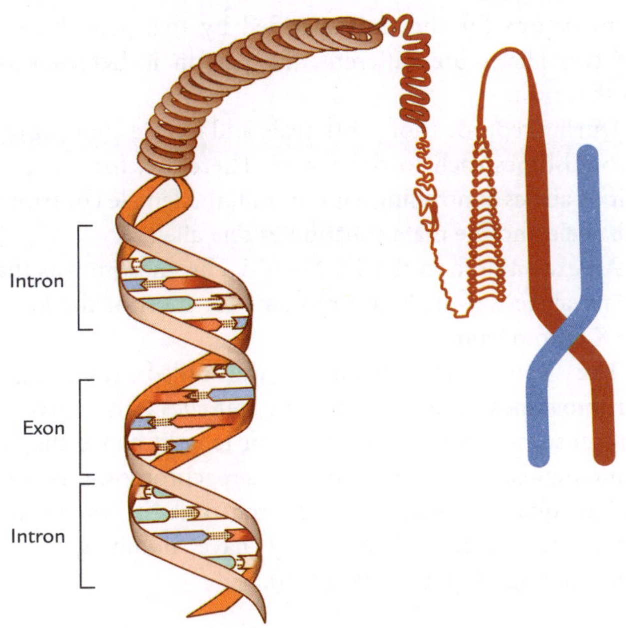

Fig. 17.14 Structure of a gene.

Types

These are as under:

1. *Structural genes*, which code for specific amino acid sequence in a protein.
2. *Operation genes*, which allow transcription.
3. *Regulator genes*, which inhibit protein synthesis.
4. *Dominant genes*, which are able to express their traits.
5. *Recessive genes*, which are able to express only in homozygous state.
6. *Sex-linked genes*, which are abnormal genes located on X or Y chromosomes.
7. *Jumping genes* (transposons), which can jump to and fro within single chromosome or an adjacent one.

Functions of Genes

1. Maintain the genetic specificity of an individual.
2. Play a key role in transmission of traits from the parents to the offspring.
3. Synthesize various proteins and enzymes of the cell.

N.B.

Genes synthesize protein through transcription from DNA and RNA, and translation from RNA to protein.

LOCATION OF GENES

Each gene occupies a specific **locus** on a chromosome. Both chromosomes of a given pair contain similar genes. The two chromosomes of a pair are homologous and genes occupying the same locus on homologous chromosomes are called **alleles**. If the two allelic genes are identical, the person is

homozygous for the trait specified by that gene locus. If the two alleles are different, the person is **heterozygous** for that trait.

During reproduction, both male and female contribute 23 chromosomes each to the zygote. Therefore, for any given pair of alleles controlling a given trait, the female contributes one allele and the male contributes one allele.

An exception occurs with X and Y chromosomes as there are no alleles on the Y chromosome for most of the loci on the X chromosome.

The paired chromosomes are called **homologous chromosomes** (Fig. 17.15). In females, the two sex chromosomes (XX) are identical in length; hence they are homologous. In males, the two sex chromosomes (XY) are unequal in length—X chromosome is longer than short chromosome; hence they have homologous and nonhomologous parts (Fig. 17.16).

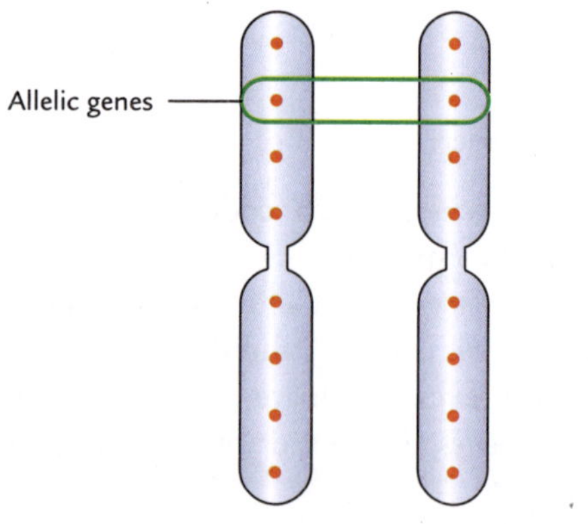

Fig. 17.15 Homologous chromosomes with allelic genes.

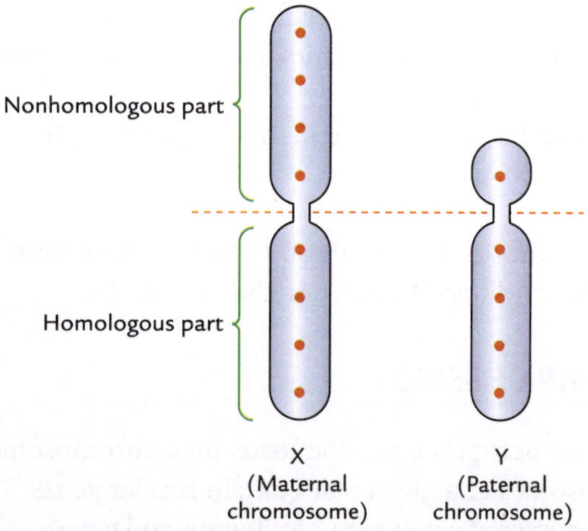

Fig. 17.16 Male sex chromosomes (XY) with homologous and nonhomologous parts.

DOMINANT AND RECESSIVE GENES

When gene produces its effect, whether it is present either upon one or upon both chromosomes of a pair of chromosome, it is called **dominant gene**. If it produces its effect only when it is present on both chromosomes, it is called **recessive gene**. Thus diseases are inherited through both dominant and recessive genes called dominant inheritance and recessive inheritance, respectively.

INHERITANCE

Inheritance is the process of transmission of characters/traits from generation to generation. The reproduction is an essential requisite for the inheritance to take place. The inheritance of traits from parents to offspring takes place through genes which carry all information about all types of traits. The genes are located in both autosomes and sex chromosomes. The inheritance occurring through genes of autosomes is called autosomal inheritance, whereas inheritance occurring through genes on sex chromosomes is called sex-linked inheritance.

AUTOSOMAL INHERITANCE

Each chromosome of a homologous pair contains genes for the same traits. For example, the ability to roll one's tongue is coded for on a single gene. Since one chromosome of each pair is inherited from the father and one from the mother, an individual has two genes controlling the ability to roll the tongue. Such paired genes are **alleles.**

The corresponding alleles contain genes concerned with same trait, but they need not be identical. As discussed earlier, an individual may have two identical forms of gene (*homozygous*) or two different forms of the gene (*heterozygous*).

Thus one copy of the tongue-rolling gene may code for the ability to roll the tongue, whereas the corresponding gene on the other chromosome may code for inability to roll the tongue. Note that this example involves only two forms of the same gene. Some traits like eye color is controlled by more than one gene.

In homozygous individual, both the alleles are either dominant or recessive, but heterozygous individuals have one dominant and one recessive gene.

Punnett square: The probability of occurrence of a given genetic combination for certain traits can be predicted by Punnett square (Fig. 17.17).

TT = Tongue-roller homozygous
Tt = Tongue-roller heterozygous
Tt = Tongue-roller heterozygous
tt = Non-roller homozygous.

Some examples of autosomal dominant traits are shown in Flowchart 17.1.

		Paternal genes	
		T	t
Maternal genes	T	TT	Tt
	t	Tt	tt

Fig. 17.17 Punnett square showing probabilities of genetic combination of the tongue-rolling gene.

Autosomal traits

Dominant traits
- Achondroplasia
- Osteogenesis imperfecta
- Brachydactyly, polydactyly, syndactyly
- Pre-senile baldness in males
- Huntington's chorea
- Marfan's syndrome
- Familial hypercholesterol-aemia
- Multiple neurofibromatosis
- Diabetes insipidus

Recessive traits
- Albinism
- Acatalasia
- Phenylketonuria
- Sickle-cell anemia
- Thalassemia
- Galactosemia
- Hurler's syndrome

Flowchart 17.1 Autosomal traits.

SEX-LINKED INHERITANCE

The *Y* chromosome is shorter than the *X* chromosome. Therefore, traits coded on the nonhomologous part of X chromosome have no corresponding traits on the Y chromosome. These genes on sex chromosomes are called **sex-linked,** those on X chromosome are X-linked and those on Y chromosome are Y-linked.

X-Linked Inheritance

X-linked genes are exclusive to X chromosome. For example, the gene that codes for normal **color vision** is carried on X chromosome only. It is the dominant form of gene. There is rare faulty recessive form of this gene which codes for **red-green blindness.** If female inherits a faulty gene, she is likely to have normal gene on her, other chromosome providing normal color vision. A female carrying the faulty gene (color-blind gene), even though she is not color blind may pass the faulty gene onto her children and thus she is called a **carrier.** If the gene is faulty in the male, he will be color blind because he has only one X chromosome and so will have only one copy of the gene.

N.B.

The ability to discern red-green color depends entirely on X chromosome.

If normal gene is represented by 'C' and faulty gene is represented by 'c', the genotype possibilities are as shown in Figure 17.18.

N.B.

In order for female to be color blind for red-green color, she has to have recessive allele (color-blind gene) on both of her X chromosome (XcXc). This is possible only if her mother is a carrier (XCXc) and her father is color blind (XcY).

Clinical correlation

Hemophilia: It is a clinical condition associated with repeated episodes of severe and prolonged bleeding at any site with little trauma. It is a sex-linked condition caused by a recessive allele responsible for faulty clotting. If H represents normal clotting and h represents abnormal clotting, then males with XHy will be normal and males with Xhy will be hemophilic. The females with XhXh will also be hemophilic.

Y-linked Inheritance (Holandric inheritance)

Since males have only one Y chromosome, the gene is necessarily unpaired. Therefore if present, it will be expressed and the question of dominance and recessiveness does not arise. Further the gene will be passed from affected male to all his sons, e.g. characteristic growth of hair on the pinna of ear. This is the only Y-linked gene inheritance and hence for all practical purposes, sex-linked means X-linked.

The sex-linked traits are given in Flowchart 17.2.

		Father (Normal)	
		XC (Normal gene)	Y (Gene absent)
Mother (Carrier)	XC (Normal gene)	XCXC Normal girl	XCY Normal boy
	Xc (Color blindness gene)	XCXc Carrier girl without color blindness	XcY Color-blind boy

Fig. 17.18 Punnett square showing sex-linked inheritance.

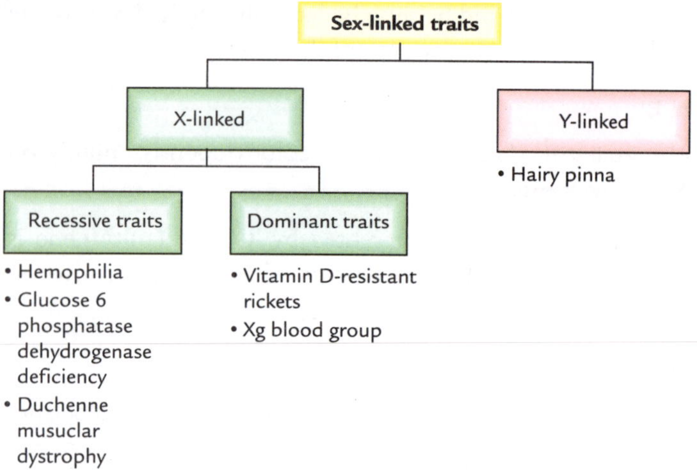

Flowchart 17.2 Sex-linked traits.

MITOCHONDRIAL INHERITANCE

The body receives all its mitochondrial DNA only from the mother, because during fertilization, mitochondria of sperm do not pass into the ovum. Consequently, diseases which occur due to mutations in the mitochondrial DNA (mtDNA) are inherited entirely through mother. The leading examples of diseases caused due to mutations in the mtDNA are:

1. **Leber's hereditary optic neuropathy (LHON):** A condition characterized by sudden onset of blindness in adults.
2. **Pearson marrow-pancreas syndrome (PMPS):** A condition characterized by a loss of bone marrow cells during childhood. It is frequently fatal.

GENETIC BASIS OF DISEASES

A large number of human diseases occur due to genetic disorders. The disorders include numerical and structural abnormalities of chromosomes and gene mutation.

DISORDERS DUE TO CHROMOSOMAL ABNORMALITIES

Disorders due to chromosomal abnormalities can be numerical or structural (Flowchart 17.3). The common disorders are discussed in detail in the following text.

Numerical Chromosomal Abnormalities Affecting Autosomes

Down's Syndrome (Mongolism) or Trisomy 21

In this disorder, there are three copies of chromosome 21 (*trisomy 21*), i.e. there is an extra chromosome 21. The karyotype of the patient is 47, XX, +21.

The trisomy 21 is of two types:

1. **Triplo-21 (nonfamilial mongolism):** It is common and the affected babies possess 47 chromosomes including two X chromosomes. It occurs during meiosis due to nondisjunction of 21st pair of chromosomes.
2. **Translocation mongolism (familial mongolism):** In this, an individual possesses 46 chromosomes. In this condition, the extra chromosome becomes attached to one of the other autosomes.

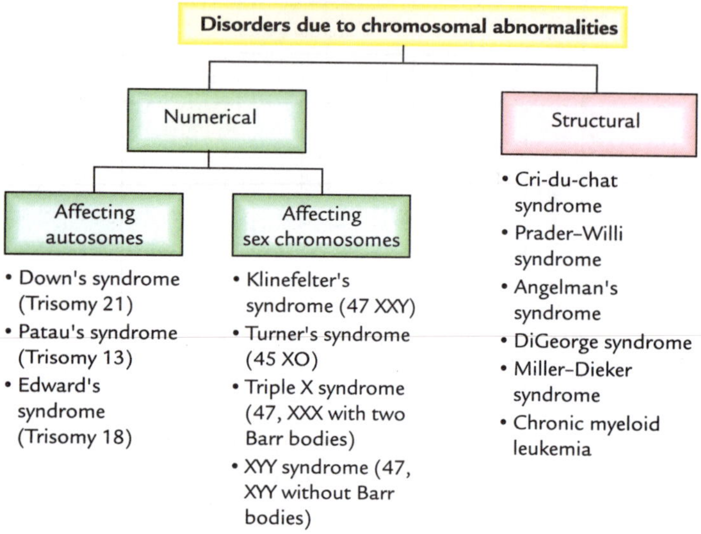

Flowchart 17.3 Disorders due to chromosomal abnormalities.

The Down's syndrome occurs in one out of every 700 births (1/700).

Majority of the mongoloid babies have 47 chromosomes with trisomy 21, but about 3% have normal 46 chromosomes with translocation of two 21 chromosomes.

Characteristic clinical features (Fig. 17.19):

The affected individuals present the following features:

1. Round face with oblique palpebral fissures and inner epicanthic folds, i.e. mongoloid facies, hence the name mongolism
2. Small nose with shallow bridge, low-set square ears
3. Short and broad hands with single transverse crease in the palm (*Simian crease*) across the bases of four fingers
4. Open mouth with long protruding tongue
5. Mental retardation (I.Q: 25 to 50)
6. Short stature with hyperflexibility of joints

N.B.

- Down's syndrome is the best known and one of the most common chromosomal abnormality in humans. It was first described by L. Down in 1886.
- Down's syndrome is the most common numerical chromosomal abnormality.
- The probability of Down's syndrome increases with the advancing age of the mother.
- The children with Down's syndrome are easy to manage as they love music. They usually die young.

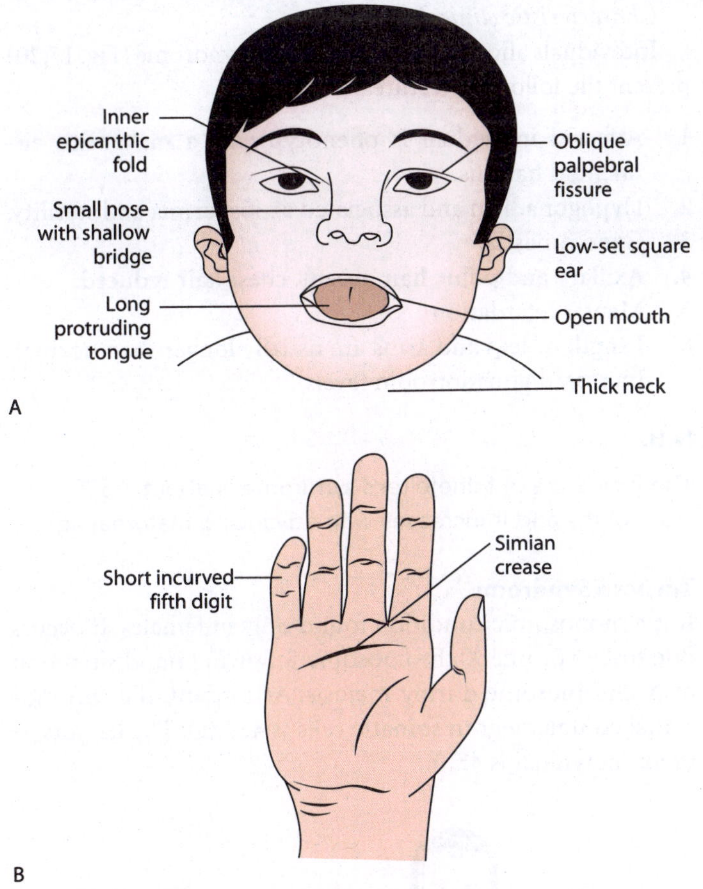

Fig. 17.19 Down's syndrome: **A,** facial features of an infant with Down's syndrome; **B,** Simian crease.

- Down's syndrome is associated with low α-*fetoprotein* levels in amniotic fluid or maternal serum.
- The children with Down's syndrome are susceptible to infection and often have associated congenital heart ab normalities.

Patau's Syndrome

In this disorder, there are three copies of chromosome 13 (*trisomy 13*).

Characteristic clinical features:

The affected children present the following features:

1. Profound mental retardation
2. Cleft-lip and cleft-palate
3. Omphalocele
4. Polydactyly

N.B.

Infants with Patau's syndrome usually die soon after birth.

Edward's Syndrome

In this disorder, there are three copies of chromosome 18 (*trisomy 18*).

Characteristic clinical features:

The affected children present the following features:

1. Elongated head with prominent occiput and low-set ears
2. Small facies with micrognathia
3. Overlapping of fingers
4. Rocker-bottom heels
5. Congenital heart defects

N.B.

Infants with Edward's syndrome usually die within few weeks after birth.

Structural Chromosomal Abnormalities Affecting Autosomes

Cri-du-chat Syndrome (Cat Cry Syndrome)

This condition is caused by a deletion in the short arm of chromosome 5 so that part of chromosome 5 is missing.

Characteristic clinical features:

The affected children present the following features:

1. Round face
2. Characteristic cat-like cry (i.e. meowing cry) of a child
3. Hypertelorism
4. Congenital heart defects
5. Microcephaly
6. Mental retardation

Prader–Willi Syndrome

This condition occurs due to microdeletion in the long arm of chromosome 15 derived from the father (i.e. *paternal imprinting*).

Characteristic clinical features:

The affected children present the following features:

1. Hyperphagia (insatiable appetite) and obesity
2. Short stature with small hands and feet
3. Hypotonia
4. Hypogonadism
5. Mild to moderate mental retardation
6. Behavioral problems such as rage, violence, etc.

Angelman's Syndrome (Happy Puppet Syndrome)

It occurs due to microdeletion of in the long arm of chromosome 15 derived from the mother (i.e. *maternal imprinting*). Angelman syndrome is the counterpart of Prader–Willi syndrome.

Characteristic clinical features:

The affected children present the following features:

1. Happy disposition with inappropriate laughter
2. Severe mental retardation (I.Q.: 5–10)
3. Ataxic gait (stiff, jerky, unsteady)
4. Seizures

DiGeorge Syndrome

It occurs due to microdeletion in the long arm of chromosome 2.

Characteristic clinical features:

The affected individuals present the following features:

1. Immunodeficiency, due to absence of thymus
2. Hypocalcemia, due to absence of parathyroid
3. Hypertelorism
4. Low-set prominent ears with micrognathia

Miller–Dieker Syndrome

It is caused by a microdeletion in the short arm of chromosome 17.

Characteristic clinical features:

The affected children present the following features:

1. Lissencephaly (smooth brain, i.e. no gyri)
2. Microcephaly with high and furrowing forehead

N.B.

Infants suffering from Miller–Dieker syndrome die at an early age. This syndrome should not be mistakenly diagnosed in case of premature infants whose brain have not yet developed an adult pattern of gyri (gyri begin to appear normally at about 28 weeks after birth).

Chronic Myeloid Leukemia

It is caused by a reciprocal translocation between chromosome 9 and chromosome 22. This is referred to as the **Philadelphia chromosome**. It is found in blood or bone marrow cells.

As a result of translocation, the **abl gene** on chromosome 9 fuses with **bcr gene** on chromosome 22, thus forming **abl/bcr oncogene** which transforms, hematopoietic precursor cells.

Characteristic clinical features:

Increased number of granulocytes in all stages of maturation and many mature neutrophils.

N.B.

Patients of chronic myeloid leukemia with negative Philadelphia chromosome have poor response to chemotherapy. It seems likely that the presence of Philadelphia chromosome is the result rather than the cause of the disease.

CHROMOSOMAL ABNORMALITIES AFFECTING SEX CHROMOSOMES

Klinefelter's Syndrome

It is a trisomic condition found only in males. It is caused by nondisjunction of XX chromosome during gametogenesis. As a result, the chromosomal complement in somatic cells is XXY. The individual is phenotypically a male but is sex-chromatin (Barr body) positive due to presence of an extra X chromosome. The karyotype of the individual is 47, XXY.

Characteristic clinical features:

Individuals affected with Klinefelter's syndrome (Fig. 17.20) present the following features:

1. Affected individual is phenotypically a male with eunuchoid habitus.
2. Hypogonadism and associated azoospermia and sterility.
3. Gynecomastia.
4. Axillary and pubic hair absent, chest hair reduced.
5. Mental retardation.
6. Length of legs and arms are usually longer than normal.
7. Increased gonadotropin levels.

N.B.

The incidence of Klinefelter's syndrome is about 1:500 male births and it increases with advancing maternal age.

Turner's Syndrome

It is a monosomic condition found only in females. It occurs due to loss of one X chromosome following nondisjunction of X chromosome during meiosis. As a result, the chromosomal complement in somatic cells is 45, XO. The karyotype of an individual is 45, X.

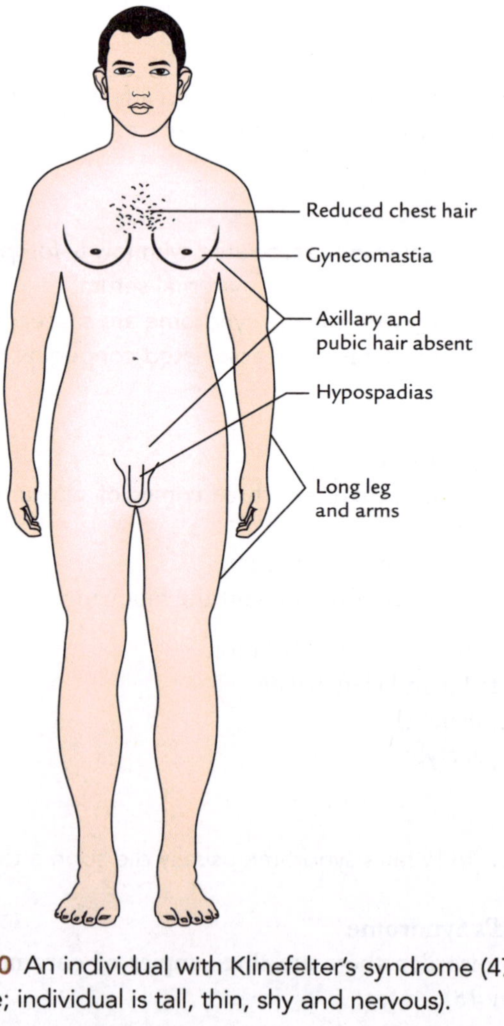

Fig. 17.20 An individual with Klinefelter's syndrome (47, XXY karyotype; individual is tall, thin, shy and nervous).

Characteristic clinical features:

The affected individuals present the following features (Fig. 17.21):

1. Affected individual is phenotypically a female.
2. Short stature, webbing of neck (due to delayed maturation of lymphatics).
3. Shield-chest with pinpoint nipples.
4. Bilateral cubital valgus.
5. Low-set ears.
6. Infantile external genitalia.
7. Gonadal dysgenesis associated with amenorrhea.
8. Coarctation of aorta.

N.B.

The incidence of Turner's syndrome is 2 : 3000 female births. This syndrome is the common cause of *primary amenorrhea*. In 75% of Turner's patients, the X chromosome is maternal in origin. Turner's syndrome is the only viable monosomy in human beings.

The key differences between Klinefelter's and Turner's syndromes are presented in Table 17.4.

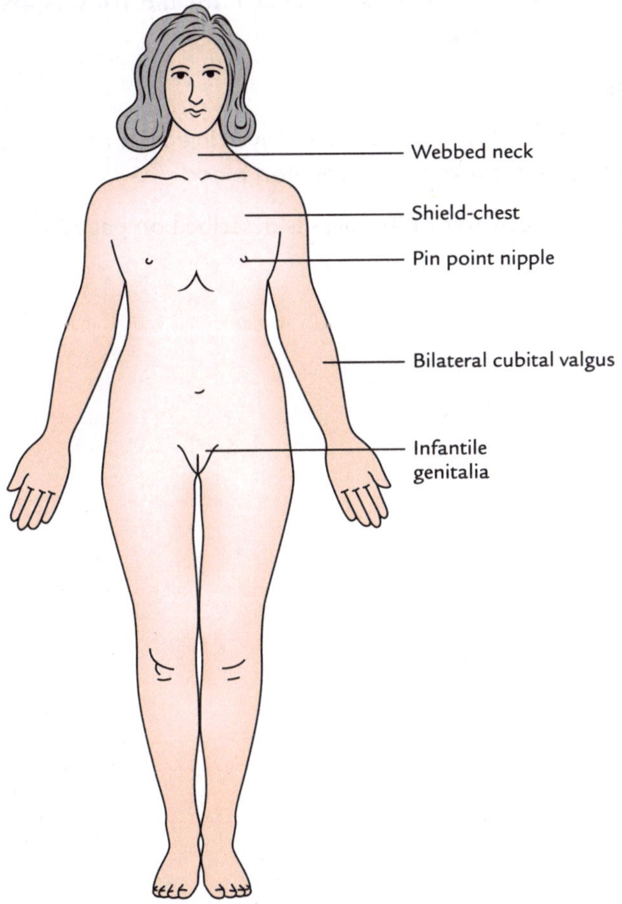

Fig. 17.21 An individual with Turner's syndrome (45 XO karyotype).

Table 17.4 Differences between Klinefelter's and Turner's syndromes

Klinefelter's syndrome	Turner's syndrome
Trisomic condition found only in males	Monosomic condition found only in females
Chromosomal complement in somatic cells is 47 XXY	Chromosomal complement in somatic cells is 45 XO
Affected individuals are phenotypically males	Affected individuals are phenotypically females
Long stature	Short stature

Super Female or Triple X Syndrome

It occurs due to fertilization of XX-containing oocyte by an X-containing sperm (gymnosperm). The karyotype shows 47 chromosomes. The individual is phenotypically a female with two Barr bodies, hence referred to as '**super female**'. The chromosome complement in somatic cell is 47 XXX.

Characteristic clinical features:

The affected individuals present the following features:

1. Female phenotype
2. Some degree of mental retardation
3. Scanty menses
4. Infantile personality

SINGLE GENE INHERITED DISEASES

Autosomal Dominant Inheritance

The diseases caused by autosomal dominant inheritance need only one defective copy of the gene from either parent, e.g. Huntington's disease.

Huntington's Disease (HD)

The HD is a fatal neurodegenerative disorder caused by autosomal dominant mutation. The HD-gene is located on the short arm of chromosome 4. The inheritance of mutant HD-gene causes cell death of neurons in the caudate nucleus and putamen which leads to a disease called **Huntington's chorea**. Death follows about 5–10 years after the symptoms make their first appearance.

Characteristic clinical features:

The affected individuals present the following features:

1. Involuntary chorea (dance-like) movements of limbs
2. Mood disturbances
3. Swift grimaces and sudden movements of head
4. Progressive loss of mental activity

Autosomal Recessive Inheritance

A disease that occurs due to autosomal recessive inheritance affects only those individuals who receive two copies of the defective gene one from each parent, e.g. **cystic fibrosis**.

Cystic Fibrosis (CF)

It is caused by autosomal recessive mutation. The CF-gene is located on the long arm of chromosome 7.

It causes production of abnormally thick secretion of mucous by epithelial cells lining the respiratory and gastrointestinal tracts, particularly in the first one.

Characteristic clinical features:

The affected individuals present the following features:

1. Obstruction of respiratory airways
2. Recurrent respiratory infections

X-Linked Recessive Inheritance

In X-linked recessive inheritance, the disease is usually observed only in the males because males have only one X chromosome.

The females may also be affected, but rarely. In females, one X chromosome is inactivated to form a Barr body. The choice of whether the maternally derived or paternally derived X chromosome is deactivated is a random and permanent event. If X chromosome with normal gene is deactivated, the female has one X chromosome with the abnormal gene and will, therefore, be affected by the disease.

The examples of X-linked recessive inherited diseases are: Duchenne muscular dystrophy (DMD), hemophilia and red-green color blindness.

Duchenne Muscular Dystrophy

It is a hereditary disease of skeletal muscle which usually affects males. The DMD is caused by X-linked recessive mutation. The DMD gene is located on the short arm of chromosome X. The DMD gene encodes for a protein called dystrophin which anchors the actin (cytoskeleton) of skeletal muscle cells to the extracellular matrix. Thus, mutation of DMD gene destroys the ability of dystrophin to anchor actin to the extracellular matrix. Consequently, the skeletal muscles become progressively weak from early childhood, and by the time the individual reaches adolescence, he/she becomes completely immobile.

Characteristic clinical features:

The affected individuals present the following features:

1. Progressive muscle weakness and wasting
2. Premature death due to cardiac and respiratory failure

Hemophilia

The hemophilia results due to deficiency or dysfunction of a clotting factor VIII. It occurs due to mutation of X-linked recessive gene located on one X chromosome, which is responsible for clotting factor VIII.

Characteristic clinical features:

The affected individuals present the following features:

1. Excessive bleeding, particularly from gums, but virtually no tissue is exempted.
2. When bleeding follows trauma, it is characteristically prolonged.
3. Bleeding tendency may range form mild to severe.
4. Excessive bleeding is unusual until the baby is about 6 months old.

N.B.

The treatment of hemophilia involves injection of missing clotting factor taken from donated blood.

The red-green color blindness is described on page 241.

Golden Facts to Remember

➢ Father of Genetics	Gregor Johann Mendel (discovered fundamental laws of inheritance in 1865)
➢ Correct structure of DNA was first deduced by	James Watson and Francis Crick (1953)
➢ Structural unit of DNA	Gene
➢ The term 'gene' was first coined by	Johannsen (1909)
➢ Unit of inheritance	Gene
➢ Number of genes in human genome	50,000–100,000
➢ Most important intermediary molecule for gene expression	RNA
➢ Best known and most common chromosomal abnormality	Down's syndrome (trisomy 21)
➢ Only viable monosomy in human beings	Turner's syndrome (45, XO)
➢ Most common translocation in chromosomes of human beings	Robertsonian translocation
➢ Commonest hereditary bleeding disorder	Hemophilia
➢ Commonest X-linked gene disorder	Red-green color blindness
➢ Most important process required for inheritance	Reproduction
➢ Most X-linked disorders are recessive condition *except*	Vitamin D-resistant rickets which is a X-linked dominant condition
➢ Only known condition which is Y-linked	Hairy pinna in male
➢ In all living organisms, the genetic information is stored in DNA *except*	In some viruses (RNA viruses) in which the genetic information is stored in RNA
➢ All cells in the body contain 46 chromosomes *except*	Gametes (sex cells) which contain 23 chromosomes

Multiple Choice Questions

1. **Each nucleotide consists of all of the following subunits *except:***
   (a) A molecule of deoxyribose sugar
   (b) A molecule of ribose sugar
   (c) A molecule of nitrogenous base
   (d) A molecule of phosphate

2. **All of the following nitrogenous bases are present in a DNA molecule *except:***
   (a) Adenine
   (b) Thymine
   (c) Uracil
   (d) Guanine

3. **Select the *incorrect statement* about the chromosomes:**
   (a) Each chromosome presents a primary constriction called centromere
   (b) Number of chromosomes is not constant in a species
   (c) Each somatic cell contains 23 pairs of chromosomes
   (d) Females have two X chromosomes (XX) in each somatic cell

4. **Select the *incorrect statement* about the Barr body:**
   (a) Structurally, it represents a X chromosome which is genetically inactive
   (b) Generally, it is located on the outer surface of nuclear membrane
   (c) The number of Barr bodies in a cell is equal to the total number of X chromosome minus one
   (d) In neurons, it appears as a small dark body opposite the nucleolus

5. **Select the *correct statement* about the karyotyping:**
   (a) Chromosomes are arranged in seven groups, referred to by letters A to G
   (b) Chromosomes of group A and F are submetacentric
   (c) Chromosome of group D and group G are metacentric
   (d) X chromosome belongs to group G and Y chromosome belongs to group C

6. **Clinical conditions caused by trisomy include all of the following *except:***
   (a) Patau's syndrome
   (b) Down's syndrome
   (c) Klinefelter's syndrome
   (d) Cri-du-chat syndrome

7. **Clinical features of Down's syndrome include all *except:***
   (a) Oblique palpebral fissures with epicanthic folds
   (b) Presence of simian crease
   (c) Long protruding tongue
   (d) Long legs and arms

8. **Select the *incorrect statement* about the Klinefelter's syndrome:**
   (a) It is a trisomic condition found only in females
   (b) The affected individual is sex-chromatin positive
   (c) The affected individual has increased level of gonadotrophin
   (d) Lengths of legs and arms are usually longer than normal

9. **Which of the following clinical condition is caused by monosomy?**
   (a) Klinefelter's syndrome
   (b) Turner's syndrome
   (c) Down's syndrome
   (d) Cri-du-chat syndrome

10. **Select the *incorrect statement* about the X-linked recessive inheritance:**
    (a) It usually affects the males
    (b) It usually affects the females
    (c) It may affect the females rarely
    (d) Females act as carrier

Answers

1. *b*, **2.** *c*, **3.** *b*, **4.** *b*, **5.** *a*, **6.** *d*, **7.** *d*, **8.** *a*, **9.** *b*, **10.** *b*

Index

N

O

P

Q

R

S

T

U

V

W

X

Y

Z

NOTES

NOTES

NOTES

NOTES

NOTES

NOTES